AF183871

Managing Maternal Chronic Diseases for a Healthy Pregnancy

Ibrahim Karaca
Editor

Managing Maternal Chronic Diseases for a Healthy Pregnancy

Springer

Editor
Ibrahim Karaca
Department of Gynecology and Obstetrics
Bakircay University
Izmir, Türkiye

ISBN 978-3-032-15220-6 ISBN 978-3-032-15221-3 (eBook)
https://doi.org/10.1007/978-3-032-15221-3

© The Editor(s) (if applicable) and The Author(s), under exclusive license to Springer Nature Switzerland AG 2026

This work is subject to copyright. All rights are solely and exclusively licensed by the Publisher, whether the whole or part of the material is concerned, specifically the rights of translation, reprinting, reuse of illustrations, recitation, broadcasting, reproduction on microfilms or in any other physical way, and transmission or information storage and retrieval, electronic adaptation, computer software, or by similar or dissimilar methodology now known or hereafter developed.
The use of general descriptive names, registered names, trademarks, service marks, etc. in this publication does not imply, even in the absence of a specific statement, that such names are exempt from the relevant protective laws and regulations and therefore free for general use.
The publisher, the authors and the editors are safe to assume that the advice and information in this book are believed to be true and accurate at the date of publication. Neither the publisher nor the authors or the editors give a warranty, expressed or implied, with respect to the material contained herein or for any errors or omissions that may have been made. The publisher remains neutral with regard to jurisdictional claims in published maps and institutional affiliations.

This Springer imprint is published by the registered company Springer Nature Switzerland AG
The registered company address is: Gewerbestrasse 11, 6330 Cham, Switzerland

If disposing of this product, please recycle the paper.

I dedicate this book to my beloved wife, Assoc. Prof. Dr. Suna Yıldırım Karaca, who has always stood by my side, and to my dearest daughters, Nisa and Umay Naz, who are my greatest sources of inspiration. Their love, support, and presence have been the most powerful driving forces on this journey.

Preface

Medicine is not merely the art of treating diseases; it is also the responsibility of guiding human life, improving quality of life, and laying the foundations for healthy generations. This responsibility is perhaps most profoundly felt during pregnancy—a process that is not only physiological but also psychological, social, and even societal in nature. For women with chronic diseases, this period becomes even more complex, requiring the coordinated efforts of not only obstetricians but also specialists from various medical disciplines.

This book titled *Managing Maternal Chronic Diseases for a Healthy Pregnancy* was born precisely from this need. It offers a comprehensive perspective on the clinical management of chronic diseases during pregnancy. Far beyond a conventional medical textbook, it stands as a product of our university's academic solidarity, a reflection of our commitment to knowledge, and a concrete example of our interdisciplinary collaboration.

This work holds the distinction of being the first comprehensive scientific publication prepared under the institutional framework of Bakırçay University Faculty of Medicine. Under my editorial leadership in the field of obstetrics and gynecology, esteemed academicians from internal medicine, cardiology, urology, general surgery, pulmonary medicine, anesthesiology, neurology, dermatology, rheumatology, and many other specialties have contributed wholeheartedly to this project. The strong collaboration among faculty members from different departments within our university has imbued this book not only with scientific depth but also with symbolic significance.

Moreover, this work has also benefited from the valuable contributions of academics from various universities and healthcare institutions across Türkiye, further enriching its multidisciplinary foundation. Our goal is for this book to become one of the most up-to-date resources on the management of chronic diseases during pregnancy.

Another important aspect of this book is its accessibility not only to healthcare professionals but also to expectant mothers who are motivated to understand their health more deeply. For this reason, it serves not only as an academic reference but also as a guide that strengthens physician-patient communication, informs clinical decisions, and contributes to healthier pregnancies.

I would like to take this opportunity to sincerely thank all the authors who contributed to this work, particularly the esteemed faculty members of Bakırçay University Faculty of Medicine, as well as the academic staff from other disciplines and the university administration for their support throughout the process. This work, born out of academic productivity, teamwork, and scientific responsibility, stands as an inspiring starting point for our future publications.

Sincerely,

Izmir, Turkey Ibrahim Karaca

Contents

Contributors

Seda Karaca Adıyeke, MD Izmir Bakircay University, Faculty of Medicine, Department of Ophthalmology, Izmir, Turkey

Aslı Akdöner, MD Dokuz Eylul University, Faculty of Medicine, Department of Obstetrics and Gynecology, Izmir, Turkey

Sabahattin Anıl Arı, MD Faculty of Medicine, Department of Obstetrics and Gynecology, Izmir Bakircay University, Izmir, Türkiye

Aysu Ayrancı, MD Izmir Bakircay University, Faculty of Medicine, Department of Chest Diseases, Izmir, Turkey

Mücahit Furkan Balcı, MD Izmir Torbali State Hospital, Department of Obstetrics and Gynecology, Izmir, Turkey

Şeyda Ceylan Arı, MD Ege University, Faculty of Medicine, Department of Anaesthesiology and Reanimation, Izmir, Turkey

Yeliz Çiftçi, MD Izmir Bakircay University, Faculty of Medicine, Department of Neurology, Izmir, Turkey

Bayram Çolak, MD Izmir Bakircay University, Faculty of Medicine, Department of General Surgery, Izmir, Turkey

Ezgi Demir, DDS Ege University, Faculty of Dentistry, Department of Endodontics, Izmir, Turkey

Vedat Gerdan, MD Izmir Bakircay University, Faculty of Medicine, Department of Rheumatology, Izmir, Turkey

Mustafa Ozan Horsanalı, MD Izmir Bakircay University, Faculty of Medicine, Department of Urology, Izmir, Turkey

Suna Yıldırım Karaca, MD Izmir Bakircay University, Faculty of Medicine, Department of Obstetrics and Gynecology, Izmir, Turkey

Eyüp Kebabçı, MD Izmir Bakircay University, Faculty of Medicine, Department of General Surgery, Izmir, Turkey

İlker Kızıloğlu, MD Izmir Bakircay University, Faculty of Medicine, Department of General Surgery, Izmir, Turkey

Pelin Koca, MD Izmir Bakircay University, Faculty of Medicine, Department of Medical Pharmacology, Izmir, Turkey

Oktay Şenöz, MD Izmir Bakircay University, Faculty of Medicine, Department of Cardiology, Izmir, Turkey

Filiz Meryem Sertpoyraz, MD Izmir Bakircay University, Faculty of Medicine, Department of Physical Medicine and Rehabilitation, Izmir, Turkey

Meltem Türkmen, MD University of Health Sciences, Faculty of Medicine, Department of Dermatology, Izmir, Turkey

Onur Yavuz, MD Dokuz Eylul University, Faculty of Medicine, Department of Obstetrics and Gynecology, Izmir, Turkey

Chapter 1
Beyond Expectations: The Astonishing Physiology of Motherhood

Suna Yıldırım Karaca

1.1 Introduction

Pregnancy is a unique state in which almost all maternal systems undergo profound and temporary changes. These physiological adaptations are essential to maintain maternal health, support fetal growth, and prepare the mother for labor and delivery. Maternal physiology is remodeled so that the mother can meet her own metabolic needs while also sustaining the fetus. These changes ensure adequate oxygen, nutrient delivery, and waste removal through the placenta. The changes that occur usually return to normal within the first 6–8 weeks after delivery.

1.2 Genital Tract Changes in Pregnancy

Before pregnancy, the uterus weighs 60–80 g, its internal volume is approximately 10–15 mL, and its dimensions are 6 × 3.5 × 2 cm. During pregnancy, it reaches a weight of about 1150 g, a volume of 5 L, and dimensions of 20 × 25 × 22.5 cm [1, 2]. This enlargement occurs mainly due to hypertrophy of muscle cells and stretching, while the formation of new muscle fibers is limited [1, 3, 4]. In the very early stages of pregnancy, uterine growth is primarily influenced by estrogen; after the 12th week, the effect of mechanical stretching becomes more pronounced. Beyond

S. Y. Karaca (✉)
Izmir Bakircay University, Faculty of Medicine, Department of Obstetrics and Gynecology, Izmir, Turkey
e-mail: suna.karaca@bakircay.edu.tr

© The Author(s), under exclusive license to Springer Nature Switzerland AG 2026

I. Karaca (ed.), *Managing Maternal Chronic Diseases for a Healthy Pregnancy*,
https://doi.org/10.1007/978-3-032-15221-3_1

the 20th week, rather than hypertrophy, enlargement of the uterine cavity and pressure from the products of conception become the main contributors [3, 4]. With advancing gestation, the corpus uteri thickens more than the cervix, and toward the end of pregnancy the lower uterine segment develops. By the 12th week, the uterus is large enough to rise out of the pelvis; by the 20th week, it reaches the level of the umbilicus; by the 36th week, it extends to the xiphoid process; and near term, it usually descends slightly.

In a term pregnant woman lying supine, the enlarged uterus can compress the aorta and inferior vena cava, thereby reducing venous return to the heart and decreasing cardiac output. Consequently, symptoms such as dizziness, pallor, and sweating may occur. For this reason, after mid-pregnancy, it is recommended that women avoid lying flat on their back and instead adopt the left lateral decubitus position.

During pregnancy, due to the vasodilatory effects of estrogen, progesterone, and relaxin on the uterine arteries, as well as decreased vascular resistance, uteroplacental blood flow increases progressively and reaches 450–650 mL/min near term [2]. As the uterus enlarges, the spiral arteries lengthen and become coiled, leading to increased shear stress. These changes provide optimal blood supply to the placenta; if insufficient, intrauterine growth restriction and preeclampsia may develop.

Approximately one month after fertilization, increased vascularity, diffuse edema, and hypertrophy and hyperplasia of the cervical glands lead to softening and cyanosis of the cervix. The cervical columnar glands show marked proliferation, often accompanied by eversion. The cervical canal is sealed by a mucus plug, which is rich in cytokines and serves as an important immunological barrier. When examined microscopically, cervical mucus does not crystallize due to high progesterone levels and therefore does not exhibit the fern pattern.

During pregnancy, endocervical gland hyperplasia and hypersecretion are common. This condition may complicate the interpretation of Pap smears due to atypical glandular cell appearances.

Pregnancy also results in softening of the vulva, perineal muscles, and connective tissues. Increased vascularity leads to hyperemia, which is most evident in the vagina. The vaginal mucosa thickens, its color takes on a bluish hue, and squamous epithelial cell hypertrophy occurs. Increased vaginal and cervical secretions produce a thick, white discharge. Vaginal pH remains acidic (3.5–6.0); however, the risk of vulvovaginal candidiasis rises 10- to 20-fold during pregnancy [2].

Ovulation does not occur in pregnancy. The corpus luteum is the primary source of progesterone until the 6th–7th week of gestation, after which the placenta assumes this role. Relaxin secretion, however, continues until delivery. The stromal-stimulating effect of progesterone may cause extrauterine decidual reactions on the ovarian surface and peritoneum, which are prone to bleeding.

Relaxin, secreted mainly by the corpus luteum, placenta, and decidua throughout pregnancy, influences renal hemodynamics, lowers plasma osmolality, and facilitates connective tissue remodeling in the genital tract to prepare for delivery. It also contributes to the structural adaptation of uterine arteries.

1.3 Pregnancy and Metabolic Changes

In the third trimester of pregnancy, the basal metabolic rate increases by approximately 15–20% [1, 2]. The additional caloric requirements during pregnancy are estimated at 85 kcal/day in the first trimester, 285 kcal/day in the second trimester, and 475 kcal/day in the third trimester [1, 5]. One of the most striking physiological changes in pregnancy is weight gain. The recommended weight gain is 11.5–16 kg in singleton pregnancies and 16–20 kg in twin pregnancies. However, the recommended gain should be adjusted according to the pre-pregnancy body mass index (BMI) [5, 6]. During pregnancy, dietary protein is utilized more efficiently; therefore, maternal muscle breakdown is not required to meet fetal protein needs, reflecting nitrogen conservation [2].

Pregnancy is characterized by mild fasting hypoglycemia, postprandial hyperglycemia, and hyperinsulinemia [1, 2]. Pregnant women are more prone to ketosis, particularly during fasting or prolonged periods without food. Accelerated lipolysis and reduced carbohydrate availability promote rapid development of ketosis, sometimes referred to as accelerated starvation of pregnancy [7]. Peripheral insulin resistance increases during pregnancy; latent diabetes may become clinically apparent, or pre-existing diabetes may worsen. This insulin resistance is primarily mediated by elevated levels of estrogen, progesterone, human placental lactogen, and cortisol [8].

Although glomerular filtration of glucose increases in pregnancy, tubular reabsorption decreases only minimally. The renal threshold for glucosuria drops to around 155 mg/dL, and physiological glucosuria (~150 mg/dL) is observed in approximately half of pregnant women [2, 9]. All lipid fractions rise during pregnancy, including triglycerides, total cholesterol, VLDL, HDL, LDL, apolipoproteins, phospholipids, and free fatty acids. Total plasma lipid levels increase significantly and progressively after the 24th week, with the most prominent elevations in triglycerides, cholesterol, and free fatty acids. HDL rises during early pregnancy, while LDL predominates in late pregnancy [10].

Leptin is secreted primarily by adipose tissue and partly by the placenta; thus, maternal serum leptin levels increase during pregnancy in correlation with placental weight. Levels especially rise in the second trimester and remain elevated until term, reaching 2–4 times pre-pregnancy values. Leptin plays an important role in fetal growth and development, and elevated maternal levels have been associated with preeclampsia and gestational diabetes [11, 12]. Ghrelin, secreted by the placenta, also increases during pregnancy, peaking in mid-gestation and gradually declining toward term. Ghrelin contributes to fetal growth, and deficiency has been linked to gestational diabetes [12, 13].

Micronutrient metabolism is also significantly altered during pregnancy. Among these, vitamin D deficiency is particularly common. Supplementation with 15 μg/day (600 IU) is considered sufficient throughout pregnancy and lactation. From the early stages of pregnancy, increased tubular reabsorption leads to water retention, resulting in an additional 6.5 L of body fluid. Edema is therefore a normal finding in pregnancy and does not indicate pathology [14, 15].

During pregnancy, glomerular filtration of sodium and potassium increases, but tubular reabsorption also rises markedly. As a result, approximately 1000 mEq of sodium and 300 mEq of potassium are retained. However, due to expanded plasma volume, serum sodium and potassium concentrations decrease slightly (by ~0.5 mEq/L). Serum osmolality also decreases during pregnancy [9, 15]. Total serum calcium concentration declines, while ionized calcium levels remain unchanged. The reduction in total calcium is attributed to plasma volume expansion, increased glomerular filtration (leading to hypercalciuria), and maternal–fetal calcium transfer. In contrast, magnesium levels decrease significantly, while phosphate levels remain stable [16].

Both maternal and fetal thyroid hormone production increase during pregnancy. Due to increased renal clearance, iodine requirements rise, and supplementation is recommended in normal pregnancies. However, routine supplementation of selenium, fluoride, or zinc is not necessary [17, 18].

In nonpregnant women, the daily folic acid requirement is 50–100 μg/day, whereas during pregnancy it increases to 400–800 μg/day. Requirements are higher in multiple pregnancies, hemolytic anemia, Crohn's disease, alcoholism, and inflammatory skin disorders. Folic acid prophylaxis reduces the incidence of neural tube defects (NTDs) from 4000 to 3000 cases per year [19]. More than half of folate deficiency cases during pregnancy originate from inadequate pre-pregnancy intake. Therefore, it is recommended that all women of reproductive age take 400 μg of folic acid daily, beginning at least 8–10 weeks before conception and continuing through the first trimester. In women with a history of NTDs in previous pregnancies, supplementation should be increased to 4 mg/day instead of 400 μg/day [19, 20]. Daily folate intake is preferable to multivitamin supplementation. For most vitamins, dietary intake is sufficient. Vitamin B12 levels decrease during pregnancy, largely due to reduced transcobalamin concentrations. In cases of preconceptional vitamin B12 deficiency, the risk of NTDs may increase [21].

1.4 Hematological Changes and Iron Metabolism

During pregnancy, blood volume increases by approximately 1600–1700 mL (40–45%). This rise begins in the first trimester, and by the 12th week of gestation, blood volume is about 15% higher than pre-pregnancy levels. The rate of increase is more rapid during the second trimester, slows in the third trimester, and eventually plateaus toward term [22, 23].

The increase in blood volume results from the expansion of both plasma and red blood cell (erythrocyte) mass, although the majority is due to plasma volume (about 1200 mL). Erythrocyte volume increases by only about 450 mL, reaching its peak in the third trimester. Erythropoietin levels rise during pregnancy, leading to mild erythroid hyperplasia in the bone marrow and a slight increase in reticulocyte counts [23, 24].

Because most of the increase occurs in plasma, physiological anemia develops as a result of hemodilution, despite enhanced erythropoiesis. Consequently, hemoglobin concentration and hematocrit gradually decline during pregnancy. In the second half of gestation, hemoglobin levels below 11 g/dL are generally considered anemia, while values below 9 g/dL indicate true iron deficiency anemia [25]. Pregnancy is also associated with leukocytosis (white blood cell counts up to 15,000/μL; during labor, up to 25,000/μL). Due to hemodilution, increased platelet consumption, and splenic enlargement, platelet counts may decrease slightly in pregnancy [26].

Iron requirements rise substantially during pregnancy. In a normal singleton pregnancy, approximately 1000 mg of additional iron is needed: 300 mg for the fetus and placenta, 500 mg for maternal erythropoiesis, and about 200 mg to compensate for blood loss. During the second trimester, the rapidly expanding plasma volume and increased iron demand for erythropoiesis lead to accelerated depletion of iron stores unless maternal reserves are adequate. In most cases, these demands cannot be met by maternal iron stores alone [27, 28].

A normal diet provides about 14 mg/day of iron, of which only 5–10% is absorbed. In pregnant women, absorption increases up to 40%. However, because the daily requirement is approximately 6–7 mg/day, iron supplementation is often necessary [29, 30].

At the beginning of pregnancy, amenorrhea and relatively low iron demand may cause serum iron and ferritin levels to increase. From mid-pregnancy onward, however, both serum iron and ferritin levels decline. Iron is transported in plasma bound to transferrin and stored in tissues as ferritin. A serum ferritin level below 10–15 mg/L in a pregnant woman indicates iron deficiency anemia.

In pregnant women without anemia, supplementation is not required during the first 4 months. After this period, preventive supplementation with 30 mg of elemental iron per day is recommended (equivalent to 150 mg ferrous sulfate, 100 mg ferrous fumarate, or 300 mg ferrous gluconate). For optimal absorption, iron should be administered in the ferrous form.

1.5 Coagulation System Changes in Pregnancy

Pregnancy is characterized by a hypercoagulable state. Levels of several clotting factors (e.g., fibrinogen, factors VII, VIII, and X) increase significantly, while natural anticoagulants such as Protein C, Protein S, and antithrombin undergo functional alterations. This shift favors clot formation, which is beneficial in reducing the risk of hemorrhage during delivery, but it also increases the maternal risk of thromboembolic events [31, 32].

During pregnancy, both coagulation and fibrinolytic activities rise; however, a balance is maintained between the two systems to preserve hemostasis. Fibrinogen (factor I) levels increase by approximately 50%. While pre-pregnancy levels range from 200 to 400 mg/dL, they may rise to as high as 600 mg/dL during pregnancy. This elevation largely accounts for the increased erythrocyte sedimentation rate observed in pregnancy [33].

Levels of plasminogen activator inhibitors 1 and 2 (PAI-1, PAI-2) increase, resulting in reduced activity of tissue plasminogen activator (tPA). Consequently, fibrinolytic activity becomes relatively insufficient during pregnancy [34]. In addition, thrombin generation progressively increases throughout gestation and does not return to preconception levels until approximately 1 year after delivery [35].

1.6 Cardiovascular System Changes in Pregnancy

1.6.1 Anatomical Positioning of the Heart and Cardiac Output Changes

As the gravid uterus enlarges, the diaphragm is elevated, causing the heart to shift upward and laterally to the left. This results in a displaced apical impulse and may produce benign auscultatory findings such as systolic murmurs. The elevated diaphragm pushes the heart upward, causes anterior rotation, and shifts the left border laterally. Due to these positional changes, a slight left axis deviation may be observed on ECG. However, the criteria for left ventricular hypertrophy are not met during pregnancy, despite the increase in body mass [36, 37].

Cardiac functional changes become evident by the 8th week of pregnancy. Cardiac output begins to increase as early as the 5th week, rises progressively throughout gestation, and remains elevated at around 6 L/min. Overall, cardiac output increases by 30–50% during pregnancy, with the maximum rise occurring within 10–30 min after delivery. The increase in heart rate is thought to be mediated by the positive inotropic effects of estrogen. Heart rate rises by approximately 10–20 beats per minute, reaching nearly 100 beats per minute [38, 39].

1.6.2 Systemic Vascular Resistance (SVR) Changes

Despite the increase in cardiac output, systemic vascular resistance decreases due to hormonal influences such as progesterone, prostaglandins, and nitric oxide. This vasodilation enhances uteroplacental perfusion [40].

1.6.3 Hemodynamic Function Changes

Although cardiac output rises during pregnancy, stroke volume index and left ventricular systolic function remain unchanged. Thus, pregnancy cannot be considered a sustained "high-output" state. Maternal blood volume increases substantially to meet the metabolic demands of both the mother and fetus. Plasma volume rises by approximately 40–50%, while red blood cell mass increases to a lesser extent (20–30%). This disproportion results in the physiological anemia of pregnancy, in which hemoglobin and hematocrit values appear reduced despite an absolute rise in red cell mass. Such adaptation improves placental perfusion and facilitates oxygen delivery [22, 23].

1.6.4 Blood Pressure Changes

Maternal blood pressure tends to decrease slightly during the first and second trimesters, reflecting the decline in systemic vascular resistance. By the third trimester, however, blood pressure typically returns to pre-pregnancy levels. The lowest values are reached around 24–26 weeks, with the reduction being more pronounced in diastolic pressure. Thereafter, blood pressure gradually rises and approaches pre-pregnancy levels by term [41].

The fall in blood pressure is attributable to reduced peripheral resistance despite increased cardiac output. Postural changes also influence arterial pressure; values in the sitting position are lower compared with those in the lateral recumbent position. During pregnancy, several hormonal changes further impact cardiovascular and renal physiology. Levels of renin, angiotensin II, and aldosterone increase significantly, contributing to sodium and water retention and thereby expanding plasma volume. Additionally, concentrations of prostaglandins E2 (PgE2) and I2 (PgI2) rise, exerting vasodilatory effects that counterbalance the expanded blood volume and help maintain adequate uteroplacental perfusion. In contrast, levels of atrial natriuretic peptide remain largely unchanged throughout pregnancy [42].

1.6.5 Venous Return and Supine Hypotensive Syndrome

The enlarged uterus may compress the inferior vena cava when the mother lies supine, reducing venous return to the heart. This can result in supine hypotensive syndrome, characterized by dizziness, pallor, or even syncope. Symptoms are relieved when the mother assumes the left lateral position [43].

1.7 Respiratory System Changes in Pregnancy

Many pregnant women experience a sensation of breathlessness, or physiological dyspnea of pregnancy, which is usually mild and related to increased ventilatory drive. This must be distinguished from pathological dyspnea, which may indicate underlying cardiopulmonary disease and requires clinical evaluation [44].

During pregnancy, increased basal oxygen consumption, elevated progesterone levels (which reduce pulmonary vascular resistance), outward expansion of the ribs, and elevation of the diaphragm by 2–4 cm contribute to several changes in respiratory function and lung capacities [45, 46].

Respiratory parameters show significant alterations in pregnancy, with increases in tidal volume, inspiratory capacity (5–10%), and minute ventilation (~40%), accompanied by enhanced oxygen uptake, elevated peak expiratory flow rate, and higher arterial oxygen tension (PaO_2). Conversely, total lung capacity decreases by ~5%, functional residual capacity by 20–30%, residual volume by 20–25%, and expiratory reserve volume by 15–20%, primarily as a result of diaphragmatic elevation [47].

The rise in tidal volume leads to a slight decrease in arterial pCO_2. Maternal hyperventilation induces a state of mild, compensated respiratory alkalosis. As a compensatory response, serum bicarbonate (HCO_3^-) decreases to 20–22 mEq/L, while plasma pH increases slightly to about 7.45 (alkalemia) [48].

This rise in pH shifts the oxygen dissociation curve to the left, increasing maternal hemoglobin's affinity for oxygen and reducing its oxygen release capacity. However, the increase in pH also stimulates a rise in erythrocyte 2,3-diphosphoglycerate (2,3-DPG) levels, which shifts the curve back to the right and restores balance. Consequently, the maternal hyperventilation-induced reduction in pCO_2 facilitates the transfer of CO_2 from the fetus to the mother, while simultaneously enhancing oxygen transfer from the mother to the fetus [49].

1.8 Renal and Urinary System Changes in Pregnancy

During pregnancy, kidney size increases slightly, with both kidneys demonstrating an approximate 30% increase in volume. The renal pelvis capacity, normally around 10 mL, may reach up to 60 mL. Due to the pressure of the gravid uterus and dextrorotation, hydronephrosis and hydroureter occur more frequently on the right side. About 5% of pregnant women develop asymptomatic bacteriuria, and if left untreated, 20–30% of these cases may progress to pyelonephritis [50–52].

Beginning at around the 12th week of gestation, the bladder trigone is elevated, bladder sensitivity increases, bladder capacity decreases, urethral length shortens, and intraurethral pressure rises. Consequently, at least half of women experience urinary incontinence in the third trimester [53, 54].

1.8.1 Renal Filtration and Reabsorption

Glucose Glomerular filtration increases, while tubular reabsorption decreases slightly, leading to impaired glucose reabsorption and glucosuria (up to 150 mg/dL) [9].

Protein Due to hyperfiltration and reduced tubular reabsorption, proteinuria may occur, particularly after the second trimester. Physiological proteinuria rarely exceeds 300 mg/day [55].

Calcium Hypercalciuria is commonly observed in pregnancy. The glomerular filtration rate (GFR) increases by about 50%, and creatinine clearance rises by approximately 30%. Serum creatinine decreases by around 25%, rarely exceeding 0.9 mg/dL. Urea levels also decline by about 25%. Serum uric acid initially decreases (~25%) but rises later in pregnancy [56].

Daily urine output increases by approximately 25%, and nocturia becomes common as a result of enhanced renal perfusion and hyperfiltration. Relaxin contributes to increased GFR and renal blood flow during pregnancy. Consequently, serum levels of creatinine, urea, and uric acid fall below those seen in nonpregnant states. Thus, even "normal" pre-pregnancy values may indicate impaired renal function in pregnancy [57, 58]. Frequent urination and nocturia are common, largely due to elevated renal blood flow, increased GFR, and bladder compression by the uterus. Although these are usually physiological, they should be distinguished from urinary tract infections, which are also more prevalent in pregnancy [59].

1.9 Gastrointestinal System Changes

During pregnancy, several gastrointestinal adaptations occur, largely mediated by hormonal influences, particularly progesterone and estrogen. Progesterone causes relaxation of smooth muscle, including the lower esophageal sphincter, predisposing pregnant women to gastroesophageal reflux and heartburn. Gastric emptying is slightly delayed, and intestinal motility is reduced, leading to a higher risk of constipation [60, 61].

Hormonal changes, especially the combined effects of progesterone and estrogen, also slow gallbladder emptying and alter bile composition, thereby increasing the risk of gallstone formation. Liver function tests demonstrate certain physiological alterations: serum alkaline phosphatase rises due to placental production, while most other liver enzymes remain within normal limits, making it important to distinguish these changes from pathological hepatic conditions of pregnancy [62].

Nausea and vomiting (*emesis gravidarum*) occur in about 60% of pregnant women, usually peaking around the 10th week and resolving by the 16th week. Gingival hypertrophy and hyperemia may also develop, making the gums more prone to bleeding. This condition, known as *pregnancy gingivitis*, typically regresses postpartum. Additionally, vascular gum lesions called *epulis* (pyogenic granuloma) may appear and generally resolve spontaneously after delivery. Pregnancy itself does not predispose women to dental caries, and salivary volume remains unchanged [63].

Progesterone-induced smooth muscle relaxation reduces bowel motility. Relaxation of the lower esophageal sphincter leads to gastroesophageal reflux (*pyrosis*). Gastric acid secretion decreases, whereas mucus production increases, which helps explain why active peptic ulcers are rare in pregnancy. Gastric secretions, however, slightly increase gastric volume. Gastric emptying time remains unchanged, except during labor, when it becomes prolonged. Progesterone-induced colonic relaxation slows motility, increasing water and salt absorption and predisposing to constipation. Constipation, combined with elevated venous pressure, contributes to the development of hemorrhoids. The spleen may enlarge by about 50% [64, 65].

Gallstone formation is more common during pregnancy due to reduced gallbladder contractility, bile stasis, and increased bile concentration. The most frequent type is cholesterol gallstones [66].

Regarding liver function tests, AST, ALT, and GGT decrease slightly, as does bilirubin. In contrast, serum alkaline phosphatase (ALP) doubles due to placental production, and bromsulfophthalein (BSP) clearance decreases [67].

1.9.1 Pregnancy and the Liver

There is no evidence of true hepatomegaly in pregnancy; any upward displacement of the liver is due to the enlarging uterus, particularly in the third trimester. Hepatomegaly in pregnancy should therefore be considered pathological until proven otherwise. Hepatic blood flow remains unchanged, with about 25–33% of cardiac output directed to the liver.

Plasma proteins: Serum albumin decreases by 20–40%, leading to reduced colloid osmotic pressure. Total plasma protein concentration also declines, whereas α1- and α2-globulins increase. Serum alpha-fetoprotein (AFP), originating from the fetus rather than the mother, rises progressively during pregnancy and serves as an important screening marker for congenital anomalies [68].

Under the influence of estrogen, hepatic protein synthesis increases, particularly for coagulation factors VII, VIII, IX, and X, while fibrinolysis decreases—contributing to the hypercoagulable state of pregnancy. Estrogen also enhances hepatic synthesis of triglycerides, cholesterol, and various binding globulins and upregulates cytochrome P450 enzyme activity. Levels of ceruloplasmin, transferrin, thyroxine-binding globulin, and corticosteroid-binding globulin all increase. Meanwhile, AST, ALT, GGT, and bilirubin decrease, whereas serum ALP rises due to placental production [69, 70].

1.10 Endocrine System Changes

The pituitary gland is the most enlarged endocrine organ during pregnancy, increasing in volume by approximately 135%. This growth is primarily due to an increase in lactotroph cells, while the numbers of gonadotroph and somatotroph cells decrease. The populations of corticotroph and thyrotroph cells remain unchanged [71].

During normal pregnancy, prolactin levels rise significantly in parallel with estrogen synthesis, reaching up to tenfold higher than baseline by term. After delivery, prolactin levels remain elevated in breastfeeding women, though they gradually decline overall. In early lactation, pulsatile increases in prolactin secretion occur in response to suckling. By contrast, prolactin levels remain unchanged in nonpregnant women. In pregnancy, prolactin induces DNA synthesis and mitotic activity in alveolar epithelial and pre-secretory alveolar cells, thereby ensuring glandular development. It also stimulates RNA synthesis in these cells and promotes the production of galactopoietic proteins such as casein, lactalbumin, and lactoglobulin, along with lipid synthesis. Prolactin levels begin to rise as early as the 5th week of gestation, peak around week 20, and remain elevated until delivery [72, 73].

1.10.1 Thyroid Gland in Pregnancy

The thyroid gland enlarges during pregnancy due to glandular hyperplasia and increased vascularity. High estrogen levels stimulate thyroxine-binding globulin (TBG) production, which rises rapidly in the first trimester, peaks between weeks 6 and 9, and then plateaus until term. Total thyroxine (T4) levels increase in parallel with TBG and plateau after week 18. Free T4 shows a slight transient increase in early pregnancy, secondary to hCG stimulation, but returns to normal levels by mid-pregnancy. Total triiodothyronine (T3) rises until week 18 and then plateaus, while free T3 remains essentially unchanged. TRH levels do not vary during pregnancy, but placental TRH may cross to the fetal pituitary and stimulate TSH release. TSH levels may be slightly suppressed in early pregnancy due to hCG, but they generally remain within the normal range compared with nonpregnant women [17, 74].

1.10.2 Parathyroid Hormone and Calcium Homeostasis

Plasma parathyroid hormone (PTH) concentrations decrease during the first trimester but progressively increase until term, most likely as a response to reduced maternal calcium levels. Elevated estrogen levels block the bone-resorptive effects of PTH, which in turn stimulates further increases in circulating PTH. Consequently, pregnancy is characterized by a state of physiological hyperparathyroidism [75].

In pregnant women, calcitonin levels rise significantly. Maternal serum levels of 1,25-dihydroxyvitamin D3 also increase due to placental production of PTH and PTH-related protein (PTHrP), enhancing calcium absorption from the gastrointestinal tract, particularly during the third trimester [16, 76].

1.10.3 Adrenal and Gonadal Hormones

In early pregnancy, adrenocorticotropic hormone (ACTH) levels are low, but in later weeks both ACTH and free cortisol increase. Maternal serum total cortisol levels rise primarily due to increased transcortin (cortisol-binding globulin). Although adrenal cortisol synthesis is enhanced, the principal reason for elevated maternal cortisol levels is reduced metabolic clearance, which decreases by about half [77].

Aldosterone levels also increase during pregnancy, contributing to trophoblast development and placental growth. Deoxycorticosterone levels may rise up to 15-fold. Antidiuretic hormone (vasopressin) remains unchanged. Maternal serum androstenedione and testosterone levels increase; however, because most are converted to estrogen in the trophoblast, no masculinizing effect occurs in the fetus. In contrast, maternal serum and urinary DHEA-S levels decline due to placental conversion into estrogens [78–80].

1.11 Immunological System Changes

Physiological leukocytosis is common in pregnancy, with a mild to moderate rise in white blood cell count, particularly neutrophils [81]. In addition, immunologic adaptations occur that allow the semi-allogeneic fetus to survive within the maternal body. These include an increase in regulatory T cells (Tregs) and a shift from Th1-dominant (cell-mediated, pro-inflammatory) immunity toward Th2-dominant (humoral, anti-inflammatory) responses. This Th1/Th2 balance shift, together with other mechanisms, underlies maternal–fetal immune tolerance, ensuring fetal survival while maintaining sufficient maternal defense against infections [82, 83].

To prevent rejection of the semi-allogeneic fetal graft, certain humoral and cellular immune responses are suppressed during pregnancy. In particular, suppression of Th1-dependent immunity plays a crucial role in maintaining gestation. This explains why Th1-dependent autoimmune diseases (such as rheumatoid arthritis, multiple sclerosis, and Hashimoto's thyroiditis) often enter remission during pregnancy. Meanwhile, Th2 activity increases, leading to enhanced secretion of cytokines such as IL-4, IL-6, and IL-13. In pregnancies lacking adequate Th1 immunosuppression, the risk of preeclampsia development is higher [84, 85].

Pregnancy is both a proinflammatory and anti-inflammatory state, comprising three distinct immunological phases:

- *Early pregnancy*: A proinflammatory phase, essential for implantation and placentation.
- *Second half of pregnancy*: An anti-inflammatory phase, allowing fetal growth and development.
- *Parturition*: A proinflammatory phase once again, facilitating labor through inflammatory activation in the myometrium [86].

Despite the rise in leukocyte count, leukocyte-dependent chemotaxis functions are suppressed from the second trimester onward. The exact mechanism remains unclear but is thought to be related to progesterone- and relaxin-mediated suppression of neutrophil activation. This functional impairment of leukocytes may account for both the remission of autoimmune diseases and the increased susceptibility to infections observed during pregnancy [87].

1.12 Musculoskeletal System

Pregnancy is characterized by progressive lordosis, with the maternal center of gravity shifting forward. The mobility of the sacroiliac, sacrococcygeal, and pubic joints also increases [88].

The hormone relaxin, secreted mainly by the corpus luteum and placenta, rises during pregnancy and promotes softening and relaxation of connective tissue. This adaptation prepares the pelvis and birth canal for delivery [89].

1.12.1 Pelvic Joints and Ligaments

The symphysis pubis and sacroiliac joints become more flexible during pregnancy, facilitating childbirth but sometimes causing discomfort or joint instability [90].

1.12.2 Lumbar and Sacral Pain

Low back and sacral pain are common complaints in pregnancy, arising from a combination of hormonally mediated ligamentous relaxation, altered biomechanics, and increased mechanical load. Although usually benign, such pain can significantly impair maternal quality of life [91, 92].

1.13 Central Nervous System

During pregnancy, blood flow in the middle and posterior cerebral arteries decreases, particularly in late gestation. Many women experience mild impairments in concentration, attention, and memory performance [93].

Due to increased aqueous humor outflow, intraocular pressure decreases. Corneal thickness increases slightly, while corneal sensitivity decreases. Changes in corneal hydration and curvature may cause transient refractive alterations; however, overall visual function is not significantly affected. Physiological corneal changes, including increased thickness and curvature secondary to fluid retention, may contribute to blurred vision and contact lens intolerance [94, 95].

1.13.1 Sleep Patterns in Pregnancy

Pregnancy is associated with increased sleep disturbances and altered sleep architecture, changes that may persist into the postpartum period [96]. Headache is also a common symptom. The course of migraine often improves, particularly in the second and third trimesters, likely due to stable estrogen levels; however, in some women, migraine may persist or even worsen. Any new-onset or severe headache warrants careful evaluation to exclude secondary causes such as pre-eclampsia [97].

1.13.2 Mood and Emotional State in Pregnancy

Pregnancy is frequently accompanied by mood fluctuations, including heightened emotional sensitivity, irritability, and anxiety. While often physiological, these changes may predispose some women to perinatal mood disorders, underscoring the importance of monitoring maternal mental health [98, 99].

1.14 Skin

1.14.1 Hyperpigmentation

More than 90% of pregnant women develop hyperpigmentation. Brownish spots of varying size and distribution may appear on the face and neck, known as chloasma (*melasma* or the "mask of pregnancy"). Increased pigmentation of the areolae and genital regions is also common. Hyperpigmentation along the midline of the abdomen is called the *linea nigra*. Most of these pigmentary changes regress after delivery. Their development is associated with elevated melanocyte-stimulating hormone (MSH), with estrogen and progesterone exerting MSH-like effects. Ultraviolet exposure can further intensify pigmentation [100, 101].

Palmar erythema and spider angiomas (telangiectasias) are additional vascular changes. These result from increased estrogen levels and typically resolve shortly after delivery [102].

1.14.2 Striae Gravidarum

From mid-pregnancy onward, reddish, atrophic streaks (*striae gravidarum*) commonly appear on the abdomen, breasts, thighs, and buttocks. Later, they evolve into whitish, depressed scars. Risk factors include maternal weight gain, younger maternal age, and family history. Although the precise etiology remains unclear, striae gravidarum are considered benign and lack effective preventive or curative treatments [103, 104].

1.14.3 Hair, Nail, and Glandular Changes

Hair growth and cycling are altered during pregnancy. Some women may develop hirsutism, while others experience postpartum telogen effluvium (diffuse hair loss) or male-pattern alopecia after delivery. Diffuse hair thinning during pregnancy is also frequently reported [105].

Nail changes include subungual hyperkeratosis, distal onycholysis, transverse ridging, and increased brittleness and softening [106].

Pregnancy influences glandular activity as well: eccrine and sebaceous gland function increases, while apocrine gland activity decreases. Connective tissue changes are notable, with striae gravidarum being the most common. Skin tags (*molluscum fibrosum gravidarum*) may also appear [107]. Vascular changes are hallmark features of pregnancy and may include spider telangiectasia, pyogenic granuloma (*granuloma gravidarum*), palmar erythema, non-pitting edema, varicose veins, vasomotor instability, gingival hyperemia, and hemorrhoids [108]. Mucosal alterations are also observed, most notably *pregnancy gingivitis*, Chadwick's sign (bluish discoloration of the cervix and vagina), and Goodell's sign (softening of the cervix). Diastasis Recti: This refers to the separation of the rectus abdominis muscles due to stretching of the abdominal wall during pregnancy [109].

1.15 Mammary Gland Adaptations in Pregnancy

During early pregnancy, breast tenderness and pain are common. From the second month onward, breast volume increases and superficial veins become more prominent. The nipples enlarge, darken, and become more pronounced. By the second trimester, colostrum may be present. Hypertrophic sebaceous glands on the areola, known as Montgomery's glands, also become more prominent, and striae may develop on the breasts [110].

Breast enlargement during pregnancy results from ductal proliferation, glandular hyperplasia, fat deposition, and fluid–electrolyte retention. Although lactation requires hypothalamic and pituitary regulation, breast size itself is not directly correlated with milk production [111].

Prolactin is essential for lactation and increases progressively during pregnancy. However, milk secretion is inhibited by high levels of estrogen, progesterone, and human placental lactogen (hPL). After delivery, when these hormone levels decline, milk secretion begins. The maintenance of lactation requires suckling, which stimulates the release of both prolactin and oxytocin. Prolactin ensures milk synthesis, whereas oxytocin induces contraction of myoepithelial cells, resulting in milk ejection. In the absence of breastfeeding, prolactin levels fall and milk secretion ceases [72, 112, 113].

1.16 Drug Metabolism and Pharmacokinetics in Pregnancy

Pregnancy alters the absorption, distribution, metabolism, and excretion of drugs. Increased plasma volume and renal clearance, reduced albumin levels, and hormonal effects on hepatic enzymes all influence drug pharmacokinetics. These changes necessitate careful consideration when prescribing medications during pregnancy [114–117].

Physiological Changes Masking Disease
Many normal adaptations of pregnancy resemble pathological findings. For example:

- Dyspnea may reflect physiological hyperventilation rather than underlying cardiopulmonary disease.
- Edema is often a result of plasma volume expansion but may also indicate preeclampsia.
- Tachycardia may be a benign response to increased cardiac output, yet it can mimic arrhythmias or thyroid dysfunction.

Recognizing these distinctions is critical to avoid misdiagnosis or delayed identification of true pathology.

Understanding the normal physiological adaptations of pregnancy is essential for accurate diagnosis and appropriate management. These adaptations ensure maternal survival and optimal fetal growth, but they may also mimic or mask pathological conditions. Distinguishing between physiological changes and true disease is therefore a critical skill in obstetric practice.

For example, physiological dyspnea, edema, or tachycardia must not be misinterpreted as cardiopulmonary disease, while genuine complications such as preeclampsia, thromboembolism, or cardiac pathology should not be overlooked. A solid understanding of maternal physiology enables clinicians to differentiate normal adaptations from pathological states, guiding timely interventions and preventing unnecessary treatments.

Ultimately, awareness of these changes is a cornerstone of safe obstetric care, helping clinicians optimize maternal health, protect fetal well-being, and improve overall pregnancy outcomes.

References

1. Cunningham FG, Leveno KJ, Bloom SL, Dashe JS, Hoffman BL, Casey BM, et al. Williams obstetrics. 25th ed. New York: McGraw-Hill; 2018.
2. Gabbe SG, Niebyl JR, Simpson JL, et al. Obstetrics: normal and problem pregnancies. 8th ed. Philadelphia: Elsevier; 2020.
3. Burton GJ, Jauniaux E. Physiology and pathology of the uteroplacental circulation. J Thromb Haemost. 2018;16(9):1907–17.
4. Pijnenborg R, Brosens I. Uteroplacental development and its disorders. In: Reece EA, Hobbins JC, editors. Clinical obstetrics: the fetus and mother. 3rd ed. Oxford: Wiley-Blackwell; 2016. p. 215–30.
5. Institute of Medicine (US), National Research Council (US) Committee to Reexamine IOM Pregnancy Weight Guidelines. Weight gain during pregnancy: reexamining the guidelines. Washington, DC: National Academies Press; 2009.
6. Rasmussen KM, Yaktine AL, editors. Nutrition during pregnancy. Washington, DC: National Academies Press; 2009.
7. Felig P, Lynch V. Starvation in human pregnancy: hypoglycemia, hypoinsulinemia, and hyperketonemia. Science. 1970;170(3961):990–2.
8. Catalano PM, Shankar K. Obesity and pregnancy: mechanisms of short term and long term adverse consequences for mother and child. BMJ. 2017;356:j1.
9. Cheung KL, Lafayette RA. Renal physiology of pregnancy. Adv Chronic Kidney Dis. 2013;20(3):209–14.
10. Herrera E, Ortega-Senovilla H. Lipid metabolism during pregnancy and its implications for fetal growth. Curr Pharm Biotechnol. 2014;15(1):24–31.
11. Henson MC, Castracane VD. Leptin in pregnancy: an update. Biol Reprod. 2006;74(2):218–29.
12. Briana DD, Malamitsi-Puchner A. The role of adipocytokines in fetal growth. Ann N Y Acad Sci. 2010;1205:82–7.
13. Fuglsang J, Møller N, Ørskov H, Fisker S, Ovesen P. Ghrelin and pregnancy: association with maternal growth hormones, insulin, and glucose. Metabolism. 2005;54(5):574–9.
14. Lindheimer MD, Roberts JM, Cunningham FG. Chesley's hypertensive disorders in pregnancy. 4th ed. San Diego: Academic Press; 2015.
15. Davison JM, Dunlop W. Renal hemodynamics and tubular function in normal human pregnancy. Kidney Int. 1980;18(2):152–61.
16. Kovacs CS. Calcium and bone metabolism in pregnancy and lactation. J Clin Endocrinol Metab. 2001;86(6):2344–8.
17. Glinoer D. The regulation of thyroid function in pregnancy: pathways of endocrine adaptation from physiology to pathology. Endocr Rev. 1997;18(3):404–33.
18. World Health Organization. Assessment of iodine deficiency disorders and monitoring their elimination. 3rd ed. Geneva: World Health Organization; 2007.
19. Czeizel AE, Dudas I. Prevention of the first occurrence of neural-tube defects by periconceptional vitamin supplementation. N Engl J Med. 1992;327(26):1832–5.
20. De-Regil LM, Peña-Rosas JP, Fernández-Gaxiola AC, Rayco-Solon P. Effects and safety of periconceptional folate supplementation for preventing birth defects. Cochrane Database Syst Rev. 2015;(12):CD007950.
21. Molloy AM, Kirke PN, Troendle JF, et al. Maternal vitamin B12 status and risk of neural tube defects in a population with high neural tube defect prevalence and no folic acid fortification. Pediatrics. 2009;123(3):917–23.
22. Hytten FE, Paintin DB. Increase in plasma volume during normal pregnancy. J Obstet Gynaecol Br Emp. 1963;70:402–7.
23. Pritchard JA. Changes in the blood volume during pregnancy and delivery. Anesthesiology. 1965;26:393–9.

24. Means RT Jr. Erythropoietin physiology in pregnancy. Am J Obstet Gynecol. 1995;172(2 Pt 1):497–500.
25. Centers for Disease Control and Prevention (CDC). Recommendations to prevent and control iron deficiency in the United States. MMWR Recomm Rep. 1998;47(RR-3):1–29.
26. Boehlen F, Hohlfeld P, Extermann P, Perneger TV, de Moerloose P. Platelet count at term pregnancy: a reappraisal of the threshold. Obstet Gynecol. 2000;95(1):29–33.
27. Bothwell TH. Iron requirements in pregnancy and strategies to meet them. Am J Clin Nutr. 2000;72(1 Suppl):257S–64S.
28. Milman N. Iron and pregnancy—a delicate balance. Ann Hematol. 2006;85(9):559–65.
29. Hallberg L, Brune M, Rossander L. Iron absorption in man: ascorbic acid and dose-dependent inhibition by phytate. Am J Clin Nutr. 1989;49(1):140–4.
30. Peña-Rosas JP, De-Regil LM, Garcia-Casal MN, Dowswell T. Daily oral iron supplementation during pregnancy. Cochrane Database Syst Rev. 2015;(7):CD004736.
31. Brenner B. Haemostatic changes in pregnancy. Thromb Res. 2004;114(5–6):409–14.
32. James AH. Pregnancy and thrombotic risk. Crit Care Med. 2010;38(2 Suppl):S57–63.
33. Stirling Y, Woolf L, North WR, Seghatchian MJ, Meade TW. Haemostasis in normal pregnancy. Thromb Haemost. 1984;52(2):176–82.
34. Lockwood CJ. Pregnancy-associated changes in the hemostatic system. Clin Obstet Gynecol. 2006;49(4):836–43.
35. Østerud B, Bjørklid E. The role of monocytes in atherogenesis. Physiol Rev. 2003;83(4):1069–112.
36. Clapp JF, Capeless EL. Cardiovascular function before, during, and after the first and subsequent pregnancies. Am J Cardiol. 1997;80(11):1469–73.
37. Robson SC, Hunter S, Boys RJ, Dunlop W. Serial study of factors influencing changes in cardiac output during human pregnancy. Am J Phys. 1989;256:H1060–5.
38. Sanghavi M, Rutherford JD. Cardiovascular physiology of pregnancy. Circulation. 2014;130(12):1003–8.
39. Meah VL, Cockcroft JR, Backx K, Shave R, Stohr EJ. Cardiac output and related haemodynamics during pregnancy: a series of meta-analyses. Heart. 2016;102(7):518–26.
40. Schobel HP, Fischer T, Heuszer K, Geiger H, Schmieder RE. Preeclampsia—a state of sympathetic overactivity. N Engl J Med. 1996;335(20):1480–5.
41. Hermida RC, Ayala DE, Iglesias M. Circadian rhythm of blood pressure in pregnant women. Hypertension. 2001;38(3):736–42.
42. Conrad KP. Emerging role of relaxin in the maternal adaptations to normal pregnancy: implications for preeclampsia. Semin Nephrol. 2011;31(1):15–32.
43. Kerr MG, Scott DB, Samuel E. Studies of the inferior vena cava in late pregnancy. Br Med J. 1964;1:532–3.
44. Weinberger SE, Weiss ST, Cohen WR, Weiss JW, Johnson TS. Pregnancy and the lung. Am Rev Respir Dis. 1980;121(3):559–81.
45. Jensen D, Duffin J, Lam YM, Webb KA, O'Donnell DE. Physiological mechanisms of hyperventilation during human pregnancy. Respir Physiol Neurobiol. 2008;161(1):76–86.
46. Hegewald MJ, Crapo RO. Respiratory physiology in pregnancy. Clin Chest Med. 2011;32(1):1–13.
47. Milne JA. The respiratory response to pregnancy. Postgrad Med J. 1979;55(643):318–24.
48. Kaminsky DA, Irvin CG. Respiratory physiology of pregnancy. In: Fishman AP, Elias JA, Fishman JA, et al., editors. Fishman's pulmonary diseases and disorders. 5th ed. New York: McGraw-Hill; 2015. p. 2601–9.
49. LoMauro A, Aliverti A. Respiratory physiology of pregnancy: physiology masterclass. Breathe. 2015;11(4):297–301.
50. Rasmussen PE, Nielsen FR. Hydronephrosis during pregnancy: a literature survey. Eur J Obstet Gynecol Reprod Biol. 1988;27(3):249–59.
51. Gilstrap LC, Ramin SM. Urinary tract infections during pregnancy. Obstet Gynecol Clin N Am. 2001;28(3):581–91.

52. Kazemier BM, Schneeberger C, de Miranda E, et al. Costs and effects of screening and treating low risk women with a singleton pregnancy for asymptomatic bacteriuria, the ASB study. BMC Pregnancy Childbirth. 2012;12:52.
53. Mørkved S, Bø K. Prevalence of urinary incontinence during pregnancy and postpartum. Int Urogynecol J Pelvic Floor Dysfunct. 1999;10(6):394–8.
54. Sangsawang B, Sangsawang N. Stress urinary incontinence in pregnant women: a review of prevalence, pathophysiology, and treatment. Int Urogynecol J. 2013;24(6):901–12.
55. Lindheimer MD, Davison JM. Renal physiology in normal pregnancy. In: Lindheimer MD, Roberts JM, Cunningham FG, editors. Chesley's hypertensive disorders in pregnancy. 2nd ed. New York: Churchill Livingstone; 1999. p. 263–81.
56. Smith MC, Moran P, Ward MK, Davison JM. Assessment of glomerular filtration rate during pregnancy using the MDRD formula. BJOG. 2008;115(1):109–12.
57. Conrad KP. Renal hemodynamics during pregnancy in animals and humans. Kidney Int. 1984;26(2):116–25.
58. McCormick KL, Robillard JE. Renal and cardiovascular adjustments during pregnancy. Semin Nephrol. 1984;4(3):190–201.
59. Schnarr J, Smaill F. Asymptomatic bacteriuria and symptomatic urinary tract infections in pregnancy. Eur J Clin Investig. 2008;38(Suppl 2):50–7.
60. Richter JE. Gastroesophageal reflux disease during pregnancy. Gastroenterol Clin N Am. 2003;32(1):235–61.
61. Carbone F, Pizzi C, Lapucci C, et al. Gastrointestinal and liver physiology in pregnancy: clinical implications. Expert Rev Gastroenterol Hepatol. 2021;15(8):849–60.
62. Bacq Y, Zarka O, Bréchot JF, et al. Liver function tests in normal pregnancy: a prospective study of 103 pregnant women and 103 matched controls. Hepatology. 1996;23(5):1030–4.
63. Laine MA. Effect of pregnancy on periodontal and dental health. Acta Odontol Scand. 2002;60(5):257–64.
64. Wald A, Van Thiel DH, Hoechstetter L, et al. Effect of pregnancy on gastrointestinal transit. Dig Dis Sci. 1982;27(11):1015–8.
65. Snooks SJ, Swash M, Mathers SE, Henry MM. Effect of pregnancy on the pelvic floor: a 5-year follow-up. Br J Surg. 1990;77(12):1358–60.
66. Everson GT. Pregnancy and gallstones. Hepatology. 1993;17(1):159–61.
67. Riely CA, Latham PS, Donaldson WE. Bromsulfophthalein metabolism in normal human pregnancy. Gastroenterology. 1979;76(2):333–8.
68. Haddow JE, Palomaki GE, Knight GJ, et al. Prenatal screening for open neural tube defects and Down's syndrome. N Engl J Med. 1992;327(9):588–93.
69. Lockitch G. Clinical biochemistry of pregnancy. Crit Rev Clin Lab Sci. 1997;34(1):67–139.
70. Khosla N, Black M. Liver disease in pregnancy. In: Schiff ER, Maddrey WC, Sorrell MF, editors. Schiff's diseases of the liver. 9th ed. Philadelphia: Lippincott Williams & Wilkins; 2003. p. 1391–410.
71. Scheithauer BW, Kovacs K, Randall RV, Ryan N. Pituitary gland in pregnancy: morphologic and immunocytologic study. Mayo Clin Proc. 1984;59(12):835–41.
72. Grattan DR. The hypothalamo-prolactin axis. J Neuroendocrinol. 2020;32(1):e12859.
73. Freeman ME, Kanyicska B, Lerant A, Nagy G. Prolactin: structure, function, and regulation of secretion. Physiol Rev. 2000;80(4):1523–631.
74. Korevaar TIM, Medici M, Visser TJ, Peeters RP. Thyroid disease in pregnancy: new insights in diagnosis and clinical management. Nat Rev Endocrinol. 2017;13(10):610–22.
75. Kovacs CS, Kronenberg HM. Maternal-fetal calcium and bone metabolism during pregnancy, puerperium, and lactation. Endocr Rev. 1997;18(6):832–72.
76. Ardawi MS, Nasrat HA, BA'Aqueel HS. Calcium-regulating hormones and parathyroid hormone-related peptide in normal human pregnancy and postpartum: a longitudinal study. Eur J Endocrinol. 1997;137(4):402–9.
77. Lindsay JR, Nieman LK. The hypothalamic–pituitary–adrenal axis in pregnancy: challenges in disease detection and treatment. Endocr Rev. 2005;26(6):775–99.

78. Quinkler M, Stewart PM. Hypertension and the cortisol-cortisone shuttle. J Clin Endocrinol Metab. 2003;88(6):2384–92.
79. Pepe GJ, Albrecht ED. Actions of placental and fetal adrenal steroid hormones in primate pregnancy. Endocr Rev. 1995;16(5):608–48.
80. Diczfalusy E. Endocrine functions of the human fetoplacental unit. Fed Proc. 1964;23:791–8.
81. Krause PJ, Ingardia CJ, Pontius LT. Physiologic leukocytosis of pregnancy. N Engl J Med. 1987;316(22):1424–6.
82. Aluvihare VR, Kallikourdis M, Betz AG. Regulatory T cells mediate maternal tolerance to the fetus. Nat Immunol. 2004;5(3):266–71.
83. Saito S, Nakashima A, Shima T, Ito M. Th1/Th2/Th17 and regulatory T-cell paradigm in pregnancy. Am J Reprod Immunol. 2010;63(6):601–10.
84. Somerset DA, Zheng Y, Kilby MD, Sansom DM, Drayson MT. Normal human pregnancy is associated with an elevation in the immune suppressive CD25+CD4+ regulatory T-cell subset. Immunology. 2004;112(1):38–43.
85. Redman CWG, Sargent IL. Immunology of pre-eclampsia. Am J Reprod Immunol. 2010;63(6):534–43.
86. Mor G, Cardenas I. The immune system in pregnancy: a unique complexity. Am J Reprod Immunol. 2010;63(6):425–33.
87. Kourtis AP, Read JS, Jamieson DJ. Pregnancy and infection. N Engl J Med. 2014;370(23):2211–8.
88. Franklin ME, Conner-Kerr T. An analysis of posture and back pain in pregnant women. J Orthop Sports Phys Ther. 1998;28(3):133–8.
89. MacLennan AH, Nicolson R, Green RC, Bath M. Serum relaxin and pelvic pain of pregnancy. Lancet. 1986;2(8501):243–5.
90. Wu WH, Meijer OG, Uegaki K, et al. Pregnancy-related pelvic girdle pain (PPP), I: terminology, clinical presentation, and prevalence. Eur Spine J. 2004;13(7):575–89.
91. Vleeming A, Albert HB, Östgaard HC, Sturesson B, Stuge B. European guidelines for the diagnosis and treatment of pelvic girdle pain. Eur Spine J. 2008;17(6):794–819.
92. Wang SM, Dezinno P, Maranets I, Berman MR, Caldwell-Andrews AA, Kain ZN. Low back pain during pregnancy: prevalence, risk factors, and outcomes. Obstet Gynecol. 2004;104(1):65–70.
93. Zeeman GG. Neurologic complications of pre-eclampsia. Semin Perinatol. 2009;33(3):166–72.
94. Weinreb RN, Lu A, Beeson C. Maternal ocular changes during pregnancy. Surv Ophthalmol. 1984;28(3):143–53.
95. Riss B, Riss P. Corneal changes in pregnancy. Graefes Arch Clin Exp Ophthalmol. 1981;216(5):262–8.
96. Mindell JA, Jacobson BJ. Sleep disturbances during pregnancy. J Obstet Gynecol Neonatal Nurs. 2000;29(6):590–7.
97. MacGregor EA. Migraine in pregnancy and lactation: a clinical review. J Fam Plann Reprod Health Care. 2007;33(2):83–93.
98. O'Hara MW, Wisner KL. Perinatal mental illness: definition, description and aetiology. Best Pract Res Clin Obstet Gynaecol. 2014;28(1):3–12.
99. Gavin NI, Gaynes BN, Lohr KN, Meltzer-Brody S, Gartlehner G, Swinson T. Perinatal depression: a systematic review of prevalence and incidence. Obstet Gynecol. 2005;106(5 Pt 1):1071–83.
100. Martin AG, Leal-Khouri S. Physiological skin changes associated with pregnancy. Int J Dermatol. 1992;31(6):375–8.
101. Puri N, Puri A. A study on physiological changes in skin during pregnancy. Our Dermatol Online. 2012;3(1):36–40.
102. Cunningham FG, Leveno KJ, Bloom SL, et al. Williams obstetrics. 25th ed. New York: McGraw-Hill; 2018.
103. Salter SA, Kimball AB. Striae gravidarum. Clin Dermatol. 2006;24(2):97–100.

104. Osman H, Rubeiz N, Tamim H, Nassar AH. Risk factors for the development of striae gravidarum. Am J Obstet Gynecol. 2007;196(1):62.e1–5.
105. Jabbour SA. Cutaneous changes in pregnancy. Clin Dermatol. 2006;24(2):84–7.
106. Kumari R. Physiological skin changes in pregnancy: a study of 140 cases. Indian J Dermatol Venereol Leprol. 2010;76(6):714.
107. Wong RC, Ellis CN. Physiologic skin changes in pregnancy. J Am Acad Dermatol. 1984;10(6):929–40.
108. Marchitelli CE, Cecatti JG, Surita FG. Skin changes during pregnancy: a review. Rev Bras Ginecol Obstet. 2021;43(5):394–401.
109. Spitznagle TM, Leong FC, Van Dillen LR. Prevalence of diastasis recti abdominis in a urogynecological patient population. Int Urogynecol J. 2007;18(3):321–8.
110. Neville MC, Morton J. Physiology and endocrine changes underlying human lactogenesis II. J Nutr. 2001;131(11):3005S–8S.
111. Hamosh M. Breastfeeding: unraveling the mysteries of mother's milk. Medscape Womens Health. 1996;1(2):5.
112. McNeilly AS. Lactational control of reproduction. Reprod Fertil Dev. 2001;13(7–8):583–90.
113. Lawrence RA, Lawrence RM. Breastfeeding: a guide for the medical profession. 8th ed. Philadelphia: Elsevier; 2016.
114. Anderson GD. Pregnancy-induced changes in pharmacokinetics: a mechanistic-based approach. Clin Pharmacokinet. 2005;44(10):989–1008.
115. Hebert MF, Easterling TR, Kirby B, et al. Effects of pregnancy on CYP3A and P-glycoprotein activities as measured by midazolam and digoxin pharmacokinetics. Clin Pharmacol Ther. 2008;84(2):248–53.
116. Costantine MM. Physiologic and pharmacokinetic changes in pregnancy. Front Pharmacol. 2014;5:65.
117. Pariente G, Leibson T, Carls A, Adams-Webber T, Ito S, Koren G. Pregnancy-associated changes in pharmacokinetics: a systematic review. PLoS Med. 2016;13(11):e1002160.

Chapter 2
Medication Use During Pregnancy

Pelin Koca

2.1 Introduction

Pregnancy is the beginning of a new life and a critical physiological process in female reproductive biology, ensuring the continuation of the species. The gestation period usually runs 36–40 weeks, during which several physiological and biochemical alterations occur in the woman's body. Drug usage is common in pregnant women, and its incidence is increasing worldwide. The rate of pregnant women exposed to at least one prescription medication was reported as 60.3% in Denmark, 80% in Italy, 93% in France, 85% in Germany, and 64% in the United States [1–7]. It is also essential to consider the possibility of unprescribed exposure. Pregnant women are exposed to drugs in chronic problems like diabetes mellitus, hypertension, eclampsia/preeclampsia, epilepsy, asthma, psychiatric diseases, or in acute conditions such as infection, fever, trauma, or allergy. In particular, in the early days of pregnancy, women may be unaware that they are pregnant and therefore may be unintentionally exposed to drugs.

The majority of pharmaceuticals transfer to the fetus [8]. Multiple factors influence placental transfer (Table 2.1). For example, physiological changes in pregnant women alter the pharmacokinetics (absorption, distribution, metabolism, and elimination) of medication [9]. However, it is extremely difficult to identify the alterations in the pharmacokinetics of any medication and to acquire detailed information regarding fetal drug exposure. Due to ethical considerations, it is hard to conduct research on pregnant mothers and fetuses. Invasive drug level measurements (e.g., amniocentesis, cordocentesis) can provide data about fetal drug concentrations; nevertheless, they may cause significant risks to both the pregnant woman and the

P. Koca (✉)
Izmir Bakircay University, Faculty of Medicine, Department of Medical Pharmacology, Izmir, Turkey
e-mail: pelin.koca@bakircay.edu.tr

© The Author(s), under exclusive license to Springer Nature Switzerland AG 2026

I. Karaca (ed.), *Managing Maternal Chronic Diseases for a Healthy Pregnancy*,
https://doi.org/10.1007/978-3-032-15221-3_2

Table 2.1 The factors affecting drug transfer across the placenta

Placental
Placental metabolic enzymes
Uteroplacental blood flow
Expression of placental transporters
Syncytiotrophoblast integrity
Placental surface area
Placental thickness
Physical/anatomical
Maternal blood flow
Fetal blood flow
pH difference (maternal vs fetal)
Gestational age
Pharmacological
Molecular size
Lipophilicity
Ionization (pKa)
Protein binding
Maternal/fetal concentration gradient
Dose, duration, and route of administration
Placental drug interactions

fetus, requiring a careful evaluation of the benefit-to-harm ratio. The results of non-invasive methodologies (e.g., in vitro or animal research) are not always translatable to humans. In addition to these methods, data about fetal drug concentrations can be obtained through the collection of extra fluid during standard amniocentesis or from noninvasive samples of fetal meconium or hair. Nonetheless, the majority of these methods are generally not highly useful in routine practice [10]. During pregnancy, an accurate assessment is essential for managing the basic treatment requirements of the mother and to safeguard the fetus's well-being.

2.2 Physiological and Pharmacokinetic Changes in Pregnancy

Pregnancy-related physiological changes are complex and dynamic processes that influence the parameters of drug absorption, distribution, metabolism, and excretion (ADME). Adaptive modifications in the cardiovascular, renal, gastrointestinal, and endocrine systems during this period substantially affect drug metabolism in the body. For example, decreased gastrointestinal motility, nausea and vomiting, and changes in gastric pH may alter oral bioavailability and result in variations in plasma peak time. Increased cardiac output may influence hepatic blood flow and alter elimination for some pharmaceuticals. Raised plasma volume and extracellular fluid may alter drug distribution and lead to increased apparent volume of distribution of hydrophilic drugs. A mitigation in plasma albumin concentration results in an increase in the free fraction of the medication. Alterations in the transporter expression and activity, enhanced renal blood flow, elevated GFR, and modifications in the activity of enzymes involved in metabolism may influence the clearance of drugs [11, 12]. Although it was reported that the activity of CYP1A2 and CYP2C19 enzymes decreases during pregnancy, a reduction in the activity of CYP2B6, CYP2C8, CYP2C9, CYP2D6, CYP2E1, and CYP3A4 enzymes was also identified. Therefore, pregnancy is a special physiological condition in which pharmacokinetic processes are also recalibrated. However, despite these predictable physiological alterations and their impact on medication pharmacokinetics, it remains unclear whether they induce modifications in pharmacological efficacy and/or adverse effect profiles [9, 12].

2.3 Placental Transport

The placenta acts as a barrier between the mother and the fetus, providing critical functions such as supplying nutrients and oxygen to the fetus, as well as releasing hormones and mediators. As previously stated, drug use is significantly prevalent during pregnancy. However, the safe administration of drugs during gestation is severely limited due to their ability to cross the placenta. Xenobiotics reach the co-cytotrophoblast layer of the placenta by placental transport, utilizing passive diffusion, active transport, or facilitated diffusion mechanisms throughout the trophoblast cytoplasm. Xenobiotics occur both in free form and bound to plasma proteins as complexes. The free fraction of drugs can be capable of crossing the placental barrier. Binding to plasma proteins reduces placental transport. In other words, the less a drug binds to plasma proteins, the more placental passage it has [8, 13, 14]. This is due to both the size of the albumin–drug complex and the gap in albumin concentration between the mother and the fetus. The plasma albumin concentration in the fetus is higher than the maternal plasma concentration, making the passage of drugs difficult. Molecules characterized by low molecular weight and high lipophilicity easily cross from the maternal blood to the fetus. The ionization constant (pK) of drugs is also significant in placental transport, as it affects the solubility of the drug in body pH. Drugs having weak basic characteristics pass more easily into the fetal circulation, which is comparatively acidic than that of the mother. Membrane transporters involved in placental transfer are also crucial for fetal exposure [8, 9, 15].

2.3.1 Passive Diffusion

The primary and typical mechanism for placental drug transport is passive diffusion. Transport occurs passively, adhering to the concentration gradient and without necessitating energy. In particular, low molecular weight and lipophilic drugs can pass to the fetus through passive diffusion; however, changes in passive diffusion capacity may occur due to alterations in placental structure and function throughout gestation. For instance, the placental barrier is thicker during early weeks of pregnancy but may become thinner in the later weeks, thereby facilitating increased passage of substances [8, 13, 14].

2.3.2 Active Transport

In contrast to passive diffusion, it requires energy and transpires against the concentration gradient, moving from locations with low to high density. Placental cells, especially the syncytiotrophoblast layer, contain various carrier proteins. These proteins assist the selective transport of drugs, nutrients, and metabolites to the fetus. Transport proteins are categorized into two groups as efflux and influx transporters. Influx transporters such as SLC22A4 (OCTN1), SLC22A5 (OCTN2), SLC22A9 (OAT4), and SLC15A1 (PEPT1) facilitate the transfer of essential substances from the maternal blood into the placental cells. Efflux transporters such as P-glycoprotein (P-gp), breast cancer resistance protein (BCRP), and multidrug resistance-associated proteins (MRPs) prevent transport of some medications and chemicals from maternal circulation to the fetal circulation. They provide protective functions for the fetus. The expression of placental carriers varies depending on the medications used by the mother, hormone levels, and environmental factors [8, 13, 14].

2.3.3 Facilitated Diffusion

Facilitated diffusion is a transport method in which molecules utilize specific carriers or channels without using energy, in contrast to passive diffusion. The large molecules that need to move down the concentration gradient but cannot penetrate the lipid layer are transported through facilitated diffusion. This mechanism provides the regulated transfer of nutrients and certain drugs that are critical for the growth and development of the fetus [8, 13, 14].

Placental Metabolism

The placenta is also an organ that metabolizes medicines before their transfer to the fetus. Placental enzymes structurally modify pharmaceuticals. They can transform them into inactive, active, or toxic metabolites or activate prodrugs. This mechanism primarily functions as a protective barrier for the fetus, significantly limiting the detrimental effects of the medication. Placental metabolism appears in two phases: Phase I and Phase II. In phase I reactions, drug molecules undergo oxidation and/or reduction and/or hydrolysis. During this phase, cytochrome p450 enzymes (especially CYP1A1, CYP19A1), dehydrogenases, and epoxide hydrolases are involved. Phase II metabolism aims to enhance the hydrophilicity of the drug.

Enzymes such as UDP-glucoryltransferase (UGT), sulfotransferases (SULT), and glutathione S-transferase (GST) facilitate conjugation reactions for this purpose. The capacity of placental metabolism may vary between individuals. The week of pregnancy during which the exposure occurs, along with the specific drug administered, its dosage, and the duration of treatment, can alter fetal exposure capacity. Therefore, fetal drug exposure is influenced by all of these factors [8, 9, 16].

2.4 An Overview of Teratology and Teratogenic Mechanisms

A human teratogen is defined as an agent that alters the growth or structure of the developing embryo or fetus, resulting in birth abnormalities [17]. The term "teratology" was first introduced by Isidore Geoffroy Saint-Hilaire (1805–1861). Teratology is the scientific field that investigates the causes, mechanisms, and patterns of abnormal development [18]. In 1941, Norman Gregg, an ophthalmologist, was the first to identify a human teratogen: maternal rubella infection during pregnancy, which caused a triad of defects (cataracts, heart malformations, and deafness) in the infants [19].

Throughout human history, the term "teratogenicity" has been understood and interpreted differently. In ancient texts written in cuneiform on clay belonging to the Chaldean people who lived in southern Mesopotamia around the ninth century BC, congenital malformations and the speculations associated with this condition. A historical trajectory beginning with mystical and supernatural interpretations has led to the modern understanding of teratology, shaped by a series of key milestones. Over time, this concept has evolved through its historical development into a more systematic and scientific framework. Camille Dareste (1822–1899), a French zoologist, was a leading scientist who applied the experimental approach to the concept of teratology [20]. The first animal studies were conducted to investigate the mechanisms of anomalies by Dareste. He stated that neural tube defects were inadequate closure of the neural tube rather than bursting of the closed neural tube [21].

The thalidomide disaster is undoubtedly one of the greatest tragic events in the history of health. Thalidomide, a sedative agent synthesized by CIBA in 1954 and marketed in 1957, has been widely used as an antiemetic in pregnant women in over 50 countries. It has resulted in infants being born with various congenital malformations, especially phocomelia [22, 23]. The thalidomide disaster has increased public awareness of teratogenicity and has provided a new perspective for evaluating drug safety in the perinatal period. In the post-thalidomide era, Wilson (1973) defined teratology as a science that focused on the adverse effects of the environment on developing systems (germ cells, embryos, fetuses, and immature individuals) and presented the "Principles of Teratology" (Table 2.2). Wilson's principles remain a fundamental guide in comprehending and investigating the effects of teratogenic agents [18, 24, 25]. Teratology is important to ensure the safety of drug use in pregnancy. The use of drugs during pregnancy is a growing concern due to the heightened teratogenic risk [26].

Table 2.2 Wilson's six principles of teratology [24]

1.	Susceptibility to teratogenesis depends on the genotype of the conceptus and the manner in which this interacts with environmental factors.
2.	Susceptibility to teratogenic agents varies with the developmental stage at the time of exposure.
3.	Teratogenic agents act in specific ways (mechanisms) on developing cells and tissues to initiate abnormal embryogenesis (pathogenesis).
4.	The final manifestations of abnormal development are death, malformation, growth retardation, and functional disorder.
5.	The access of adverse environmental influences to developing tissues depends on the nature of the influences (agent).
6.	Manifestations of deviant development increase in degree as dosage increases from the no-effect to the totally lethal level.

Teratogenic Mechanisms of the Medication

The mechanisms that may induce teratogenic effects of pharmaceuticals are as follows:

(a) *Folate antagonism*: Pharmacological agents that interfere with folic acid metabolism, such as methotrexate, valproic acid, carbamazepine, and phenytoin, can impact processes such as DNA synthesis, methylation, and cellular division, leading not only to anomalies such as neural tube defects but also to cardiovascular defects, oral clefts, and urinary tract defects [27–29].

(b) *Neural Crest Cell Disruption*: Retinoic acid, ethanol, and some epileptics may interfere with the migration and differentiation of neural crest cells during embryonic development, resulting in craniofacial anomalies such as cleft lip/palate, heart defects, and various neurocrest syndromes [27, 30, 31].

(c) *Endocrine Disruption*: Under physiological conditions, embryo development depends on the balance between maternal and fetal hormones. Drugs such as diethylstilbestrol, antithyroids, and glucocorticoids can disrupt developmental processes by affecting this fragile equilibrium. They can influence organ development and the reproductive system [27].

(d) *Oxidative Stress*: Embryos are particularly sensitive to oxidative stress during the organogenesis period. Thalidomide, phenytoin, and antineoplastic agents induce oxidative damage at the cellular level, increasing reactive oxygen species (ROS) and potentially harming fundamental cellular components such as DNA, proteins, and lipids, tissue dysplasia, and disruption of organogenesis. They may result in birth defects, including skeletal and extremity malformations, neural tube defects, cleft lip/palate, and cardiac anomalies [27, 32, 33].

(e) *Vascular Disruption*: Circulation to the tissue is essential for the formation of healthy embryonic/fetal tissue. Complications may occur associated with the uterine–placental unit, placental–fetal unit, or fetal vascular system deterioration.

Conditions such as hypo/hyper-perfusion, hypoxia, and obstruction influence tissue development. Vasoactive substances such as misoprostol, ergotamine, and pseudoephedrine reduce fetal blood flow. Peripheral vasculature is predominantly impacted, leading to terminal extremity malformations, skeletal anomalies, hydranencephaly/porencephaly, gastroschisis, and small bowel atresia [27, 34].

(f) *Specific Receptor- or Enzyme-Mediated Teratogenesis*: Pharmaceuticals such as angiotensin-converting enzyme inhibitors (ACEIs), angiotensin II receptor antagonists (ARBs), and non-steroidal anti-inflammatory drugs (NSAIDs) disrupt embryonic development by binding to certain specific receptors and/or may have teratogenic effects [27].

2.5 Evaluating Possible Teratogenic Risks Associated with Medications

Certain pharmaceuticals and chemicals can traverse the embryo/fetus and cause developmental disorders, structural anomalies, or functional disorders. The assessment of teratogenic risk associated with medication use during pregnancy necessitates a multidisciplinary approach, integrating pharmacology, clinical medicine, embryology, and toxicology. The clinician should always consistently assess the benefit-to-harm ratio for both the mother and the fetus and evaluate possible fetal risks with the consequences of untreated maternal disease [22]. For instance, although β-adrenoceptor agonists and corticosteroids may slightly increase the baseline risk, their use during pregnancy is justified in asthmatic women, as poorly controlled asthma itself poses significant risks to both the fetus and the mother. On the other hand, oral isotretinoin for acne treatment should be discontinued well before conception. Isotretinoin exposure during early pregnancy is significantly associated with the risk of fetal malformations and neurological disorders [15]. Assessing teratogenic risk is often complex, as it relies on numerous aspects. These are classified under the main topics: variables related to the administration of the medication, evaluating the data, genetic susceptibility, and confounding factors [22, 35, 36]

- *Variables related to the administration of the medication*
  - *Time of administration*
  - *Dosage, duration, and route of administration*
  - *Monotherapy* vs. *polytherapy*
- *Evaluating the data*
- *Genetic susceptibility*
- *Confounding factors*

2.5.1 *Variables Related to the Administration of the Medication*

Time of Administration

The preimplantation period involves the timeframe from conception to implantation (0–1 week). During this phase, if there is any drug exposure, the fetus is either unaffected or, in the case of a teratogenic effect, the pregnancy results in miscarriage. Consequently, it is referred to as the "all-or-none period." The embryonic (organogenesis) period (3–8 weeks) is the most sensitive period to teratogens. During this period, differentiation in the organ system develops, resulting in teratogen exposure potentially causing structural anomalies. The fetal period (9–40 weeks) is characterized by the growth of developed organs and their functional development. Teratogenic exposure during this period may result in dysfunction of organs, growth retardation, and neurodevelopmental problems [22, 36, 37]. The teratogenic risk profile of ACE inhibitors (ACEIs) varies depending on the trimester of exposure. While the evidence for increased risk in the first trimester is inconclusive, substantial data support that ACEI exposure during the second and third trimesters can lead to severe fetal abnormalities, particularly affecting renal development [38].

Dosage, Duration, and Route of Administration

The probability of teratogenic effects is often dose-dependent; the risk rises with increasing dosage. Valproic acid treatment during pregnancy has demonstrated a dose-dependent impact on cognitive impairment [39]. Similarly, the risk of teratogenicity escalates with prolonged treatment duration; short-term use may sometimes not present a teratogenic risk [22, 36, 40]. The route of administration of the substance exposure is also important for assessing teratogenic risk. The possibility of the drug reaching systemic circulation and affecting the fetus varies depending on the route of administration. It has been shown that the use of topical retinoids does not increase the risk of major and minor congenital malformations, spontaneous abortion, low birth weight, stillbirth, or prematurity in the fetus [41–43]. However, systemic retinoid use is also known to cause teratogenic effects such as facial, skull, cardiovascular, nervous system, and thymus abnormalities [44, 45]. Consequently, it is recommended that women who are planning pregnancy or are pregnant should be treated with the lowest possible dose and duration [22, 36].

Monotherapy Versus Polytherapy

The concomitant use of multiple drugs increases the risk of drug–drug interactions. One drug may increase or decrease the effect of another drug or increase the risk of side effects or teratogenic effects. Consequently, it is advisable for women who are planning pregnancy or are pregnant to switch to monotherapy if possible [22, 36, 46, 47]. Tomson et al. showed that high-dose (1500 mg/day) valproic acid use during pregnancy increased the risk of major malformations in combination use (24.0% for monotherapy, 31.0% for VPA + lamotrigine) [48].

2.5.2 Evaluating the Data

The absence of data on the effects of drugs in pregnancy is a significant problem. Conducting randomized controlled trials in pregnant women is challenging due to ethical issues. Thus, following a drug's market release, the potential teratogenic risk is generally unknown. Over 90% of the US Food and Drug Administration (FDA)-approved drugs do not have sufficient teratogenic information. Although the literature provides sufficient data regarding certain drugs, this information is either inaccessible or challenging to adapt to clinical practice. Therefore, it is critical for the physician to comprehend the interpretation of experimental studies, human studies (case reports, epidemiological studies), and meta-analyses in the assessment of potential teratogenic risk. The clinician must evaluate both the prevailing scientific evidence and the health conditions and requirements of the mother and infant while making recommendations [22, 35, 49]. Animal studies cannot be extrapolated to humans. High maternal toxicity in the animal study may result in nonspecific developmental disorders in the offspring. Case reports are particularly important for reporting teratogenic effects from rare teratogenic effects, but they cannot provide absolute risk estimates. Since randomized controlled studies cannot be conducted in pregnant women, observational cohort and case–control studies, which are epidemiological studies, are actually the main study types that provide data in this field. Cohort studies might not achieve sufficient sample size to identify rare anomalies. In case–control studies, drug exposures of mothers of infants with congenital anomalies are compared to those of unexposed mothers of healthy infants. Case–control studies are planned retrospectively and are susceptible to the risk of recall bias. A meta-analysis improves sample size and provides more statistical power [22, 49].

The analysis and interpretation of information obtained from data sources is crucial. The baseline risk of major congenital anomalies is approximately 3%. The potential of the medicine, whether administered or intended for use, to elevate this risk should be assessed optimally based on the available information. The sample sizes of studies in the literature, their research designs (e.g., case reports, meta-analyses), potential risks of bias, absolute risk assessments regarding congenital anomalies, the presence of confounding factors such as maternal comorbidities, and the consistency of findings across different studies should be critically evaluated. Furthermore, it should be noted that the association between drug exposure and observed anomalies should not be directly interpreted as causal [35]. Teratology information services, such as OTIS, ENTIS, and Medicaid, perform multicenter prospective studies. National teratology health databases may provide valuable data for assessing teratogenic risk [49]. Public perception of the potential teratogenic risk of medications is high [50–53]. Exaggerating the teratogenic potential of a drug may cause both the physician and the pregnant woman to unnecessarily avoid potentially effective treatment options. Understanding the reasons behind this overestimation is essential for optimizing treatment planning.

2.5.3 Genetic Susceptibility

Interindividual genetic variations may alter the potential teratogenic effects of in utero drug exposure on the fetus. Genetic differences may affect drug pharmacokinetics, target receptor binding, or fetal tissue sensitivity, resulting in increased or decreased teratogenic risk. For example, polymorphisms in the MTHFR gene, which is involved in folate metabolism, may increase the risk of neural tube defects as a result of exposure to antiepileptic drugs. Similarly, mutations in the GSPT1 and GSTT1 genes may affect fetal lung development by altering the effects of drugs such as paracetamol through oxidative stress mechanisms [54, 55].

2.5.4 Confounding Factors

Pregnancy is not a special situation that is only seen in healthy women. The heightened risk of congenital malformations during pregnancy in women with chronic diseases is not always attributable to drug exposure; this risk may also be due to the underlying disease itself. In addition to comorbidities, factors such as increased body mass index, tobacco/alcohol use, hypertension, diabetes mellitus, maternal conditions such as epilepsy, folate deficiency, lifestyle characteristics, parity, socioeconomic status, and history of malformations in previous pregnancies may also independently increase the risk of fetal malformations, regardless of medication exposure [22, 26, 36, 56]. When assessing potential teratogenic risk, confounding factors should be evaluated individually for each pregnant woman. Additionally, when evaluating data, it is essential to consider whether confounding factors have been accounted for or not.

2.6 Pregnancy Risk Categories for Medication Use

After the thalidomide disaster, risk categories for drug use in pregnancy were first developed in 1978 by Farmaceutiska Specialiteteri Sverige (FASS) (Table 2.3). The FASS classification system includes four groups (A, B, C, and D). The potential teratogenic risk of the drug increases from category A to category D. The Australian Medicines Evaluation Commission produced the ADEC (B1, B2, B3, and X) classification in 1989. In 1979, the FDA developed a classification system comprising five groups (A, B, C, D, and X) and implemented a variety of measures to mitigate the risks of teratogenicity associated with drugs. These categories have become mandatory to include in the prescribing information of the drug. This process, which commenced with the prescribing information of drugs in the 1970s, continued with medication guides and Risk

Table 2.3 Categorization of the risk of drug use during pregnancy

Category	Assessment summary
	FASS *(Farmaceutiska Specialiteteri Sverige)*
A	Drugs widely used by pregnant women without any observed reproductive harm, supported by retrospective studies.
B	Drugs used by a few pregnant women without observed reproductive harm; animal data varies (B1, B2, B3).
B1	Animal studies show no fetal damage or other deleterious effects on the reproductive process.
B2	Animal studies are inadequate or lacking, but no evidence of damage or other deleterious effects on the reproductive process.
B3	Animal studies show an increased incidence of fetal damage or other deleterious effects on the reproductive process. The clinical significance of these results in humans is uncertain.
C	Medicinal products suspected to cause harmful pharmacological effects without direct teratogenicity; animal research may indicate risks whose significance for humans is uncertain.
D	Medicinal products known or suspected to cause directly or indirectly fetal malformations or permanent damage in humans.
	FDA *(U.S. Food and Drug Administration)*
A	Controlled human studies show no fetal risk, and the possibility of fetal damage appears negligible.
B	Animal studies have shown no fetal risk, or observed animal risk has not been confirmed in human studies; however, adequate and well-controlled studies in pregnant women are lacking.
C	Animal studies have shown fetal risk, and no human studies; use only if the potential benefit justifies the potential risk to the fetus.
D	Human studies have demonstrated fetal risk; use may be acceptable in pregnant women only if the potential benefits outweigh the risks.
X	Pharmaceutical agents with demonstrated fetal abnormalities or risks in humans or animals, where the potential risk clearly outweighs any benefit; contraindicated in pregnant women.
	ADEC (Australian Drug Evaluation Committees)
A	Extensive clinical use in pregnant women has not demonstrated an increased risk of fetal malformations or other harmful effects, indicating established safety in pregnancy.
B	Although clinical exposure in pregnant women and women of childbearing age is limited, current human data do not indicate an increased risk of fetal malformations or adverse outcomes. Consequently, risk evaluation primarily relies on toxicological and reproductive studies in animals, which inform subclassification within this category.
B1	Limited human exposure with no observed fetal harm; animal studies have not shown evidence of an increased occurrence of fetal risk.
B2	Animal studies are inadequate and lacking; however, available data have not demonstrated an increased incidence of fetal risk, the relevance of which to humans remains uncertain.

(continued)

Table 2.3 (continued)

Category	Assessment summary
B3	Animal studies demonstrate increased incidence of fetal damage; however, the clinical significance of these findings in humans remains.
C	Drugs that may cause, or be suspected of causing, reversible pharmacological effects in the fetus or neonate without causing abnormalities.
D	Drugs associated with an increased risk of human fetal malformations or irreversible damage; may also adverse pharmacological effects.
X	Drugs with a high risk of causing permanent fetal harm; contraindicated in pregnancy or when pregnancy is possible.

Minimization Action Plans (RiskMAP) in the 1990s. In addition, the FDA has mandated that pharmaceutical companies implement Risk Evaluation and Mitigation Strategies (REMSs) for drugs known to have high teratogenicity risks. REMSs aim to prevent the uncontrolled use of these drugs during pregnancy. REMS programs include steps such as educational materials, patient registration systems, birth control requirements, pregnancy tests, and limited drug distribution.

Over time, clinicians have observed that there are some challenges and limitations in interpreting the FDA pregnancy categories (A-X). In response, FDA officials established a forum to discuss these problems, as well as to consider criticisms and evaluations of the classification system [57–60].

- The categories provide an oversimplified narrative.
- There is a prevalent perception that risk increases linearly from category A to X.
- The categories are excessively generalized; the potential teratogenic risks of drugs in the same group are assumed to be similar.
- The effects of important factors such as dose, duration, and time of use are ignored or perceived as unimportant.
- The distinction between animal and human studies is not emphasized enough.

In 2015, the FDA established the Pregnancy and Lactation Labeling Rule (PLLR), a regulation designed to update and improve the labeling of medications used during pregnancy and breastfeeding. New labeling requires narrative notes in three categories of pregnancy, lactation, and females and males of reproductive potential. The main difference from the A-X letter category is the addition of the "females and males of reproductive potential" section. The pregnancy section includes the headings "Risk Summary," "Clinical Consideration," and "Background Data" [35, 61–63]. Table 2.4 presents information on the contents of the new classification system.

Table 2.4 Overview of the New FDA Pregnancy Labeling Rule (PLLR)

Section	Content
Risk summary	Potential teratogenic risk in humans is evaluated. A conclusion is drawn regarding whether the risk is increased. If increased risk is observed in human data, a detailed narrative is provided. If the drug is not systemically absorbed, fetal exposure is considered unlikely. If systemically absorbed, human data are presented first, followed by animal data.
Clinical considerations	Information on inadvertent exposure is provided. Risks of untreated maternal disease for both mother and fetus are explained. Dose adjustments including dosage, timing, and duration during pregnancy are described. Pregnancy-specific or increased frequency adverse effects are discussed. Potential neonatal issues postpartum and necessary medical interventions are detailed. If the drug is used during labor, effects on the mother, fetus, and labor process are assessed.
Background data	Study type is specified. Dosage, duration, and timing of treatment are explained. Beneficial and adverse outcomes are reported. Human data are presented first, followed by animal data. Animal species used in studies are identified, and the equivalent human doses are provided.

2.7 Key Resources for Teratogenic Risk Assessment in Pregnancy

The decision-making process regarding the use of drugs during pregnancy requires careful consideration of safety for both the mother and the fetus. Therefore, it is crucial to identify sources that provide up-to-date and reliable information on the safety profile of drugs in pregnancy. Different countries and institutions have developed various systems and databases to classify the teratogenic risks of drugs. Table 2.5 summarizes the main sources of information and classification systems for the use of drugs during pregnancy.

Table 2.5 Useful information sources on drug use during pregnancy

Research Databases
WoS, Scopus, PubMed, Embase, Cochrane Library, Google Scholar
Books
Briggs GG, Freeman RK. Drugs in Pregnancy and Lactation: A Reference Guide to Fetal and Neonatal Risk.
Schaefer C, Peters P, Miller RK. Drugs During Pregnancy and Lactation
Teratology Information Services/Networks
UKTIS (UK Teratology Information Service) (https://www.uktis.org)
OTIS/MotherToBaby (Organization of Teratology Information Specialists) (https://mothertobaby.org)
ENTIS (European Network of Teratology Information Services) (https://www.entis-org.eu)
Motherisk (Canadian Teratology Information Service)[a]
Electronic Databases/Digital Sources
Micromedex (https://www.ibm.com/products/micromedex)
Reprotox (https://reprotox.org)
TERIS (Teratology Information System) (https://deohs.washington.edu/teris/)
Lexicomp (https://www.entis-org.eu)
UpToDate (https://www.uptodate.com)
Embryotox (https://www.embryotox.de/)
TOXBASE (https://www.toxbase.org)

[a]Motherisk was discontinued in 2019 and is no longer maintained or updated

References

1. Lacroix I, Hurault C, Sarramon MF, Guitard C, Berrebi A, Grau M, Albouy-Cossard C, Bourrel R, Elefant E, Montastruc JL, Damase-Michel C. Prescription of drugs during pregnancy: a study using EFEMERIS, the new French database. Eur J Clin Pharmacol. 2009;65(8):839–46.
2. Daw JR, Hanley GE, Greyson DL, Morgan SG. Prescription drug use during pregnancy in developed countries: a systematic review. Pharmacoepidemiol Drug Saf. 2011;20(9):895–902.
3. Andrade SE, Gurwitz JH, Davis RL, Chan KA, Finkelstein JA, Fortman K, McPhillips H, Raebel MA, Roblin D, Smith DH, Yood MU, Morse AN, Platt R. Prescription drug use in pregnancy. Am J Obstet Gynecol. 2004;191(2):398–407.
4. Mitchell AA, Gilboa SM, Werler MM, Kelley KE, Louik C, Hernández-Díaz S, National Birth Defects Prevention Study. Medication use during pregnancy, with particular focus on prescription drugs: 1976–2008. Am J Obstet Gynecol. 2011;205(1):51.e1–8.
5. Smolina K, Hanley GE, Mintzes B, Oberlander TF, Morgan S. Trends and determinants of prescription drug use during pregnancy and postpartum in British Columbia, 2002–2011: a population-based cohort study. PLoS One. 2015;10(5):e0128312.
6. Fortinguerra F, Belleudi V, Poggi FR, Bortolus R, Puccini A, Solfrini V, Stella P, Trotta F. Medication prescriptions before, during and after pregnancy in Italy: a population-based study. Ann Ist Super Sanita. 2021;57(3):249–58.
7. Thunbo MØ, Vendelbo JH, Witte DR, Larsen A, Pedersen LH. Maternal demographic patterns in medication use during pregnancy: a nationwide register study. Basic Clin Pharmacol Toxicol. 2025;136(4):e70020.
8. Kotta-Loizou I, Pritsa A, Antasouras G, Vasilopoulos SN, Voulgaridou G, Papadopoulou SK, Coutts RHA, Lechouritis E, Giaginis C. Fetus exposure to drugs and chemicals: a holistic overview on the assessment of their transport and metabolism across the human placental barrier. Diseases. 2024;12(6):114.

9. Gong C, Bertagnolli LN, Boulton DW, Coppola P. A literature review of changes in phase II drug-metabolizing enzyme and drug transporter expression during pregnancy. Pharmaceutics. 2023;15(11):2624.
10. Hudson RE, Metz TD, Ward RM, McKnite AM, Enioutina EY, Sherwin CM, Watt KM, Job KM. Drug exposure during pregnancy: current understanding and approaches to measure maternal-fetal drug exposure. Front Pharmacol. 2023;14:1111601.
11. Berezowska M, Sharma P, Pilla Reddy V, Coppola P. Physiologically based pharmacokinetic modelling of drugs in pregnancy: a mini-review on availability and limitations. Fundam Clin Pharmacol. 2024;38(3):402–9.
12. Pariente G, Leibson T, Carls A, Adams-Webber T, Ito S, Koren G. Pregnancy-associated changes in pharmacokinetics: a systematic review. PLoS Med. 2016;13(11):e1002160.
13. Goetzl L, Darbinian N, Merabova N, Devane LC, Ramamoorthy S. Gestational age variation in human placental drug transporters. Front Pharmacol. 2022;13:837694.
14. Mao Q, Chen X. An update on placental drug transport and its relevance to fetal drug exposure. Med Rev (2021). 2022;2(5):501–11.
15. Yates LM, Thomas SHL. Prescribing medicines in pregnancy. In: Randall MD, editor. Clinical pharmacology. 7th ed. London: Elsevier; 2016. p. 438–43.
16. Syme MR, Paxton JW, Keelan JA. Drug transfer and metabolism by the human placenta. Clin Pharmacokinet. 2004;43(8):487–514.
17. Alwan S, Chambers CD. Identifying human teratogens: an update. J Pediatr Genet. 2015;4(2):39–41.
18. Ujházy E, Mach M, Navarová J, Brucknerová I, Dubovický M. Teratology – past, present and future. Interdiscip Toxicol. 2012;5(4):163–8.
19. Gregg NM. Congenital cataract following German measles in the mother. Trans Ophthalmol Soc Aust. 1941;3:35–46.
20. DeSesso JM. The arrogance of teratology: a brief chronology of attitudes throughout history. Birth Defects Res. 2019;111(3):123–41.
21. Dareste C. Recherches sur la Production Artificielle des Monstruosités, ou Essais de Tératogénie Expérimentale. Paris: C Reinwald; 1876.
22. Kaplan YC, Erol-Coşkun H. Safety parameters and risk categories used for psychotropic drugs in pregnancy and lactation. In: Uguz F, Orsolini L, editors. Perinatal psychopharmacology. Cham: Springer; 2019. p. 37–53.
23. Franks ME, Macpherson GR, Figg WD. Thalidomide. Lancet. 2004;363(9423):1802–11.
24. Wilson J. Current status of teratology: general principles and mechanisms derived from animal studies. In: Wilson J, Fraser F, editors. Handbook of teratology. 4 vols. New York: Plenum Press; 1977. p. 47–74.
25. Friedman JM. The principles of teratology: are they still true? Birth Defects Res A Clin Mol Teratol. 2010;88(10):766–8.
26. Dukare SG, Wagh AB, Waje MR. Understanding teratogenicity in pregnancy: a comprehensive review. Int J Creat Res Thoughts. 2024;12(4):e9–e20.
27. van Gelder MM, van Rooij IA, Miller RK, Zielhuis GA, de Jong-van den Berg LT, Roeleveld N. Teratogenic mechanisms of medical drugs. Hum Reprod Update. 2010;16(4):378–94.
28. Hernández-Díaz S, Werler MM, Walker AM, Mitchell AA. Folic acid antagonists during pregnancy and the risk of birth defects. N Engl J Med. 2000;343(22):1608–14.
29. Fathe K, Palacios A, Finnell RH. Brief report: novel mechanism for valproate-induced teratogenicity. Birth Defects Res A Clin Mol Teratol. 2014;100(8):592–7.
30. Cerrizuela S, Vega-Lopez GA, Aybar MJ. The role of teratogens in neural crest development. Birth Defects Res. 2020;112(8):584–632.
31. Karunamuni GH, Ma P, Gu S, Rollins AM, Jenkins MW, Watanabe M. Connecting teratogen-induced congenital heart defects to neural crest cells and their effect on cardiac function. Birth Defects Res C Embryo Today. 2014;102(3):227–50.
32. Zaken V, Kohen R, Ornoy A. The development of antioxidant defense mechanism in young rat embryos in vivo and in vitro. Early Pregnancy (Cherry Hill). 2000;4(2):110–23.

33. Sahambi SK, Hales BF. Exposure to 5-bromo-2′-deoxyuridine induces oxidative stress and activator protein-1 DNA binding activity in the embryo. Birth Defects Res A Clin Mol Teratol. 2006;76:580–91.
34. Gilbert-Barness E, Van Allen MI. Vascular disruptions. In: Gilbert-Barness E, Kapur RP, Siebert JR, Potter EL, editors. Potter's pathology of the fetus, infant and child. Philadelphia: Mosby Elsevier; 2007. p. 176–212.
35. Kaplan YC. Klinik farmakolog gözüyle gebelikte ilaç kullanımına yaklaşım. In: Üstün Y, editor. Gebelik öncesi danışmanlık el kitabı. 1. baskı ed. Ankara: Türkiye Maternal Fetal Tıp ve Perinatoloji Derneği Yayınları; 2018. p. 65–72.
36. Alwan S, Grant KS. Maternal medication use in pregnancy: a narrative review on assessing and communicating the "risk" of birth defects to the patient. Pharmacoepidemiology. 2024;3(4):336–49.
37. Kaplan YC, Kelekçi S, Demir Ö. Risk evaluation, risk communication and perinatal evaluation in pregnancies with drug exposure. Nobel Medicus. 2015;11:14–21.
38. Schaefer C. Angiotensin II-receptor-antagonists: further evidence of fetotoxicity but not teratogenicity. Birth Defects Res A Clin Mol Teratol. 2003;67:591–4.
39. Meador KJ, Baker GA, Browning N, Cohen MJ, Bromley RL, Clayton-Smith J, Kalayjian LA, Kanner A, Liporace JD, Pennell PB, Privitera M, Loring DW, NEAD Study Group. Fetal antiepileptic drug exposure and cognitive outcomes at age 6 years (NEAD study): a prospective observational study. Lancet Neurol. 2013;12(3):244–52.
40. Inselman AL, Slikker W Jr. Is there a safe dose of a medication associated with birth defects? In: Kavlock RJ, editor. Teratology primer. 3rd ed. Reston: Teratology Society; 2015.
41. Kaplan YC, Ozsarfati J, Etwel F, Nickel C, Nulman I, Koren G. Pregnancy outcomes following first-trimester exposure to topical retinoids: a systematic review and meta-analysis. Br J Dermatol. 2015;173(5):1132–41.
42. Panchaud A, Csajka C, Merlob P, Schaefer C, Berlin M, De Santis M, Vial T, Ieri A, Malm H, Eleftheriou G, Stahl B, Rousso P, Winterfeld U, Rothuizen LE, Buclin T. Pregnancy outcome following exposure to topical retinoids: a multicenter prospective study. J Clin Pharmacol. 2012;52(12):1844–51.
43. Jick SS, Terris BZ, Jick H. First trimester topical tretinoin and congenital disorders. Lancet. 1993;341(8854):1181–2.
44. Lammer EJ, Chen DT, Hoar RM, Agnish ND, Benke PJ, Braun JT, Curry CJ, Fernhoff PM, Grix AW Jr, Lott IT, et al. Retinoic acid embryopathy. N Engl J Med. 1985;313(14):837–41.
45. Browne H, Mason G, Tang T. Retinoids and pregnancy: an update. Obstet Gynaecol. 2014;16(1):7–11.
46. Kluger BM, Meador KJ. Teratogenicity of antiepileptic medications. Semin Neurol. 2008;28(3):328–35.
47. Thunbo MØ, Vendelbo JH, Volqvartz T, Witte DR, Larsen A, Pedersen LH. Polypharmacy in polymorbid pregnancies and the risk of congenital malformations-a systematic review. Basic Clin Pharmacol Toxicol. 2022;130(3):394–414.
48. Tomson T, Battino D, Bonizzoni E, Craig J, Lindhout D, Perucca E, Sabers A, Thomas SV, Vajda F, EURAP Study Group. Dose-dependent teratogenicity of valproate in mono- and polytherapy: an observational study. Neurology. 2015;85(10):866–72.
49. Källén BA. Methodological issues in the epidemiological study of the teratogenicity of drugs. Congenit Anom (Kyoto). 2005;45(2):44–51.
50. Shroukh WA, Steinke DT, Willis SC. Risk management of teratogenic medicines: a systematic review. Birth Defects Res. 2020;112(20):1755–86.
51. Petersen I, McCrea RL, Lupattelli A, Nordeng H. Women's perception of risks of adverse fetal pregnancy outcomes: a large-scale multinational survey. BMJ Open. 2015;5(6):e007390.
52. Pole M, Einarson A, Pairaudeau N, Einarson T, Koren G. Drug labeling and risk perceptions of teratogenicity: a survey of pregnant Canadian women and their health professionals. J Clin Pharmacol. 2000;40(6):573–7.

53. Czeizel AE. The estimation of human teratogenic/fetotoxic risk of exposures to drugs on the basis of Hungarian experience: a critical evaluation of clinical and epidemiological models of human teratology. Expert Opin Drug Saf. 2009;8(3):283–303.
54. Gomes JDA, Olstad EW, Kowalski TW, Gervin K, Vianna FSL, Schüler-Faccini L, Nordeng HME. Genetic susceptibility to drug teratogenicity: a systematic literature review. Front Genet. 2021;12:645555.
55. Gomes JDA, Kowalski TW, Fraga LR, Macedo GS, Sanseverino MTV, Schuler-Faccini L, Vianna FSL. The role of ESCO2, SALL4 and TBX5 genes in the susceptibility to thalidomide teratogenesis. Sci Rep. 2019;9(1):11413.
56. Källén B. The problem of confounding in studies of the effect of maternal drug use on pregnancy outcome. Obstet Gynecol Int. 2012;2012:148616.
57. Kaplan YC, Can H, Demir Ö, Karadaş B, Yılmaz İ, Temiz TK. İlaçların gebelikte kullanımlarına dair risk iletişiminde yeni dönem: FDA gebelik risk kategorileri değişiyor. Turkiye Aile Hekim Derg. 2014;18(4):195–8.
58. Frederiksen MC. The new FDA pregnancy labeling requirements for drugs. J Midwifery Womens Health. 2011;56:303–7.
59. Feibus KB. FDA's Proposed Rule for Pregnancy and Lactation Labeling: improving maternal child health through well-informed medicine use. J Med Toxicol. 2008;4:284–8.
60. Brucker MC, King TL. The 2015 US Food and Drug Administration pregnancy and lactation labeling rule. J Midwifery Womens Health. 2017;62(3):308–16.
61. Källén B. Drugs in pregnancy – the dilemma of labeling. Ther Innov Regul Sci. 1999;33(4):1135–43.
62. Sarayani A, Albogami Y, Thai TN, Smolinski NE, Patel P, Wang Y, Nduaguba S, Rasmussen SA, Winterstein AG. Prenatal exposure to teratogenic medications in the era of Risk Evaluation and Mitigation Strategies. Am J Obstet Gynecol. 2022;227(2):263.e1–263.e38.
63. Byrne JJ, Saucedo AM, Spong CY. Evaluation of drug labels following the 2015 pregnancy and lactation labeling rule. JAMA Netw Open. 2020;3(8):e2015094.

Chapter 3
Mastering the Art of Pregnancy Nutrition

Sabahattin Anıl Arı

3.1 Introduction

Successful fetal growth and development throughout pregnancy depend on the mother's physiological adjustments and evolving nutritional demands. Moreover, increasing evidence suggests that the intrauterine environment, shaped by maternal nutrition and metabolic conditions, can induce epigenetic alterations that regulate gene expression. These modifications may have lasting effects, influencing disease susceptibility during childhood and later in adulthood [1]. Pioneering studies of individuals who experienced in-utero exposure to the Dutch famine during World War II offer persuasive evidence that prenatal environmental conditions can exert lasting influences on health in adulthood [2].

Although the relationship between certain nutrients, such as folic acid, and specific pregnancy outcomes, including the prevention of neural tube defects, has been clearly established, many aspects of maternal nutrition remain insufficiently understood. These stem from the considerable difficulties in executing rigorous clinical studies in pregnant populations. Several factors complicate research on maternal nutrition, including limited knowledge about how diet affects fetal development during key stages of pregnancy. Other difficulties stem from ongoing physiological changes, variations in maternal adaptation, unreliable dietary reporting, and the ethical or practical constraints of performing randomized studies in pregnant women. It is also challenging to isolate the effects of single nutrients in a mixed diet, and there are no animal models that can fully reproduce human pregnancy [3].

S. A. Arı (✉)
Faculty of Medicine, Department of Obstetrics and Gynecology, Izmir Bakircay University, Izmir, Türkiye
e-mail: sabahattinanil.ari@bakircay.edu.tr

© The Author(s), under exclusive license to Springer Nature Switzerland AG 2026

I. Karaca (ed.), *Managing Maternal Chronic Diseases for a Healthy Pregnancy*, https://doi.org/10.1007/978-3-032-15221-3_3

3.2 Dietary Principles for Optimal Obstetric Outcomes

A balanced pregnancy diet should include a broad range of nutrient-rich foods, featuring colorful vegetables like dark green, red, and orange types, together with legumes (beans, peas, lentils), fruits, whole grains, and starchy vegetables. Dairy products, lean meats, poultry, and eggs supply quality protein, while seafood, nuts, seeds, and soy products offer additional protein and beneficial fats, particularly polyunsaturated fatty acids from plant oils and fish.

Excessive energy intake is common during pregnancy and may contribute to unfavorable maternal and fetal outcomes. Therefore, dietary guidance should emphasize the selection of nutrient-dense, high-quality foods while limiting the consumption of highly processed products and sugar-sweetened beverages with minimal nutritional value. Reducing or eliminating ultra-processed foods is particularly important to lower the intake of added sugars, saturated fats, and sodium. Furthermore, caffeine, widely consumed in modern diets, should be restricted to no more than 300 mg per day.

3.3 Dietary Requirements

3.3.1 Energy Intake

During the first trimester, a pregnant individual's daily energy requirements are generally equivalent to those of a nonpregnant person. During the second and third trimesters, a pregnant individual's energy requirements are modified according to various factors such as maternal age, body height, weight prior to conception, stage of gestation, and level of physical activity. The additional caloric needs during pregnancy differ according to pre-pregnancy BMI. Individuals with a low BMI may require an extra 300 kcal per day, while those with a normal BMI may need around 200 kcal. For individuals who are overweight, the increase is approximately 150 kcal daily, whereas those with obesity may require a reduction of about 50 kcal per day [4].

3.3.2 Macronutrients

Protein In the second and third trimesters, a daily protein intake of about 1.1 g/kg of body weight is recommended for pregnant women [5]. Across both pregnant and nonpregnant populations, protein should contribute roughly 10% to 35% of total caloric intake.

High-quality protein sources include lean meats, poultry, eggs, seafood, legumes such as lentils, peas, and beans, along with soy-based products, nuts, and seeds. The consumption of highly processed or cured meats should be minimized. For women whose protein intake already meets recommended levels, consuming extra protein offers no proven benefit and may increase the likelihood of unfavorable outcomes, such as giving birth to low-birth-weight or SGA babies [6].

Carbohydrates and Dietary Fiber During pregnancy, the daily carbohydrate requirement rises to approximately 175 g [7]. For both pregnant and nonpregnant adults, carbohydrates should contribute between 45% and 65% of total caloric intake. In addition, a daily fiber intake of about 28–36 g is recommended, as adequate fiber, when combined with sufficient fluid consumption, can help alleviate or prevent constipation, a common complaint during pregnancy.

Fats Fats are recommended to make up 20–35% of total calories during pregnancy, and saturated fats should stay below 10%. Expectant mothers should include essential fatty acids daily, around 13 g of linoleic acid (omega-6) and 1.4 g of alpha-linolenic acid (omega-3) [5]. Choosing unsaturated, heart-healthy fats instead of saturated ones is strongly advised.

Within a healthy dietary pattern, fats should primarily be obtained from plant-based oils, particularly olive oil, and nuts, complemented by consuming fish two to three times per week. Fish and other seafood serve as the main sources of omega-3 long-chain polyunsaturated fatty acids (n-3 LCPUFAs), notably docosahexaenoic acid (DHA) and eicosapentaenoic acid (EPA). DHA is essential for fetal neurodevelopment and retinal maturation, and regular maternal seafood intake has been associated with improved cognitive performance in children [5]. Moreover, the anti-inflammatory properties of omega-3 polyunsaturated fatty acids (n-3 PUFAs) may contribute to lowering the risk of preterm birth and slightly prolonging gestational duration [8].

Achieving the recommended daily intake of 200–300 mg of DHA depends on the type and amount of seafood consumed. For instance, this requirement can typically be met by eating sardines twice weekly or sea bass/gilt-head bream three to four times per week. However, individuals who are pregnant or planning pregnancy should steer clear of deep-sea fish known to accumulate mercury or other pollutants.

For pregnant women whose dietary intake of seafood is inadequate, the recommended 200–300 mg of DHA per day can be obtained from n-3 long-chain polyunsaturated fatty acid (LCPUFA) supplements or fortified food products. Foods such as enriched eggs, milk, and yogurt are valuable alternative sources, and several prenatal multivitamin formulations also include DHA, often in combination with eicosapentaenoic acid (EPA).

3.3.3 Micronutrients

Ideally, essential nutrients should be obtained mainly from a well-balanced diet composed of nutrient-dense, fortified, and minimally processed whole foods and beverages. Nevertheless, in Türkiye, the consumption of key micronutrients, particularly calcium, vitamin D, folate, and iron, routinely remains below the recommended dietary allowances [9].

Iron Iron is essential for fetal brain growth, placental development, and the normal rise in maternal red blood cell volume. Worldwide, iron deficiency is the most common nutritional problem and the main cause of anemia [10]. The World Health Organization advises daily oral supplementation with 30–60 mg of elemental iron during pregnancy [11]. For pregnant individuals diagnosed with iron deficiency anemia, characterized by hemoglobin levels below 11 g/dL during the first or third trimester, or under 10.5 g/dL in the second trimester, alongside reduced serum ferritin concentrations (<40 ng/mL), it is recommended to administer additional iron at doses ranging from 30 to 120 mg daily until anemia is resolved [12].

Calcium Throughout pregnancy, around 30 g of calcium are required to ensure proper fetal skeletal formation, with the highest demand occurring during the third trimester. This quantity accounts for only a small fraction of total maternal calcium stores and can be mobilized from these reserves when necessary. During pregnancy, both intestinal calcium absorption and renal calcium conservation progressively increase to meet fetal needs [13]. Among women with inadequate dietary calcium intake, supplementation has been shown to lower the risk of hypertensive disorders in pregnancy [14]. In the United States, pregnant and breastfeeding women are advised to consume 1000–1300 mg of calcium daily, depending on age, with average intake levels around 1090 mg per day. However, approximately one in five pregnant women consumes less than 800 mg/day from dietary sources alone [15].

Vitamin D In the United States, the recommended daily intake of vitamin D during pregnancy is 600 international units (IU) [5]. Worldwide, vitamin D deficiency is highly prevalent, affecting an estimated 40–98% of pregnant women [16]. The primary natural source of vitamin D is cutaneous synthesis following exposure to sunlight, as few foods naturally contain significant amounts of the vitamin. Consequently, dietary intake alone is often inadequate. Among supplemental forms, vitamin D_3 is more efficiently converted into its active metabolites and has been demonstrated to elevate serum 25-hydroxyvitamin D levels more effectively than vitamin D_2.

Folic Acid Strong evidence shows that taking folic acid can prevent about 70% of neural tube defects, including both first occurrences and recurrences. It is recommended that women begin taking 400 μg of folic acid daily at least 1 month prior to conception and continue through the first trimester. For those at elevated risk, such as individuals with a previous NTD-affected pregnancy or those using antiepileptic drugs, the advised dosage increases to 4 mg per day.

Choline Choline is essential for the formation of the fetal central nervous system and for supporting cognitive development [17]. Low choline intake during pregnancy is linked to about twice the risk of neural tube defects [18]. It is recommended that pregnant women get roughly 450 mg of choline daily from both diet and supplements. However, NHANES data indicate that average intake is only about 319 mg per day, and fewer than one in ten women meet the target level [19]. During pregnancy, the best sources of choline come from animal foods such as eggs, meat, poultry, fish, and dairy. Because plant-derived foods, including legumes, Brussels sprouts, broccoli, and spinach, contain much smaller amounts, vegetarian or vegan individuals should adopt alternative dietary approaches or consider supplementation [3].

Zinc Zinc is a vital micronutrient involved in numerous physiological functions, including fetal growth and neural development. Although biologically important, evidence from a meta-analysis of 25 randomized controlled trials indicates that zinc supplementation does not produce significant improvements in perinatal outcomes [20]. The recommended dietary allowance for zinc during pregnancy ranges from 11 to 12 mg per day. Pregnant women in the United States get around 10.3 mg of zinc a day from food, and this amount increases to about 18.4 mg when supplements are included. Still, nearly 11% do not reach the recommended intake [15]. The best dietary sources of zinc are animal foods like meat, poultry, and seafood, especially oysters, crab, and lobster. Grains and legumes also contain zinc, but much of it is poorly absorbed due to phytates that interfere with mineral uptake [5].

Iodine Iodine is a crucial trace element necessary for the production of thyroid hormones. Deficiency during pregnancy can result in unfavorable outcomes, including maternal and fetal or neonatal hypothyroidism. Both the World Health Organization and the American Thyroid Association recommend a daily intake of 250 mg of iodine during pregnancy and lactation to maintain optimal thyroid function in the mother and fetus [21]. The recent decline in iodine intake has been associated with greater reliance on processed foods and increased use of noniodized salts, such as sea salt, which generally contain minimal iodine. Although initiating table salt consumption is not required for those who avoid it, pregnant women are encouraged to use iodized salt when seasoning foods and to include iodine-rich options, such as cooked seafood, in their diet to ensure adequate intake [3].

Vitamin B12 A systematic review has shown that low maternal plasma concentrations of vitamin B12, particularly in women with overt deficiency, are linked to an elevated risk of preterm birth [22]. Conversely, a randomized clinical trial from Nepal, where 71% of 800 participants were deficient, found that daily supplementation with 50 μg of vitamin B12 during pregnancy did not result in measurable clinical benefits [23]. In the United States, pregnant women are advised to take 2.6 μg of vitamin B12 daily, with the requirement rising slightly to 2.8 μg while breastfeeding [5]. Most pregnant women in the United States meet or exceed these requirements, with an average intake of approximately 5.6 μg per day, more than twice the recommendation. In cases of deficiency, supplementation is required: parenteral administration is preferred for malabsorption, whereas oral supplementation suffices for those with dietary insufficiency and normal absorption. Because vitamin

B12 is found exclusively in animal foods like meat, fish, poultry, eggs, and dairy, people following vegetarian or vegan diets are more likely to develop a deficiency and are advised to take suitable supplements.

Vitamin A Vitamin A is vital for cellular proliferation, fetal organogenesis, and skeletal formation, and it also contributes to immune regulation, fetal visual development, and maintenance of maternal eyesight [24]. For women who already have enough vitamin A, taking extra supplements provides no proven benefit and can increase the risk of toxicity. On the other hand, mild deficiency, particularly in the third trimester when fetal growth is most rapid, can make pregnant women more prone to night blindness [25]. Maternal vitamin A requirements rise slightly in pregnancy, with the recommended intake increasing to 750–770 μg retinol equivalents (2500–2560 IU) compared to 700 μg (≈2330 IU) for nonpregnant women [5]. In the United States, average vitamin A consumption among pregnant women is approximately 696 μg retinol equivalents from food alone and 1283 μg when supplements are included [15].

Most prenatal multivitamins contain vitamin A, typically provided as beta-carotene (provitamin A). Including foods like dairy, fish, eggs, carrots, leafy greens, broccoli, melon, and squash in the daily diet usually ensures an adequate vitamin A intake. However, liver should be avoided because of its extremely high vitamin A concentration. Intakes exceeding 10,000 IU per day (≈3000 μg retinol) are known to be teratogenic [26]. Pregnant individuals should generally avoid taking multivitamins or prenatal supplements containing more than 5000 IU (1500 mcg retinol equivalents) of vitamin A, unless they have a severe deficiency. Therefore, vitamin A supplementation should not exceed 5000 IU (≈1500 μg retinol equivalents) unless severe deficiency is confirmed. Notably, beta-carotene, the predominant form used in prenatal formulations, has not been associated with teratogenic risk, unlike preformed vitamin A types such as retinol and retinyl esters [27].

Vitamin E Reviewing data from multiple randomized trials, researchers found that taking vitamin E during pregnancy, alone or combined with vitamin C or other nutrients, did not meaningfully affect the risk of stillbirth, premature birth, preeclampsia, or low birth weight [28].

Vitamin C According to a 2015 review of clinical trials, taking vitamin C during pregnancy, either by itself or with other nutrients, showed no clear positive or negative effect on pregnancy or newborn health outcomes [29]. The review found that vitamin C did not help prevent stillbirth, premature birth, preeclampsia, or low birth weight. However, another meta-analysis reported that in women who smoked during pregnancy, vitamin C improved newborn lung function, specifically forced vital capacity and expiratory flow, indicating it may help protect against tobacco exposure before birth [30].

Vitamin B6 Vitamin B6, or pyridoxine, acts as a coenzyme in more than a hundred enzyme reactions, helping the body metabolize proteins, carbohydrates, and fats, and supporting neurotransmitter production. Most pregnant women achieve adequate intake levels [15]. According to a Cochrane review, there is no substantial evidence supporting the clinical benefits of routine vitamin B6 supplementation during pregnancy [31]. Nevertheless, pyridoxine has proven useful in managing mild to moderate nausea and vomiting associated with pregnancy.

References

1. Barker DJP, Thornburg KL. The obstetric origins of health for a lifetime. Clin Obstet Gynecol. 2013;56(3):511–9.
2. Roseboom T, de Rooij S, Painter R. The Dutch famine and its long-term consequences for adult health. Early Hum Dev. 2006;82(8):485–91.
3. Nutrition in pregnancy: Dietary requirements and supplements – UpToDate [Internet]. [cited 2025 May 6]. Available from: https://www.uptodate.com/contents/nutrition-in-pregnancy-dietary-requirements-and-supplements
4. Dietary Reference Intakes for Energy. Dietary reference intakes for energy [Internet]. 2023 Jan 1 [cited 2025 May 6]; 1–526. Available from: https://pubmed.ncbi.nlm.nih.gov/36693139/
5. Snetselaar LG, De Jesus JM, Desilva DM, Stoody EE. Dietary guidelines for Americans, 2020–2025: understanding the scientific process, guidelines, and key recommendations. Nutr Today. 2021;56(6):287.
6. Blumfield ML, Collins CE. High-protein diets during pregnancy: healthful or harmful for offspring? Am J Clin Nutr. 2014;100(4):993–5.
7. Board I of M (US) F and N. Dietary reference intakes. 1998;
8. Middleton P, Gomersall JC, Gould JF, Shepherd E, Olsen SF, Makrides M. Omega-3 fatty acid addition during pregnancy. Cochrane Database Syst Rev. 2018;2018(11):CD003402.
9. Akgun S PGAEKGKEKSOHYNKSCNAFKZ. Türkiye Beslenme ve Saglik Arastirmasi (TBSA). Ankara: T.C. Saglik Bakanligi Halk Sagligi Genel Mudurlugu, Yayin No. 1132; 2019.
10. McLean E, Cogswell M, Egli I, Wojdyla D, De Benoist B. Worldwide prevalence of anaemia, WHO vitamin and mineral nutrition information system, 1993–2005. Public Health Nutr. 2009;12(4):444–54.
11. Daily iron and folic acid supplementation during pregnancy [Internet]. [cited 2025 May 6]. Available from: https://www.who.int/tools/elena/interventions/daily-iron-pregnancy
12. Earl R, Woteki CE. Iron deficiency anemia: recommended guidelines for the prevention, detection, and management among U.S. children and women of childbearing age. In: Earl R, Woteki CE, editors. . Washington (DC): National Academies Press; 1993.
13. Hacker AN, Fung EB, King JC. Role of calcium during pregnancy: maternal and fetal needs. Nutr Rev. 2012;70(7):397–409.
14. Hofmeyr GJ, Lawrie TA, Atallah ÁN, Torloni MR. Calcium supplementation during pregnancy for preventing hypertensive disorders and related problems. Cochrane Database Syst Rev. 2018;2018(10):CD001059.
15. Bailey RL, Pac SG, Fulgoni VL, Reidy KC, Catalano PM. Estimation of total usual dietary intakes of pregnant women in the United States. JAMA Netw Open. 2019;2(6):e195967.
16. Van Schoor NM, Lips P. Worldwide vitamin D status. Best Pract Res Clin Endocrinol Metab. 2011;25(4):671–80.
17. Derbyshire E, Obeid R. Choline, neurological development and brain function: a systematic review focusing on the first 1000 days. Nutrients. 2020;12(6):1–32.
18. Obeid R, Derbyshire E, Schön C. Association between maternal choline, fetal brain development, and child neurocognition: systematic review and meta-analysis of human studies. Adv Nutr. 2022;13(6):2445–57.

19. Wallace TC, Fulgoni VL. Usual choline intakes are associated with egg and protein food consumption in the United States. Nutrients. 2017;9(8):839.
20. Carducci B, Keats EC, Bhutta ZA. Zinc supplementation for improving pregnancy and infant outcome. Cochrane Database Syst Rev. 2021;2021(3):CD000230.
21. Harding KB, Peña-Rosas JP, Webster AC, Yap CMY, Payne BA, Ota E, et al. Iodine supplementation for women during the preconception, pregnancy and postpartum period. Cochrane Database Syst Rev. 2017;2017(3):CD011761.
22. Rogne T, Tielemans MJ, Chong MFF, Yajnik CS, Krishnaveni GV, Poston L, et al. Associations of maternal vitamin B12 concentration in pregnancy with the risks of preterm birth and low birth weight: a systematic review and meta-analysis of individual participant data. Am J Epidemiol. 2017;185(3):212–23.
23. Chandyo RK, Kvestad I, Ulak M, Ranjitkar S, Hysing M, Shrestha M, et al. The effect of vitamin B12 supplementation during pregnancy on infant growth and development in Nepal: a community-based, double-blind, randomised, placebo-controlled trial. Lancet. 2023;401(10387):1508–17.
24. Vitamin A supplementation during pregnancy [Internet]. [cited 2025 May 6]. Available from: https://www.who.int/tools/elena/interventions/vitamina-pregnancy
25. Maia SB, Souza ASR, Caminha MDFC, da Silva SL, Cruz R d SBLC, Dos Santos CC, et al. Vitamin a and pregnancy: a narrative review. Nutrients. 2019;11(3):681.
26. Mccauley ME, van den Broek N, Dou L, Othman M. Vitamin A supplementation during pregnancy for maternal and newborn outcomes. Cochrane Database Syst Rev. 2015;2016(3):CD008666.
27. Mathews-Roth MM. Lack of genotoxicity with beta-carotene. Toxicol Lett. 1988;41(3):185–91.
28. Rumbold A, Ota E, Hori H, Miyazaki C, Crowther CA. Vitamin E supplementation in pregnancy. Cochrane Database Syst Rev. 2015;2016(3):CD004069.
29. Rumbold A, Ota E, Nagata C, Shahrook S, Crowther CA. Vitamin C supplementation in pregnancy. Cochrane Database Syst Rev. 2015;2016(3):CD004072.
30. Wang L, Wei L, Wang Z, Ren X, Yang F, Sun L. A meta-analysis of the effects of vitamin C supplementation for pregnant smokers on the pulmonary function of their offspring. BMC Pregnancy Childbirth. 2024;24(1):184.
31. Salam RA, Zuberi NF, Bhutta ZA. Pyridoxine (vitamin B6) supplementation during pregnancy or labour for maternal and neonatal outcomes. Cochrane Database Syst Rev. 2015;2016(3):CD000179.

Chapter 4
A Holistic Approach to Pregnancy and Heart Health

Oktay Şenöz

4.1 Introduction

The incidence of cardiovascular disease in pregnant women ranges from 1% to 4% [1]. The age of pregnancy is progressively rising. World Atlas indicates that in the ten countries with the highest average age at first pregnancy, fertility ranges from 28.8 to 31.2 years [2]. As maternal age increases, along with an associated increase in cardiovascular risk factors, and considering that women with congenital heart disease undergo surgery in childhood and then experience pregnancy in maturity, this incidence is expected to rise over time [3]. Hypertensive diseases are the most prevalent cardiovascular disorders during pregnancy, affecting 5–10% of pregnancies. Congenital heart disease is the most prevalent cardiovascular disease (CVD) during pregnancy in Western countries, ranging from 75% to 82%, whereas rheumatic valve disease is prominent in other parts of the world, representing 56–89% of all CVDs during pregnancy. Cardiomyopathies in pregnancy are rare, but they represent the most serious causes of cardiovascular complications during pregnancy [4]. The primary cause of mortality during pregnancy is preexisting or pregnancy-acquired cardiovascular diseases [1].

4.2 Physiological Adaptations to Pregnancy

Pregnancy causes changes in the cardiovascular system to meet the increasing metabolic demands of the mother and fetus. Plasma volume and cardiac output (CO) increase to 40–50% above baseline by the 32nd week of pregnancy, with 75% of

O. Şenöz (✉)
Izmir Bakircay University, Faculty of Medicine, Department of Cardiology, Izmir, Turkey
e-mail: oktay.senoz@bakircay.edu.tr

© The Author(s), under exclusive license to Springer Nature Switzerland AG 2026

I. Karaca (ed.), *Managing Maternal Chronic Diseases for a Healthy Pregnancy*,
https://doi.org/10.1007/978-3-032-15221-3_4

this increase occurring by the end of the first trimester. The increase in CO is achieved through an increase in stroke volume during the first half of pregnancy and a gradual increase in heart rate thereafter. During pregnancy, while the atrial and ventricular diameters increase, ventricular function is preserved. Women with heart disease may not be able to adapt their left ventricle (LV) and right ventricle (RV) functions to pregnancy, which can lead to impaired uteroplacental blood flow [5, 6]. During pregnancy, systemic and pulmonary vascular resistances decrease. An increase in erythrocytes is observed to a lesser extent than the plasma volume (20–30%). As a result, relative anemia is observed, and this condition is considered physiological. The risk of thromboembolism due to hypercoagulability also increases during pregnancy [7].

In the third trimester of pregnancy, the increase in uterine volume may cause pressure on the inferior vena cava. This pressure is felt more strongly, especially in the supine position. The left lateral decubitus position reduces venous pressure and increases venous return [8]. Uterine contractions, lying position, exertion, anxiety, pain, hemorrhage, and uterine involution cause significant hemodynamic changes during and after the labor process. Anesthesia, hemorrhage, and infection can cause additional cardiovascular stress. Blood pressure (BP) and CO increase during and after labor.

The increase in the activity of liver enzyme systems, glomerular filtration rate, and plasma volume, changes in protein binding, and the decrease in serum albumin levels contribute to changes in the pharmacokinetics of many drugs [9]. In conclusion, the physiological adaptations that occur during pregnancy necessitate the reevaluation and analysis of cardiac functions and clinical status.

4.3 Pre-pregnancy Counselling

All women with known cardiac or aortic disease who wish to start a pregnancy need pre-pregnancy counseling. Informed maternal decisions are very important. Not only medical conditions but also emotional and psychological issues should be considered to make individualized decisions. Especially in patients at high risk for pregnancy, the necessity of careful planning and the risks associated with pregnancy should be discussed at a young age. Additionally, it is important to pay attention to unhealthy habits such as obesity, smoking, and alcohol consumption, as these negatively affect maternal and fetal outcomes.

At least an electrocardiogram (ECG), echocardiography, and an exercise test should be performed for risk estimation in the pre-pregnancy evaluation. In the case of aortic pathology, comprehensive aortic imaging with computed tomography (CT) scan or magnetic resonance imaging (MRI) may be required [7].

4.4 Risk of Maternal Cardiovascular Complications

The risk of complications during pregnancy depends on the underlying cardiac condition, ventricular and valve function, functional class, presence of cyanosis, pulmonary artery pressures, and other factors.

To determine the maternal risk of cardiac complications during pregnancy, the woman's medical history, functional class, oxygen saturation, natriuretic peptide levels, echocardiographic evaluation of ventricular and valvular function, intrapulmonary pressures and aortic diameters, exercise capacity, and arrhythmias should be taken into account. Disease-specific risk should be determined using the modified World Health Organization (mWHO) classification (Table 4.1) [7].

4.5 Risk of Obstetric and Offspring Complications

In women with heart disease, there is an increased risk of complications related to pregnancy, such as premature delivery, preeclampsia, and postpartum hemorrhage. In newborns of pregnant women with heart disease, complications are observed in 18–30% of cases, and the neonatal mortality rate is between 1% and 4% [1].

In women with moderate or high complication risk during pregnancy (mWHOII–III, III, and IV), pre-pregnancy, pregnancy process, and delivery counseling should be conducted by a multidisciplinary team. The pregnancy heart team should include at least a cardiologist, obstetrician, and anesthesiologist [7] (Table 4.2).

4.6 Genetic Counseling During Pregnancy

Pre-pregnancy risk assessment, along with genetic counseling, is especially necessary for women with congenital heart or aortic disease. Although it may vary depending on the type of disease, it is generally accepted that the likelihood of congenital diseases being passed from mother to baby is higher than from father to baby. In pregnant women suspected of having a genetically transmitted disease, chorionic villus sampling is recommended at the 12th week of pregnancy. In women with congenital heart disease, fetal echocardiography is recommended between the 19th and 22nd weeks of pregnancy. In all pregnant women over 35 years of age, it is recommended to measure nuchal translucency at the 12th week. In particular,

Table 4.1 Physiological hemodynamic changes that occur during pregnancy

30–50% increase in plasma volume
20–30% increase in heart rate
30–50% increase in cardiac output
20–30% increase in erythrocytes

Table 4.2 Predictors of maternal and neonatal events

Predictors of maternal cardiovascular events	Predictors of neonatal events
NYHA class III/IV	NYHA class III/IV
Prior cardiac event	Cyanosis during baseline prenatal visit
Left heart obstruction (moderate to severe)	Maternal left heart obstruction
Reduced systemic ventricular systolic function (EF <40%)	Low maternal oxygen saturation (<90%)
Reduced subpulmonary ventricular function (TAPSE <16 mm)	'At birth' cyanotic heart disease
Pulmonary atrioventricular valve regurgitation (moderate to severe)	Multiple gestations
Systemic atrioventricular valve regurgitation (moderate to severe)	Use of anticoagulants throughout pregnancy
Pulmonary arterial hypertension	Multiple gestations
Cyanosis (O_2 saturation <90%)	Maternal cardiac event during pregnancy
Natriuretic peptide levels (NT-proBNP >128 pg/mL)	Smoking during pregnancy
Mechanical valve prosthesis	Cardiac medication before pregnancy
Repaired or unrepaired cyanotic heart disease	Maternal decline in cardiac output during pregnancy
Smoking history	Abnormal uteroplacental Doppler flow
Cardiac medication before pregnancy	

Predictors identified in Ref. [7]
NT-proBNP N-terminal proB type natriuretic peptide, *NYHA* New York Heart Association, *TAPSE* tricuspid annular plane systolic excursion

recommended pregnancy pathologies for genetic testing include: cardiomyopathy and channel defects, Marfan syndrome, Williams–Beuren syndrome, Alagille syndrome, Noonan syndrome, Holt–Oram syndrome, and 22q11 deletion [8].

4.7 Physiological Examination Findings in Pregnancy

In women, many symptoms that could be considered pathological outside of pregnancy, such as palpitations, dizziness, vision changes, shortness of breath, and peripheral edema, are considered normal during pregnancy. In pregnancy, the pulse is palpated more quickly, full, and bounding. Similarly, carotid pulses are felt to be faster and more pronounced. From the second trimester of pregnancy, venous pressure increases, and jugular venous distension can be observed. Innocent venous murmurs, venous hum, and mammary souffle can be heard. With the increase in cardiac output, the apical impulse becomes more pronounced, and the first heart sound becomes more pronounced. In 80% of pregnancies, the S3 sound can be physiologically heard. The pathological examination findings in pregnancy are as follows: diastolic murmurs, third-degree and higher systolic murmurs, the presence of an S4 sound, and a fixed S2 splitting [10]. Table 4.3 summarizes the physiological and pathological examination findings in pregnancy.

Table 4.3 Physiological and pathological examination findings during pregnancy

Physiological examination findings	Pathological examination findings
Rapid and jerky pulse	Diastolic murmurs
Apical beat becomes more prominent	3/6 and above systolic murmurs
S1 hardening	Fixed S2 splitting
S3 sound	S4 sound
Increased jugular venous distension	
Venous hum and mammary suffocation	

4.8 Cardiovascular Diagnostic Methods in Pregnancy

4.8.1 Electrocardiography

In most pregnant women, a 15–20 degree left axis deviation can be observed on the ECG. Other commonly observed physiological findings include temporary ST/T wave changes, negative T waves in V1 and V2, Q waves and negative T waves in lead III, and a small Q wave in lead aVF. These changes can mimic LV hypertrophy and other structural heart diseases. Holter ECG monitoring should be performed in patients with known paroxysmal/persistent arrhythmias [ventricular tachycardia (VT), AF, atrial flutter] or those reporting palpitations.

4.8.2 Echocardiography

Transthoracic echocardiography is a safe and preferred imaging method during pregnancy. This examination is a widely used, easily repeatable, inexpensive, and safe diagnostic method. It can be used for both outpatient and inpatient services, emergency services, intensive care units, and maternity wards. In pregnancy, changes in some parameters, such as mild dilation of the heart chambers, changes in the left ventricular wall thickness, and a slight increase in the valve gradient, are expected. Transesophageal echocardiography is a relatively safe method, but the risk of vomiting, aspiration, and sudden increase in intra-abdominal pressure should be considered, and it should be performed with fetal monitoring.

4.8.3 Exercise Testing

The physiological exercise test is an important part of monitoring in pregnant women with congenital heart or valve disease. In this group of patients, it should be done for pre-pregnancy evaluation. In patients with preexisting heart disease who are asymptomatic, a submaximal exercise test (80% of the estimated maximum heart rate) is recommended. There is no evidence that it increases the risk of spontaneous abortion. Dobutamine stress echocardiography is rarely used during pregnancy. If other options are available, the use of this test should be avoided.

4.8.4 Ionizing Radiation Exposure

The potential risks of fetal exposure to ionizing radiation depend on the stage of pregnancy and the absorbed dose. The risks are highest during organogenesis and the early fetal period, less in the second trimester, and lowest in the third trimester [11]. Malformations are typically associated with the central nervous system. Fetal damage generally occurs at doses >250 mGy. If it is not urgent, procedures involving radiation should be postponed at least until the completion of the major organogenesis period (>12 weeks after the last menstrual period). During the procedure, the fetus's exposure to radiation should be minimized.

4.8.5 Chest Radiography and Computed Tomography

Although the fetal dose in a chest radiograph is <0.01 mGy, it should only be performed when a diagnosis cannot be made by other methods. Lung ultrasound can be a safe and promising diagnostic tool. Computed tomography (CT) is generally not required and can be used in cases where other diagnostic tools are insufficient. If necessary, the use of low-radiation CT with 0.01–0.66 mGy is recommended.

4.8.6 Cardiac Catheterization

Cardiac catheterization for diagnostic purposes is rarely needed during pregnancy, but it may be necessary to guide interventional procedures. The average radiation exposure to the unprotected abdomen is 1.5 mGy, and less than 20% of this reaches the fetus. When cardiac catheterization is necessary during pregnancy, the radial approach is preferred. Electrophysiological study is recommended only in the presence of an arrhythmia resistant to medical treatment. The use of electroanatomical mapping systems is recommended to reduce the radiation dose.

4.8.7 Magnetic Resonance Imaging (MRI)

MRI is used when the diagnosis cannot be confirmed with other noninvasive diagnostic methods and is preferred over imaging methods based on ionizing radiation if feasible. Evidence regarding the use of gadolinium-based contrast agents during pregnancy is insufficient, and it is particularly recommended to avoid their use in the first trimester. The penetration of gadolinium-based agents into breast milk is limited, and breastfeeding can continue after the administration of such agents [12].

4.9 Timing of Cardiovascular Intervention During Pregnancy

Interventional cardiac treatments and cardiac surgery during pregnancy should only be performed in urgent cases. The most suitable timing for angiography-based procedures is after the 16th week of pregnancy. The most suitable time frame for the necessity of cardiac surgery is between the 20th and 28th weeks [13].

4.10 Delivery Methods in Pregnant Women with Cardiovascular Disease

For most pregnant women with cardiovascular disease, the most suitable method of delivery is normal vaginal delivery [14]. Spinal anesthesia-related sympatholytic activity can cause a drop in blood pressure, which may lead to serious side effects in patients with severe aortic stenosis and left ventricular outflow tract obstruction. Induction of labor with dinoprostone is contraindicated in patients with active cardiovascular disease. Similarly, methylergometrine should not be used in individuals with cardiovascular disease as it can cause vasoconstriction. Cesarean delivery is generally necessary due to obstetric reasons. In some specific cardiovascular diseases, cesarean delivery is recommended. These diseases are presented in Table 4.4. Prophylaxis for infective endocarditis during normal vaginal delivery or cesarean section is a controversial issue, and there is no clear recommendation.

4.11 Contraception Methods

Birth control pills containing ethinylestradiol have the highest risk of thrombosis. It is not recommended for use in women with thromboembolic risk. Additionally, this treatment is contraindicated in patients with known hypertension because it increases blood pressure. Birth control pills containing only progestin can be used

Table 4.4 Specific cardiovascular diseases for which cesarean delivery is recommended

Aortic dissection
Marfan syndrome (aortic diameter >45 mm)
Severe aortic stenosis
Severe left ventricular outflow tract obstruction
Advanced heart failure
Severe pulmonary hypertension
Pregnant woman receiving warfarin treatment

as a good alternative to ethinyl estradiol-containing medications due to their minimal effects on clotting factors, blood pressure, and lipid levels. Levonorgestrel-containing long-acting reversible contraception implants and intrauterine devices are among the safest and most effective contraceptive methods. Barrier methods for contraception are not completely reliable, but they reduce the risk of pelvic inflammatory disease.

4.12 Risk Classification in Pregnancy

Risk assessment during pregnancy should begin before gestation. Patients considering pregnancy should discontinue medications that may be contraindicated before pregnancy (RAAS blockers, statins, etc.). All pregnant women with cardiovascular disease should have their deliveries done at a hospital. Many scoring methods have been developed for risk stratification in pregnancy. Among these, the BACH (Boston Adult Congenital Heart), CAPREG (Cardiac Disease in Pregnancy), and WHO (World Health Organization) classifications are the most commonly used. The WHO classification is currently the most accepted and frequently used method. According to this classification, cardiovascular diseases are divided into four groups based on the potential risks that may arise during pregnancy. In the first group, there is no mortality risk, and the probability of morbidity is quite low. In the second group, there is a slight increase in the risk of mortality and morbidity. In the third group, pregnancy mortality and morbidity have significantly increased. It is recommended that the continuation of pregnancy in these patients and, if it continues, the pregnancy monitoring be carried out by a specialized team. In group four patients, pregnancy mortality and morbidity are at the highest levels. Patients in this group should be informed that pregnancy is prohibited. In pregnant patients, it should be recommended to terminate the pregnancy for the health of the mother. If the family wishes to continue the pregnancy, it should be closely monitored by a specialized team. According to the WHO classification, disease groups are provided in Table 4.5 [15, 16].

Table 4.5 Cardiovascular disease groups according to the WHO classification

Group 1	Patent ductus arteriosus
	Mitral valve prolapse
	Mild pulmonary stenosis
	Operated simple congenital diseases
	Isolated atrial and ventricular extravasations
Group 2	Most arrhythmias are in this group
	Uncorrected tetralogy of Fallot
	Uncorrected atrial and ventricular septal defect
Groups 2–3	Hypertrophic cardiomyopathy
	Mild left ventricular dysfunction
	Marfan syndrome (normal aortic diameter)
	Valve diseases other than Groups 1 and 4
	Bicuspid aorta (aortic diameter <45 mm)
Group 3	Presence of systemic right ventricle
	Fontan circulation
	Presence of mechanical heart valve
	Unrepaired cyanotic heart diseases
	Marfan syndrome (aortic diameter 40–45 mm)
	Bicuspid aorta (aortic diameter 45–50 mm)
Group 4	Severe left ventricular failure (NHYA class 3–4)
	Severe pulmonary hypertension
	Severe mitral stenosis
	Severe and symptomatic left ventricular outflow tract obstruction
	Marfan syndrome (aortic diameter >45 mm)
	Bicuspid aorta (aortic diameter >50 mm)
	Severe aortic coarctation

Patients in groups 2–3 will be evaluated in groups 2 or 3, depending on their clinical condition

Congenital heart diseases in pregnancy are examined under two groups: cyanotic (right-to-left shunt) and acyanotic (left-to-right shunt). In acyanotic patients, pregnancy is better tolerated, while in cyanotic patients, pregnancy is more risky. In some cases of acyanotic heart disease, Eisenmenger syndrome develops over time, causing the shunt to reverse, leading to a right-to-left shunt and the appearance of cyanosis. Regardless of the direction of the shunt, pregnancy is contraindicated in the presence of severe pulmonary hypertension. In pregnant women with a right-to-left shunt, peripheral resistance may decrease over time, leading to increased cyanosis. Cyanosis can cause significant problems for both the mother and the baby. Cyanosis-related elevated hematocrit can prepare the way for thrombosis and paradoxical embolism. In pregnant women with cyanosis, an oxygen saturation level below 85% indicates a poor prognosis, while a level above 90% indicates a good prognosis.

4.12.1 Acyanotic Heart Diseases

4.12.1.1 Atrial Septal Defect (ASD)

Pregnancy is well tolerated by those with a repaired atrial septal defect (ASD) (WHO risk class I). In unrepaired ASDs, thromboembolic risks have increased (5%). Atrial arrhythmias are more common, especially in unrepaired or late-closed ASDs. Percutaneous ASD closure can be performed during pregnancy, but this is rarely necessary, and the general approach is to wait until the pregnancy is completed.

4.12.1.2 Ventricular Septal Defect (VSD)

Small or repaired ventricular septal defects (VSDs) (without left heart dilation or ventricular dysfunction) are generally well tolerated during pregnancy and have a low risk of complications (WHO Class I and II). It is sufficient for patients to be evaluated for pulmonary pressures once or twice during pregnancy. Patients should be evaluated for pulmonary pressures once or twice during pregnancy.

4.12.1.3 Atrioventricular Septal Defect (AVSD)

In patients with atrioventricular septal defect, pregnancy is generally well tolerated after ASD repair (WHO risk class II–III). Arrhythmias and worsening of atrioventricular valve insufficiency during pregnancy can be seen, although rarely. The risk of heart failure is low and is only seen in those with severe valve insufficiency or left ventricular dysfunction.

4.12.1.4 Coarctation of the Aorta

Pregnancy is generally well tolerated in women after repair of aortic coarctation (CoA) (WHO risk class II). In pregnant women with unrepaired CoA and those with repaired CoA who have systemic hypertension, residual stenosis, and aortic aneurysm, the risk of dissection increases. For Re-CoA, treatment during pregnancy is possible with a percutaneous intervention (using a covered stent), but it should only be done when there is refractory hypertension and a risk to the mother or baby.

4.12.1.5 Patent Duktus Arteriozus (PDA)

In patients with a corrected or uncorrected small PDA and normal pulmonary artery pressure, pregnancy is generally well tolerated. However, in patients with a large PDA, symptoms of volume overload may be observed in the later stages of pregnancy due to increased volume load. It is recommended that this group of patients be closely monitored throughout their pregnancy [17].

4.12.1.6 Pulmonary Valve and Right Ventricular Outflow Tract Disease

Pulmonary (valvular) stenosis (PS) during pregnancy is generally well tolerated. However, if there is severe and symptomatic stenosis, it can lead to complications such as RV failure and arrhythmia. In the presence of severe and symptomatic stenosis, percutaneous valvuloplasty can be applied in cases resistant to medical treatment and bed rest.

4.12.2 Cyanotic Heart Diseases

4.12.2.1 Tetralogy of Fallot

Women with repaired tetralogy of Fallot generally tolerate pregnancy well (WHO risk class II). In 8% of repaired patients, cardiac complications may develop. These complications have generally been reported in those who used cardiac medications before pregnancy. Among these, arrhythmia is the most commonly encountered complication. Thromboembolism and endocarditis are rarer. In infants, fetal growth retardation may be observed. If right ventricular failure occurs during pregnancy, diuretic treatment should be initiated and bed rest should be recommended. In cases that do not respond to this treatment, early delivery or transcatheter valve implantation may be considered [7].

4.12.2.2 Ebstein's Anomaly

Women with uncomplicated Ebstein anomaly generally tolerate pregnancy well (WHO risk class II). The hemodynamic complications encountered during pregnancy are mostly dependent on the severity of tricuspid regurgitation (TR) and right ventricular function. Cyanosis (due to ASD/patent foramen ovale) and arrhythmias originating from accessory pathways are more commonly observed during pregnancy. In pregnant women with this anomaly, the risk of heart failure and preterm birth also increases. Adverse outcomes related to the mother and baby are directly associated with the mother's oxygen saturation.

4.12.2.3 Fontan Circulation

In pregnant women with Fontan circulation, the risk of pregnancy complications increases. These patients can have a successful pregnancy. However, these are high- or very-high-risk pregnancies (WHO risk class III or IV). In patients with left ventricular dysfunction, moderate to severe valvular pathologies, and oxygen saturation <85%, pregnancy should be prevented through preconception counseling. The risk of miscarriage in Fontan patients is quite high (30%). Additionally, prepartum and postpartum mortality is frequently observed in these pregnant women. The risk of thromboembolic complications is high in Fontan patients; therefore, therapeutic anticoagulation is recommended for patients who do not have a high risk of bleeding [7].

4.12.2.4 Corrected Transposition of the Great Arteries

If there is no additional congenital cardiovascular condition, it is generally well tolerated. Cyanosis and ventricular failure may develop with pregnancy, so they should be monitored in this regard. These patients are particularly at risk for arrhythmias, especially atrioventricular block. In these patients, agents that cause atrioventricular block should be avoided.

4.12.2.5 Pulmonary Hypertension and Eisenmenger Syndrome

The most common cause of pulmonary hypertension in pregnant women is congenital cardiovascular disease. The presence of pulmonary hypertension may pose a vital risk to both the pregnant woman and the baby. When Eisenmenger syndrome develops, pregnancy mortality increases to 50%. The presence of severe pulmonary hypertension or Eisenmenger syndrome is contraindicated for pregnancy. These patients should receive pre-pregnancy counseling to avoid pregnancy. If pregnancy has developed, termination should be recommended. Patients receiving specific medications for pulmonary hypertension before pregnancy should be completely informed about the teratogenic effects of the drugs. It has been determined that endothelin receptor antagonists are teratogenic in animals. Sildenafil and tadalafil groups of drugs have less side effects. In patients with pulmonary hypertension and Eisenmenger syndrome, the risk of pulmonary embolism increases, and anticoagulation therapy may be considered for these patients. In this group of patients, mortality is most commonly observed in the last trimester and the first 3 months postpartum. It is recommended that this group of patients be monitored in the hospital during the last trimester of pregnancy.

4.12.3 *Valvular Heart Disease*

The most commonly encountered heart valve disease in the female reproductive years is aortic bicuspid. In addition, especially in low- to middle-income countries, valve pathologies due to rheumatic heart disease are prominent. During pregnancy, due to the increase in heart rate and output, valve gradients increase by 50% [18]. Mechanical heart valve prostheses also lead to specific problems during pregnancy.

4.12.3.1 Stenotic Valve Lesions

Mitral Stenosis

Mild mitral stenosis (MS) during pregnancy is generally well tolerated. Symptoms of heart failure are observed in one-third of pregnant women with a valve area of $\leq 1.0\ cm^2$ and in half of those with a valve area of $\leq 1.5\ cm^2$. Symptoms usually begin to appear in the second trimester. Severe stenosis, advanced age, NYHA class >II, and systolic PAP >30 mmHg are the most important predictors of maternal complications. Patients with mitral stenosis who are planning pregnancy should undergo pre-pregnancy percutaneous balloon mitral valvuloplasty if they are suitable for the procedure. In the later stages of pregnancy, the risk of developing atrial fibrillation due to increased volume, which results in the risk of pulmonary edema and systemic embolism, can increase. Anticoagulation therapy should be initiated in patients who develop atrial fibrillation. In patients who develop heart failure symptoms during pregnancy, bed rest should be planned and beta-blocker and diuretic treatments should be used. In patients resistant to medical treatment, percutaneous mitral balloon valvuloplasty can be performed after the first trimester. In resistant patients who are not suitable for this treatment, surgical intervention may be considered [19].

Valvular Aortic Stenosis

Mild and moderate aortic stenosis are well tolerated during pregnancy and usually do not cause any symptoms. Less than 10% of asymptomatic patients with moderate aortic stenosis develop symptoms of heart failure. Even in patients with severe aortic stenosis who have normal exercise capacity before pregnancy, pregnancy is well tolerated. Pregnancy is not recommended for patients with pre-pregnancy symptoms and impaired left ventricular function, moderate to severe aortic stenosis, without treatment. In patients who become symptomatic during pregnancy, diuretic treatment in addition to rest is recommended. In patients resistant to medical treatment, balloon valvuloplasty is recommended [20].

Pulmonary Stenosis

Moderate and severe pulmonary stenosis with asymptomatic and normal right ventricular functions before pregnancy are well tolerated during pregnancy. It is recommended that those with symptomatic severe pulmonary stenosis be treated before pregnancy. For patients with severe pulmonary stenosis who become symptomatic during pregnancy, balloon valvuloplasty treatment can be applied [21].

4.12.3.2 Regurgitant Valve Lesions

Mitral and Aortic Regurgitation

Pre-pregnancy women with severe regurgitation and symptoms or impaired left ventricular function are at high risk for heart failure during pregnancy. Moreover, 20–25% of pregnant women with moderate or severe rheumatic mitral regurgitation develop heart failure. The prognosis depends on the severity of the valve regurgitation and the left ventricular functions. It is recommended that symptomatic patients be treated before pregnancy. In patients who become symptomatic during pregnancy, diuretic treatments should be used cautiously to reduce congestion symptoms. In patients with treatment-resistant symptoms, surgery may be necessary during pregnancy. If the fetus is sufficiently mature, it is recommended to deliver before heart surgery.

Tricuspid Regurgitation

Secondary tricuspid regurgitation (TR) is more common than primary TR. The more common causes of primary TR are endocarditis or Ebstein anomaly. Maternal risk is dependent on the severity of left-sided valvular disease or pulmonary hypertension. In pregnant women with severe symptomatic TR or right ventricular dysfunction, maternal risk increases. Even symptomatic patients with severe TR can be treated medically during pregnancy. When surgery is required for left-sided valve lesions, if there is severe TR and annular dilation (≥40 mm), surgical intervention is also indicated for the tricuspid valve.

4.12.3.3 Prosthetic Valves

When prosthetic valve implantation is inevitable in a woman who wishes to become pregnant in the future, valve selection requires performance and long-term durability. The need for anticoagulation associated with a prosthetic valve increases mortality and morbidity in both the mother and fetus. Bioprosthetic valves are more advantageous in terms of major cardiovascular events during pregnancy. Compared to mechanical valves, the risk of thrombogenicity is lower and anticoagulation is not required. However, bioprosthetic valves are at high risk of valve degeneration in young women. The need for reoperation may arise, and redo surgery has a high mortality rate. Transcatheter valve implantation (currently especially for pulmonary valves) and the Ross procedure (pulmonary autograft and pulmonary homograft in the aortic position) are other natural options to consider (k5). Desire for pregnancy is a class II indication for biological valves [22].

The durability and hemodynamic performance of mechanical prosthetic valves are better. However, the risk of thrombogenicity is higher compared to bioprostheses. In pregnancy, there is an increase in platelet adhesion, changes in coagulation factors, and a decrease in fibrinolysis. Due to these changes, the risk of valve thrombosis is higher during pregnancy. Therefore, anticoagulation therapy during pregnancy is very important. All anticoagulation treatment options can pose risks for both the mother and the baby due to the risk of bleeding. Unfractionated Heparin (UFH) and low molecular weight Heparin (LMWH) do not cross the placenta and do not have fetotoxic effects. However, the risk of valve thrombosis is higher compared to warfarin treatment. However, while warfarin treatment is more reliable in terms of valve thrombosis, it has a fetotoxic effect. Warfarin treatment can cause optic atrophy, nasal hypoplasia, epiphyseal stippling, and intellectual disability in the first trimester. However, the fetotoxic effect of using less than 5 mg of warfarin daily is quite low. If an effective INR level can be achieved with 5 mg of warfarin treatment for the mother in the first trimester, it is recommended to continue this treatment. If a higher dose of warfarin is necessary, UFH or LMWH treatment should be considered. In patients receiving UFH, the aPTT level should be adjusted to twice the normal level. DMAH is administered twice a day and requires dose adjustment based on factor Xa levels during pregnancy; 4–6 h after administering DMAH, the factor Xa level should be between 0.8 and 1.2 U/mL. If it is not possible to measure factor Xa, it is recommended not to use this treatment. Since organogenesis is complete, warfarin treatment can be safely used in the second and third trimesters. Warfarin treatment should be stopped at the 36th week, and UFH infusion therapy should be initiated. UFH infusion should continue for 4–6 h before delivery. After postpartum hemorrhage control is achieved, UFH treatment should be resumed 4–6 h later [15]. If mechanical valve thrombosis develops during pregnancy and the patient's clinical condition is stable, UFH treatment should be initiated and continued with oral anticoagulant therapy. In patients whose clinical condition is not stable, surgical treatment is indicated. In patients who cannot undergo surgery, fibrinolytic therapy may be considered.

4.12.3.4 Marfan Syndrome

Marfan syndrome is a genetically inherited connective tissue disorder. Due to the autosomal dominant inheritance, there is a 50% chance that the baby will have Marfan syndrome. The risk of aortic dilation and dissection increases during pregnancy. The aortic width of pregnant patients with Marfan syndrome needs to be evaluated in detail. If the ascending aorta is >45 mm, surgical correction before pregnancy is recommended. In patients with an aortic diameter of >45 mm during pregnancy, cesarean delivery is recommended to prevent complications [23].

4.13 Coronary Artery Disease in Pregnancy

Pregnancy increases the risk of acute myocardial infarction by 3–4 times. In addition to conventional risk factors, factors such as (pre-)eclampsia, thrombophilia, postpartum infection, and multiparity are added during pregnancy. The increase in maternal age over 40 raises the risk of AMI by 20% each year. In pregnant women, the etiology of AMI differs from that of the normal population and is generally due to non-atherosclerotic causes. The most common etiological causes are pregnancy-related spontaneous coronary artery dissection (P-SCAD) (43%), angiographically normal coronary arteries (18%), and coronary thrombosis (17%). P-SCAD occurs more frequently in the late stages of pregnancy and the early postpartum period. It usually involves the left coronary arteries [24, 25].

The treatment approach for AMI occurring during pregnancy is similar to that for the normal population. When planning treatment, a multidisciplinary approach involving gynecology and cardiology is recommended. In the case of clinical necessity, invasive intervention should not be restricted due to the side effects of ionizing radiation. However, the radiation dose should be minimized.

4.14 Peripartum Cardiomyopathy

The precise mechanism of peripartum cardiomyopathy has not been completely understood, but it is believed that inflammation and angiogenic factors play a role in its development. Some of the risk factors are multiparity, African ethnicity, smoking, diabetes, pre-eclampsia, and advanced age. It is generally associated with rapidly developing heart failure symptoms, and usually the LVEF drops below 45%. Patients may present with arrhythmia or cardiac arrest in addition to heart failure symptoms. Initial LVEF <30%, significant LV dilation (LV-end-diastolic diameter >6.0 cm), and RV involvement are indicators of poor prognosis [26, 27]. In a prospective study conducted in Turkey, the 24-month mortality rate was found to be 24%. When LVEF does not improve beyond 50–55%, the next pregnancy should be avoided. Even if LVEF completely normalizes, there is still a risk of recurrence. Therefore, preconception counseling for subsequent pregnancies is necessary [28]. Patients with symptoms of acute heart failure should be treated according to current heart failure guidelines. In patients with cardiogenic shock and those requiring mechanical circulatory support, emergency cesarean delivery is recommended regardless of the gestational week [29].

4.14.1 *Hypertrophic Cardiomyopathy*

The incidence of hypertrophic cardiomyopathy (HCM) in pregnancy is less than 1 in 1000. Women with HCM generally tolerate pregnancy well. In a recent meta-analysis, the maternal mortality rate was found to be 0.5%. The fetal death rate is around 20%. In women with high-risk criteria such as being symptomatic before pregnancy, having diastolic dysfunction, severe left ventricular outflow tract obstruction, or a history of arrhythmia, the prognosis is worse [30, 31]. In treatment, beta-blockers are preferred. When atrial fibrillation develops, cardioversion may be considered. In low-risk cases, normal vaginal delivery may be possible. In patients with severe LV outflow obstruction and severe heart failure, cesarean delivery is recommended. Epidural and spinal anesthesia should be administered carefully, especially in patients with severe LV outflow tract obstruction.

4.15 Hypertension in Pregnancy

Hypertension is the most common cardiovascular disease encountered during pregnancy and is a significant cause of morbidity and mortality for pregnant women. Hypertension in pregnancy is examined in three subgroups.

4.15.1 *Preexisting Hypertension*

It is hypertension that occurs before the 20th week of pregnancy and continues after the 40th day of pregnancy.

4.15.2 *Gestational Hypertension*

It is hypertension that occurs after the 20th week of pregnancy and resolves before the 40th day of pregnancy. Gestational hypertension with the presence of 0.3 g/day proteinuria is defined as preeclampsia. In preeclampsia, vascular pathologies, hepatocellular damage, hemolytic anemia, and pulmonary edema can also be observed. The addition of convulsions to these conditions is defined as eclampsia and is the most severe form.

4.15.3 *Superimposed Preeclampsia*

It is the addition of preeclampsia to preexisting chronic hypertension after the 20th week of pregnancy and is more severe than isolated preeclampsia. In pregnancy hypertension, whether it is chronic hypertension or gestational hypertension, the treatment initiation threshold is 140/90 mmHg. A systolic blood pressure of >160 mmHg and a diastolic blood pressure of >110 mmHg are considered a hypertensive emergency in pregnancy and should be treated in a hospital. In treatment, dihydropyridine group calcium channel blockers (preferably extended-release nifedipine), labetalol, and methyldopa are preferred as the first choice. The treatment goal should be targeted at <140/90.

4.16 Arrhythmias in Pregnancy

In pregnancy, due to hormonal and emotional changes, palpitations are frequently observed as a result of increased cardiac output and heart rate. These palpitations are generally benign, but as the pregnancy progresses, they can rarely be seen in malignant arrhythmias. In the second trimester of pregnancy, symptomatic bradycardias may be observed with a drop in blood pressure. Congenital atrioventricular blocks are generally well tolerated during pregnancy. During delivery, a temporary pacemaker may rarely need to be placed [32]. When supraventricular tachycardia (SVT) develops during pregnancy, the treatment approach is the same as in non-pregnant women. Some antiarrhythmic treatments can harm the fetus. In the treatment of supraventricular tachycardia, carotid sinus massage and other vagal maneuvers with minimal side effects are preferred first. If vagal maneuvers fail, adenosine is administered as the safest medical treatment. In SVTs that do not respond to adenosine, metoprolol or verapamil can be used. In the presence of hemodynamic instability, electrical cardioversion should be the primary choice. Atrial fibrillation (AF) is rarely seen during pregnancy, but it can develop in patients with congenital heart disease and valvular heart disease. In the medical cardioversion of acute AF, ibutilide or flecainide can be preferred primarily. In the presence of AF, anticoagulation indications are the same as in the normal population. Anticoagulant agent preferences may vary according to the trimester of pregnancy. Direct oral anticoagulants are contraindicated during pregnancy. Ventricular arrhythmias are quite rare during pregnancy, but malignant arrhythmias can occur in those with structural heart disease. The most common ventricular tachycardias originate from the right ventricular outflow tract. If there is hemodynamic instability, emergency electrical cardioversion is indicated. If hemodynamics are stable, sotalol and procainamide are primarily preferred. In patients resistant to these treatments, amiodarone can be used as the last option. In pregnancy, ICD indications are the same as in the general population. If ICD implantation is necessary, it is recommended to be performed after the 8th week and accompanied by echocardiography [33].

References

1. Siu SC, Sermer M, Colman JM, Alvarez AN, Mercier LA, Morton BC, Cardiac Disease in Pregnancy (CARPREG) Investigators. Prospective multicenter study of pregnancy outcomes in women with heart disease. Circulation. 2001;104(5):515–21.
2. Worldatlas. Countries with the oldest average mother's age at first birth. https://www.worldatlas.com/articles/countries-with-the-highest-mother-s-mean-age-atfirst-birth.html. 25 Apr 2017.
3. Elkayam U, Goland S, Pieper PG, Silverside CK. High-risk cardiac disease in pregnancy: part I. J Am Coll Cardiol. 2016;68:396–410.
4. Hilfiker-Kleiner D, Sliwa K. Pathophysiology and epidemiology of peripartum cardiomyopathy. Nat Rev Cardiol. 2014;11(6):364–70.
5. Kampman MA, Valente MA, vanMelle JP, Balci A, Roos-Hesselink JW, Mulder BJ, vanDijk AP, Oudijk MA, Jongbloed MR, vanVeldhuisen DJ, Pieper PG. Cardiac adaption during pregnancy in women with congenital heart disease and healthy women. Heart. 2016;102:1302–8.
6. Cornette J, Ruys TP, Rossi A, Rizopoulos D, Takkenberg JJ, Karamermer Y, Opic P, VandenBosch AE, Geleijnse ML, Duvekot JJ, Steegers EA, Roos-Hesselink JW. Hemodynamic adaptation to pregnancy in women with structural heart disease. Int J Cardiol. 2013;168:825–31.
7. Regitz-Zagrosek V, Roos-Hesselink JW, Bauersachs J, Blomström-Lundqvist C, Cifkova R, De Bonis M, Warnes CA. 2018 ESC guidelines for the management of cardiovascular diseases during pregnancy: the task force for the management of cardiovascular diseases during pregnancy of the European Society of Cardiology (ESC). Eur Heart J. 2018;39(34):3165–241.
8. Ouzounian JG, Elkayam U. Physiologic changes during normal pregnancy and delivery. Cardiol Clin. 2012;30(3):317–29.
9. Pieper PG. Use of medication for cardiovascular disease during pregnancy. Nat Rev Cardiol. 2015;12:718–29.
10. Sanghavi M, Rutherford JD. Cardiovascular physiology of pregnancy. Circulation. 2014;130(12):1003–8.
11. Ray JG, Vermeulen MJ, Bharatha A, Montanera WJ, Park AL. Association between MRI exposure during pregnancy and fetal and childhood outcomes. JAMA. 2016;316:952–61.
12. Sachs HC. The transfer of drugs and therapeutics into human breast milk: an update on selected topics. Pediatrics. 2013;132:e796–809.
13. Becker RM. Intracardiac surgery in pregnant women. Ann Thorac Surg. 1983;36(4):453–8.
14. Bonow RO, Mann DL, Zipes DP, Libby P. Braunwald's heart disease e-book: a textbook of cardiovascular medicine. Elsevier Health Sciences; 2011.
15. Emren Z, Emren V. Kadınlar. In: Kozan Ö, Kocabay G, Şafak Ö, editors. Kalp Kitabı cilt-2. İstanbul: Nobel tıp kitabevi; 2020. p. 1309–27.
16. Siu SC, Sermer M, Colman JM, Alvarez AN, Mercier LA, Morton BC, Cardiac Disease in Pregnancy (CARPREG) Investigators. Prospective multicenter study of pregnancy outcomes in women with heart disease. Circulation. 2011;104(5):515–21.
17. Brickner ME. Cardiovascular management in pregnancy: congenital heart disease. Circulation. 2014;130(3):273–82.
18. Samiei N, Amirsardari M, Rezaei Y, Parsaee M, Kashfi F, Hantoosh Zadeh S, Beikmohamadi S, Fouladi M, Hosseini S, Peighambari MM, Mohebbi A. Echocardiographic evaluation of hemodynamic changes in left-sided heart valves in pregnant women with valvular heart disease. Am J Cardiol. 2016;118:1046–52.

19. vanHagen IM, Thorne SA, Taha N, Youssef G, Elnagar A, Gabriel H, ElRakshy Y, Iung B, Johnson MR, Hall R, Roos-Hesselink JW, ROPAC Investigators and EORP Team. Pregnancy outcomes in women with rheumatic mitral valve disease: results from the Registry of Pregnancy and Cardiac Disease. Circulation. 2018;137:806–16.
20. Leśniak-Sobelga A, Tracz W, KostKiewicz M, Podolec P, Pasowicz M. Clinical and echocardiographic assessment of pregnant women with valvular heart diseases—maternal and fetal outcome. Int J Cardiol. 2004;94(1):15–23.
21. Hameed AB, Goodwin TM, Elkayam U. Effect of pulmonary stenosis on pregnancy outcomes—a case-control study. Am Heart J. 2007;154(5):852–4.
22. Baumgartner H, Falk V, Bax JJ, De Bonis M, Hamm C, Holm PJ, Iung B, Lancellotti P, Lansac E, Rodriguez Munoz D, Rosenhek R, Sjogren J, Tornos Mas P, Vahanian A, Walther T, Wendler O, Windecker S, Zamorano JL. 2017 ESC/EACTS guidelines for the management of valvular heart disease. Eur Heart J. 2017;38:2739–91.
23. Meijboom LJ, Drenthen W, Pieper PG, Groenink M, van der Post JA, Timmermans J, Mulder B. Obstetric complications in Marfan syndrome. Int J Cardiol. 2006;110(1):53–9.
24. Elkayam U, Jalnapurkar S, Barakkat MN, Khatri N, Kealey AJ, Mehra A, Roth A. Pregnancy-associated acute myocardial infarction: a review of contemporary experience in 150 cases between 2006 and 2011. Circulation. 2014;129:1695–702.
25. Roos-Hesselink JW, Duvekot JJ, Thorne SA. Pregnancy in high-risk cardiac conditions. Heart. 2009;95:680–6.
26. Haghikia A, Podewski E, Libhaber E, Labidi S, Fischer D, Roentgen P, Tsikas D, Jordan J, Lichtinghagen R, vonKaisenberg CS, Struman I, Bovy N, Sliwa K, Bauersachs J, Hilfiker-Kleiner D. Phenotyping and outcome on contemporary management in a German cohort of patients with peripartum cardiomyopathy. Basic Res Cardiol. 2013;108:366.
27. McNamara DM, Elkayam U, Alharethi R, Damp J, Hsich E, Ewald G, Modi K, Alexis JD, Ramani GV, Semigran MJ, Haythe J, Markham DW, Marek J, Gorcsan J III, Wu WC, Lin Y, Halder I, Pisarcik J, Cooper LT, Fett JD. Clinical outcomes for peripartum cardiomyopathy in North America: results of the IPAC study (Investigations of Pregnancy-Associated Cardiomyopathy). J Am Coll Cardiol. 2015;66:905–14.
28. Hilfiker-Kleiner D, Haghikia A, Masuko D, Nonhoff J, Held D, Libhaber E, Petrie MC, Walker NL, Podewski E, Berliner D, Bauersachs J, Sliwa K. Outcome of subsequent pregnancies in patients with a history of peripartum cardiomyopathy. Eur J Heart Fail. 2017;19:1723–8.
29. Bauersachs J, Arrigo M, Hilfiker-Kleiner D, Veltmann C, Coats AJ, Crespo-Leiro MG, DeBoer RA, vander Meer P, Maack C, Mouquet F, Petrie MC, Piepoli MF, Regitz-Zagrosek V, Schaufelberger M, Seferovic P, Tavazzi L, Ruschitzka F, Mebazaa A, SliwaK. Current management of patients with severe acute peripartum cardiomyopathy: practical guidance from the Heart Failure Association of the European Society of Cardiology Study Group on Peripartum Cardiomyopathy. Eur J Heart Fail. 2016;18:1096–105.
30. Metra M. September 2016 at a glance: pregnancy, hypertrophic cardiomyopathy, epidemiology, medical treatment. Eur J Heart Fail. 2016;18:1091–2.
31. Spirito P, Autore C. Management of hypertrophic cardiomyopathy. BMJ. 2006;332:1251–5.
32. Hidaka N, Chiba Y, Kurita T, Satoh S, Nakano H. Is intrapartum temporary pacing required for women with complete atrioventricular block? An analysis of seven cases. BJOG Int J Obstet Gynaecol. 2006;113(5):605–7.
33. Nakagawa M, Katou S, Ichinose M, Nobe S, Yonemochi H, Miyakawa I, Saikawa T. Characteristics of new-onset ventricular arrhythmias in pregnancy. J Electrocardiol. 2004;37(1):47–53.

Chapter 5
Navigating Asthma in Pregnancy: Respiratory Health for Expecting Mothers

Aysu Ayrancı

5.1 Introduction

Asthma represents the most common respiratory condition encountered in pregnancy [1], with data indicating that it occurs in roughly 2–13% of all pregnant individuals [1–3]. When asthma is not adequately controlled during pregnancy, both maternal and fetal complications may arise [4, 5]. Therefore, current clinical guidelines focus on minimizing exacerbations and achieving optimal asthma control in pregnant women to protect the health of both mother and fetus.As a chronic inflammatory disorder of the airways characterized by variable airflow limitation, asthma requires careful management during pregnancy, as poor control is associated with increased risk of adverse outcomes [6].

5.2 Epidemiology and Impact of Asthma in Pregnancy

The interaction between asthma and pregnancy is bidirectional. While inadequate asthma control contributes to increased maternal and fetal morbidity, pregnancy itself can intensify bronchial inflammation, leading to poorer asthma control and a higher likelihood of exacerbations [7].In the United States, one study reported the prevalence of asthma in pregnancy to be 8.8% [6], and since 1994, the rate has risen from 3% to 8% [6]. Similarly, about 8% of pregnant women in the United Kingdom have asthma [8], whereas the prevalence reaches 12% in Australia [9]. The clinical course of asthma during pregnancy is known to be highly variable.Approximately

A. Ayrancı (✉)
Izmir Bakircay University, Faculty of Medicine, Department of Chest Diseases, Izmir, Turkey
e-mail: aysu.ayranci@bakircay.edu.tr

© The Author(s), under exclusive license to Springer Nature Switzerland AG 2026

I. Karaca (ed.), *Managing Maternal Chronic Diseases for a Healthy Pregnancy*, https://doi.org/10.1007/978-3-032-15221-3_5

one-third of pregnant individuals with asthma experience worsening symptoms, another third see no change, and the remaining third show improvement [10]. In one study, 52–65% of those with severe asthma reported deterioration during pregnancy, compared with only 8–13% of individuals with mild disease [11]. Another investigation revealed that nearly 65% of pregnant patients had poor asthma control. Furthermore, 64.4% demonstrated incorrect inhaler technique, only 38% could differentiate between reliever and controller medications, and just 12.7% had a written asthma action plan. In addition, only 17% had spirometry within the previous 5 years, and just 3.8% owned a peak expiratory flow meter for home monitoring [12].

Research indicates that maternal asthma is associated with a higher risk of numerous complications affecting both the mother and the fetus. These include small for gestational age (SGA) births, low birth weight (LBW), congenital anomalies such as cleft lip or cleft palate, increased perinatal mortality, preterm delivery, maternal preeclampsia, gestational hypertension, gestational diabetes, antepartum hemorrhage, cesarean section, urinary tract infections, and polyhydramnios. In addition, premature rupture of membranes is particularly common in women with severe or poorly controlled asthma during pregnancy [4, 13]. Therefore, pregnant individuals with asthma should be closely followed from early pregnancy by both an obstetrician and a pulmonologist to ensure that treatment maintains adequate asthma control while safeguarding the health of both the mother and the fetus.

5.3 Physiological Changes During Pregnancy and Their Effects on Asthma

The mechanisms underlying asthma improvement or worsening during pregnancy are strongly linked to the physiological and pathological alterations that occur in this period. Mechanical factors caused by uterine enlargement and hormonal influences play a central role. As intra-abdominal and uterine pressure increases, the diaphragm is pushed upward by approximately 4–5 cm, the subcostal angle widens by about 50%, and both the transverse and anteroposterior diameters of the thoracic cage expand. These structural changes are partially compensated for by relaxation of the costal ligaments, which helps counterbalance decreased thoracic compliance. Consequently, total lung volume is reduced by around 5%, and functional residual capacity (FRC) declines by nearly 20% [14]. In addition, weight gain during pregnancy increases neck circumference and reduces the oropharyngeal airway, further contributing to dyspnea [15]. To meet the metabolic needs of the mother and fetus, pregnancy induces substantial hormonal changes, including elevated levels of progesterone, estrogen, cortisol, and prostaglandins, each of which can influence the clinical course of asthma.Progesterone enhances the sensitivity of the respiratory center to carbon dioxide, stimulating ventilation. Estrogen may reinforce this effect by increasing progesterone receptor responsiveness within the respiratory center, and together these hormones alter respiratory physiology [16]. As a result, minute ventilation rises by approximately 30–50%, primarily due to a 40% increase in tidal volume, while respiratory rate remains relatively constant. Total lung capacity (TLC), vital capacity (VC), lung compliance, and diffusing capacity for carbon monoxide (DLCO) remain largely unchanged.

Similarly, forced vital capacity (FVC), forced expiratory volume in 1 s (FEV_1), the FEV_1/FVC ratio, and peak expiratory flow rate (PEFR) show no significant differences between pregnant and nonpregnant individuals [14]. Therefore, spirometry remains a useful tool during pregnancy for evaluating dyspnea and monitoring respiratory disorders. Beyond its central respiratory effects, progesterone also promotes mucosal vasodilation and congestion, contributing to pregnancy rhinitis and increasing the likelihood of epistaxis [17]. These hormonal effects may also induce airway changes in the oropharyngeal and laryngopharyngeal regions, potentially worsening asthma symptoms during pregnancy.

Estradiol can enhance maternal innate immunity as well as both cellular and humoral adaptive immune responses. At low levels, estradiol favors $CD4^+$ Th1 cell activity and cell-mediated immunity, whereas at higher concentrations it promotes $CD4^+$ Th2 responses and humoral immunity. Progesterone, on the other hand, suppresses maternal immune function and shifts the balance between Th1 and Th2 pathways. Although cell-mediated immunity plays a greater role in respiratory viral infections, the hormonally driven shift from Th1 to Th2 during pregnancy is believed to be a major contributor to asthma pathogenesis in this period [18, 19]. Pregnancy is also characterized by a hypercortisolemic state. The placenta produces both corticotropin-releasing hormone (CRH) and adrenocorticotropic hormone (ACTH), resulting in elevated levels of free and conjugated cortisol. Increased free cortisol enhances beta-adrenergic receptor expression and promotes bronchodilation [15]. Additionally, higher levels of prostaglandin E2 (PGE2) have a protective role in asthma due to its anti-inflammatory effects, inhibition of airway smooth muscle proliferation, and bronchodilatory action. Progesterone further influences airway smooth muscle tone [16]. These hormonal changes may contribute to asthma remission during pregnancy.

In summary, the mechanical and biochemical effects of pregnancy on the maternal respiratory system are highly complex. Hormonal actions on the respiratory center, peripheral airways, and immune system can cause varying degrees of dyspnea even in pregnant individuals without asthma. For those with asthma, optimizing disease management throughout pregnancy is essential to prevent maternal hypoxemia and ensure adequate fetal oxygenation.

5.4 Interaction Between Pregnancy and Asthma

5.4.1 Effect of Pregnancy on Asthma

Anatomical, hormonal, and immunological alterations during pregnancy have a substantial influence on asthma control. Anatomical adaptations lead to increases in tidal volume (TV) and inspiratory capacity (IC), whereas functional residual capacity (FRC), total lung capacity (TLC), and vital capacity (VC) progressively decline over the course of pregnancy. In contrast, forced expiratory volume in 1 s (FEV_1), peak expiratory flow rate, and airway resistance typically remain stable.

During pregnancy, serum cortisol levels increase by approximately twofold, serum progesterone levels increase ninefold, and serum estrogen levels rise by 100- to 1000-fold. Although cortisol and progesterone are expected to exert bronchodilatory effects, their competitive affinity for glucocorticoid receptors limits the clinical significance of these effects [20]. However, progesterone may contribute to asthma exacerbations by promoting mucosal vasodilation and congestion, which can lead to rhinitis and laryngopharyngeal edema.

During pregnancy, immunological adaptations include a shift in T-helper cell balance toward a Th2-dominant profile, which may increase the likelihood of asthma exacerbations [20]. To avoid maternal immune reactions against fetal antigens, the activity of effector T cells and natural killer (NK) cells is downregulated, creating a state of immunosuppression. This immunosuppressive environment predisposes pregnant individuals to viral infections and related complications [21].In a study evaluating the effect of viral infections on asthma during pregnancy, influenza-like illness occurred in 71% of pregnant women with asthma compared to 46% of pregnant women without asthma. Rhinovirus was the most frequently detected pathogen, present in 38.5% of cases. Among pregnant individuals with asthma who contracted viral infections, one-third experienced exacerbations and another one-third reported a loss of asthma control. Furthermore, compared with the control group, pregnant women with asthma exhibited diminished interferon-λ (IFN-λ), interferon-γ (IFN-γ), and interleukin-10 (IL-10) responses [22].

In approximately 60% of patients, asthma follows a similar course in successive pregnancies as it did in the first pregnancy [23]. Allergen exposure does not appear to result in a significantly different pattern of exacerbation in pregnant women with asthma [24, 25]. Comorbid conditions such as allergic rhinitis have also been reported to follow a similar course during pregnancy in about 50% of cases [9, 10]. Some studies suggest that the sex of the fetus may influence asthma symptoms in pregnant individuals. When carrying a male fetus, pregnant women with asthma have been found to be less symptomatic and to require lower doses of inhaled corticosteroids and fewer rescue medications. This phenomenon has been attributed to fetal testosterone, which may enhance β2-adrenergic-mediated airway smooth muscle relaxation, particularly during the second trimester [26, 27].

Asthma may first appear during pregnancy, or existing asthma control may change over the course of gestation. Although it is traditionally stated that one-third of pregnant individuals with asthma improve, one-third worsen, and one-third remain stable [23], a recent case-control study found an exacerbation rate of only 18.8%—notably lower than the expected proportion [28]. In a cohort of 1739 pregnant patients with asthma, 30% of those with mild disease progressed to moderate or severe asthma, while 23% of those with severe asthma improved to a moderate level [29]. Individuals with severe or poorly controlled asthma before conception are more likely to experience worsening symptoms during pregnancy.

The highest rate of severe exacerbations typically occurs between the 29th and 36th weeks of gestation [23], although some studies suggest the second trimester carries the greatest risk [11]. In the final 4 weeks of pregnancy, asthma symptoms generally improve, and exacerbations during labor are uncommon, occurring in only about 10% of cases.

5.4.2 *Effect of Asthma on Pregnancy*

Studies evaluating the impact of asthma on pregnancy have reported widely variable findings. Nonetheless, the presence of asthma during gestation has consistently been linked to increased maternal morbidity. Asthma is a chronic inflammatory airway disorder, and it has been suggested that maternal inflammatory mediators may impair placental function and influence fetal development [19]. Although the underlying mechanisms remain poorly defined, substantial evidence indicates that pregnant individuals with asthma face a higher risk of adverse perinatal outcomes, such as impaired fetal growth, preeclampsia, and preterm birth [30].

Asthma has been associated with several serious pregnancy complications, including preeclampsia, gestational diabetes, gestational hypertension, congenital malformations such as cleft lip and cleft palate, antepartum hemorrhage, and placenta previa [4, 5]. Additionally, numerous studies have demonstrated that asthma increases the risk of preterm delivery, cesarean section, low birth weight, and neonatal mortality [30–32]. Compared with pregnant individuals without asthma, those with asthma have a 1.41-fold higher risk of preterm labor. In pregnancies affected by asthma, the likelihood of delivering a low birth weight infant increases by 46%, the risk of preterm birth rises by 22%, and the incidence of preeclampsia is elevated by 54% [30].

The proposed mechanisms for these complications include maternal hypoxia, systemic inflammation, impaired uterine smooth muscle relaxation, placental deficiency of 11β-hydroxysteroid dehydrogenase, and medication-related effects such as those associated with β_2-agonists [30, 33]. Nonetheless, these potential risks should not be viewed as contraindications to pregnancy. Multiple studies and clinical guidelines have shown that effective therapy and well-controlled asthma can substantially reduce adverse outcomes [30, 34].

In one study, pregnant individuals with asthma who were enrolled before 18 weeks of gestation and managed with monthly spirometry, fractional exhaled nitric oxide (FeNO) monitoring, and individualized treatment adjustments achieved asthma control in 80% of cases, thereby preventing many complications. However, even under optimal control, a slight but statistically significant increase in preeclampsia and small for gestational age (SGA) infants was still observed [35]. It is also important to recognize that different pregnancies in the same individual may follow distinct clinical patterns.

5.5 Diagnosis of Asthma During Pregnancy

Asthma is typically described as a chronic inflammatory disorder of the airways, presenting with recurrent respiratory symptoms—such as wheezing, dyspnea, chest tightness, and cough—and associated with variable expiratory airflow limitation that can be triggered by multiple stimuli. Confirmation of variable airflow obstruction is made by demonstrating a positive bronchodilator reversibility test, significant peak expiratory flow (PEF) variability, or a positive bronchial provocation test [34].

In pregnant individuals, asthma manifests with clinical features similar to those seen in the general population. However, it is important to note that up to two-thirds of nonasthmatic pregnant women may experience dyspnea as a result of normal physiological changes, particularly in late gestation. Consequently, a detailed medical history and comprehensive physical examination are crucial for establishing an accurate diagnosis.

Unlike in nonpregnant patients, all types of provocation testing—including bronchial challenge tests and allergy skin tests—are contraindicated during pregnancy because of the potential risk of fetal distress and maternal hypoxemia [36]. Spirometry, peak expiratory flow (PEF) monitoring, and fractional exhaled nitric oxide (FeNO) measurement are considered safe for both diagnostic and follow-up purposes in pregnant individuals. However, in cases of preeclampsia or cervical insufficiency, spirometry and PEF assessment are also contraindicated [37].

5.6 Monitoring and Follow-Up of Asthma During Pregnancy

- Asthma assessment generally involves evaluating levels of asthma control—both current symptom control and the risk of future adverse outcomes—as well as identifying treatment-related issues such as inhaler technique and medication adherence, and recognizing comorbidities that may increase symptom burden or diminish quality of life [34]. Continuous monitoring from early pregnancy is essential to maintain disease stability and identify potential complications promptly [38].
- Pregnant individuals with asthma should be followed regularly by a pulmonologist. Clinical visits should include assessment of symptom severity and pulmonary function, along with patient education on indoor and outdoor air pollution, tobacco exposure, and environmental triggers. Correct inhaler technique should be demonstrated, appropriate use of rescue medication should be reviewed, and guidance on step-up therapy at home when necessary should be provided.

Table 5.1 Components of effective asthma monitoring during pregnancy

Monthly objective assessment of asthma control
Taking a validated symptom history using standardized questionnaires (e.g., ACT, GINA, ACQ)
Spirometry or peak expiratory flow (PEF) measurement
Fetal monitoring after the 32nd week of gestation
Patient education
General asthma education for all women of childbearing age
Instruction on correct inhaler technique
Provision of a written asthma action plan
Addressing concerns about the teratogenic effects of medications and explaining the potential risks of discontinuing therapy
Avoidance of environmental triggers (e.g., pollen, mold, fungi, house dust mites, air pollution)
Smoking cessation
Management of Comorbid Conditions (e.g., gastroesophageal reflux [GERD], rhinitis, allergies)

- Monthly follow-up is recommended. If not contraindicated, spirometry or peak expiratory flow (PEF) measurements should be performed. Typical PEF values range between 380 and 550 L/min, although the optimal value varies with the individual's maximal effort. A PEF greater than 90% of a patient's personal best indicates good asthma control [36]. Additional monitoring tools during pregnancy include the Asthma Control Test (ACT), symptom diaries, and fractional exhaled nitric oxide (FeNO) measurements. In a study by Powell et al., FeNO monitoring effectively predicted exacerbation risk, guided rescue medication adjustment, and reduced exacerbation frequency [39].
- The key components of effective asthma monitoring during pregnancy are summarized in Table 5.1 [40]. According to the Global Initiative for Asthma (GINA), important recommendations for maintaining asthma control during pregnancy include the following [34]:
  - Active asthma management is more important than the potential risks of medications (Level A evidence).
  - Even if their safety profiles are not fully established, the use of existing medications is appropriate for symptom control and prevention of exacerbations (Level A evidence).
  - Discontinuation of inhaled corticosteroids (ICS) is a known risk factor for exacerbations (Level A evidence).
  - Step-down therapy is not recommended during pregnancy (Level D evidence).
  - Provide educational materials to patients.
  - Monthly follow-up is recommended.
  - Monitor and appropriately treat respiratory infections.
  - Prompt treatment of exacerbations using short-acting beta-agonists (SABAs), oxygen, and systemic corticosteroids (SCS) if necessary.

5.7 Asthma Treatment in Pregnancy

The primary goal of asthma management in pregnancy is to maintain optimal disease control by minimizing—or ideally eliminating—symptoms, preserving lung function, and reducing the likelihood of future exacerbations through appropriate pharmacologic and nonpharmacologic strategies [41].Although concerns about medication safety for both mother and fetus are common, the use of inhaled corticosteroids (ICS), short-acting β_2-agonists (SABA), short-acting anticholinergics (SAMA), long-acting β_2-agonists (LABA), montelukast, and theophylline has not been linked to a significant increase in fetal abnormalities [34, 42]. Overall, asthma medications are considered safe during pregnancy, and despite possible side effects, better maternal asthma control is associated with improved fetal outcomes [43]. Treatment should be individualized, with medication choices based on a careful risk–benefit evaluation. Therapy is recommended when the maternal benefits of controlling asthma outweigh any potential fetal risks [44].

The drugs used for asthma management during pregnancy are largely the same as those used in the general population; however, some differences exist in treatment planning. One distinction is that asthma control should be assessed monthly rather than quarterly. Additionally, step-down therapy is seldom used during pregnancy. The usual approach is to maintain the current regimen at the dose required to sustain asthma control, provided the dose is not excessively high [34]. If a patient was already receiving anti-IgE therapy or allergen immunotherapy before conception and derived benefit, continuation during pregnancy is advised. However, initiating these treatments during pregnancy is not recommended due to the risk of anaphylaxis [45].

The medications commonly used in asthma treatment and their safety profiles during pregnancy are summarized in Table 5.2 [46, 47].

5.7.1 B-Agonists

β_2-agonists are the most potent bronchodilators used in asthma management, acting on beta-adrenergic receptors to alleviate bronchospasm. Among pregnant individuals with asthma, inhaled β_2-agonists are the most frequently prescribed medications [48]. These drugs function as "rescue medications" and are divided into short-acting and long-acting classes.

Short-acting β_2-agonists (SABAs), such as salbutamol and terbutaline, are used for rapid relief during acute symptom episodes. SABAs are considered safe in pregnancy and have not been linked to congenital anomalies, low birth weight, intrauterine growth restriction, or adverse maternal or perinatal outcomes [49].

Long-acting β_2-agonists (LABAs), including formoterol and salmeterol, are used as maintenance therapy for moderate-to-severe asthma, always in combination with inhaled corticosteroids. Although long-term safety data for LABAs in pregnancy

Table 5.2 Medications used in asthma treatment and their safety profiles during pregnancy [46, 47]

Active ingredient	FDA category	Pregnancy	Delivery	Lactation	Observations/warnings
SABA (salbutamol/terbutaline)	C/C	Safe to use	Safe to use	Safe to use	Side effect profile similar to the general population. Systemic administration may cause maternal/fetal tachycardia, maternal hyperglycemia, and fetal hypoglycemia. May have tocolytic effects during labor.
LABA (formoterol/salmeterol)	C/C	Safe to use	Safe to use	Safe to use	Limited data available, but post-marketing data suggest safety. Due to greater clinical experience, salmeterol is preferred over formoterol; however, if the patient was using formoterol before pregnancy, switching is not recommended.
Ultra-LABA (olodaterol/vilanterol)	–/C	Possibly safe	Possibly safe	Possibly safe	No human data available; animal studies indicate low risk.
LAMA (tiotropium bromide)	–	Possibly safe	Possibly safe	Safe to use	Limited data during pregnancy and lactation. No teratogenic effects observed in animal studies, although high-dose fetal toxicity has been reported.
Theophylline	C	Safe to use	Safe to use	Safe to use	No teratogenic effects reported. Serum levels should be monitored. If used until late pregnancy, it may inhibit uterine contractions.
ICS (budesonide/beclomethasone/fluticasone)	B/–/–	Safe to use	Safe to use	Safe to use	At standard doses, no association with major malformations, preterm birth, or low birth weight. Treatment should be maintained at the minimum effective controller dose.
Systemic steroids (prednisolone/prednisone/hydrocortisone)	C/C/C	Possibly safe	Possibly safe	Possibly safe	Study results are conflicting. Generally considered safe, though some studies report increased risks of low birth weight, preterm birth, cleft lip ± palate, and preeclampsia.
LTRA (montelukast/zafirlukast)	B/B	Possibly safe	Possibly safe	Possibly safe	Insufficient data. Can be continued if the patient was already using it before pregnancy.
Monoclonal antibodies (omalizumab/mepolizumab/reslizumab)	B/–/–	Possibly safe	Possibly safe	Possibly safe	If omalizumab was initiated before pregnancy, it may be continued; however, initiation during pregnancy is not recommended due to potential anaphylaxis.

SABA Short-acting beta-agonist, *LABA* Long-acting beta-agonist, *Ultra-LABA* Ultra-long-acting beta-agonist, *LAMA* Long-acting muscarinic antagonist, *ICS* Inhaled corticosteroid, *LTRA* Leukotriene receptor antagonist are limited, they are recommended in step-up treatment when asthma control cannot be achieved with medium-dose inhaled corticosteroids and SABAs alone. Due to their pharmacologic and toxicologic similarity to salbutamol, both formoterol and salmeterol are considered acceptable controller options when paired with inhaled corticosteroids. Salmeterol is often preferred over formoterol because it has a longer history of use in clinical practice [50].

Most studies have not shown a significant association between β_2-agonist use and outcomes such as low birth weight or major congenital anomalies [49]. Although a few reports have suggested possible links between β_2-agonist exposure during pregnancy and adverse outcomes such as low birth weight, gastroschisis, or cleft palate [33], these results are difficult to interpret due to confounding variables. In many cases, the study populations included individuals with poorly controlled asthma who required frequent rescue medication use, making it unclear whether the adverse outcomes were related to the drugs themselves or to the underlying uncontrolled disease.

Supporting the effectiveness of β_2-agonists, a study involving 1744 nonpregnant asthma patients showed that adding a long-acting β_2-agonist (LABA) reduced exacerbation rates and short-acting β_2-agonist (SABA) use more effectively than increasing the dose of inhaled corticosteroids (ICS) alone [51]. Furthermore, Eltonsy et al. [52] found no significant difference in congenital malformations between ICS/LABA combination therapy and higher-dose ICS monotherapy. Similarly, Cossette et al. [53] reported that both ICS/LABA and low-to-moderate dose ICS regimens had no detrimental effect on perinatal outcomes.

In summary, current clinical guidelines support the use of β_2-agonists during pregnancy—both as reliever and controller medications—in combination with inhaled corticosteroids [34, 47].

5.7.2 *Inhaled Corticosteroids*

Inhaled corticosteroids (ICSs) are the foundation of asthma therapy, as they effectively reduce airway inflammation while limiting systemic adverse effects. Budesonide and beclomethasone are the preferred ICS options due to their long history of use and well-established safety profiles [46]. Among available agents, budesonide has the strongest evidence supporting safety; however, other ICS medications are also considered safe. Therefore, if a pregnant patient with well-controlled asthma is already using a different ICS, treatment should be continued without interruption. A Danish registry study of 83,043 pregnancies found no association between first-trimester glucocorticoid use and congenital malformations or cleft lip/palate [54].

Multiple studies have evaluated the efficacy and safety of ICS therapy during pregnancy. ICS use has been shown to decrease the frequency of asthma exacerbations and related hospitalizations without increasing the risk of congenital anomalies or adverse outcomes [55]. No association has been identified between ICS treatment and intrauterine growth restriction (IUGR) or other fetal abnormalities [56]. Furthermore, large-scale studies reported no teratogenic effects in the fetuses of 2014 pregnant women who used budesonide during early pregnancy [57], and no clinically relevant impact on pregnancy outcomes in a cohort of 2968 pregnant women with asthma [58]. These findings confirm that budesonide is safe for both mother and fetus.

If a patient was already using a different ICS before conception, switching is unnecessary; however, when initiating ICS therapy during pregnancy, budesonide is preferred. Because ICSs are considered safer than LABAs, treatment should begin with low- to medium-dose ICS monotherapy. If escalation is required, transitioning to a fixed-dose ICS/LABA combination is recommended [21].

5.7.3 Systemic Corticosteroids

Oral corticosteroids may be required during pregnancy to manage uncontrolled asthma or treat acute exacerbations. Data from studies including 52,038 pregnant women—238 of whom received oral corticosteroids—are available. A slight increase in the risk of isolated cleft lip with or without cleft palate during first-trimester exposure has been reported (0.3% vs. 0.1%), along with associations with preterm delivery, low birth weight, and preeclampsia [59]. While early epidemiological studies suggested a link between first-trimester corticosteroid use and cleft lip and/or palate [60], later investigations did not confirm this association [54].

Long-term systemic corticosteroid use in pregnancy has been associated with increased risks of preeclampsia, preterm birth, and low birth weight [50, 61]. However, distinguishing the effects of corticosteroids from those of severe or poorly controlled asthma is challenging. Overall, clinical guidelines stress that the dangers of inadequate asthma control are greater than the potential risks of systemic corticosteroid therapy. Therefore, systemic corticosteroids should not be withheld when clinically necessary. Prednisolone is the preferred agent during pregnancy, as approximately 90% of the drug is metabolized by the placenta, thereby reducing fetal exposure.

5.7.4 Anticholinergics

Ipratropium bromide may be used as a rescue therapy in pregnant individuals with asthma, especially in combination with salbutamol. Although no adverse maternal or fetal effects have been demonstrated, its ability to improve lung function or reduce hospital admissions has not been clearly established [62].

For patients with uncontrolled or partially controlled asthma already receiving medium- to high-dose ICS or ICS plus LABA therapy, adding tiotropium has been shown to enhance lung function and decrease exacerbation frequency [63, 64]. However, evidence regarding tiotropium use during pregnancy is limited. While animal studies have not revealed teratogenic effects, high doses have been associated with fetal toxicity and intrauterine growth restriction. Although tiotropium is classified as an FDA Category B medication, its safety and efficacy in pregnant populations are not well defined, and it should not be used as a first-line option.

5.7.5 *Theophylline*

Low-dose theophylline can be used as an alternative long-acting bronchodilator in patients with persistent asthma when inhaled corticosteroids (ICS) alone do not provide adequate control. Theophylline has not been linked to teratogenic effects or intrauterine growth restriction [65]. Because theophylline readily crosses the placenta, serum levels must be carefully monitored. Concentrations above 10 μg/mL may result in transient neonatal vomiting, tremors, and tachycardia, while levels exceeding 20 μg/mL are associated with a markedly increased risk of toxicity [50]. For this reason, theophylline levels in pregnant patients should be maintained between 5 and 12 μg/mL. Although not considered a first-line therapy for asthma during pregnancy, theophylline may be used as an alternative to LABAs in individuals who do not achieve adequate control with ICS alone.

5.7.6 *Leukotriene Receptor Antagonists*

The leukotriene receptor antagonists (LTRAs) available in Turkey—montelukast and zafirlukast—are generally less effective than inhaled corticosteroids (ICS) and are typically used as add-on therapies. When combined with ICS, LTRAs have demonstrated comparable efficacy to the addition of a LABA [66]. In a study of 1164 pregnant women using LTRAs, no increase in major congenital anomalies was observed [67]. However, another study reported higher rates of gestational diabetes, preeclampsia, maternal underweight, preterm birth, and low Apgar scores in pregnant individuals using LTRAs [68].LTRAs are classified as FDA Category B drugs. Montelukast also has a favorable safety profile during lactation. For patients who were already benefiting from LTRA therapy before pregnancy, continuation of treatment during pregnancy is recommended.

5.7.7 *Omalizumab*

Omalizumab is a recombinant monoclonal antibody that selectively binds to human immunoglobulin E (IgE). By preventing IgE from attaching to high-affinity receptors on basophils and mast cells, it inhibits cellular activation and subsequent inflammatory responses. Anti-IgE therapy is indicated in patients with moderate to severe asthma that remains uncontrolled despite medium- to high-dose inhaled corticosteroids (ICS) combined with long-acting β_2-agonists, provided the patient has an IgE level between 30–1500 IU/mL and a positive skin test to perennial allergens. In nonpregnant individuals with persistent asthma inadequately controlled on ICS, the addition of omalizumab has been shown to decrease exacerbation frequency, improve symptoms, lower hospitalization rates, and reduce corticosteroid requirements [69, 70].

The U.S. Food and Drug Administration (FDA) classifies omalizumab as a Category B medication in pregnancy. Although clinical experience remains limited, available data are reassuring. In the EXPECT study—a prospective, observational trial—191 pregnant patients who received at least one dose of omalizumab during pregnancy or within 8 weeks prior to conception were monitored. The rates of major congenital anomalies, preterm birth, and low birth weight were comparable to those seen in other pregnant women with asthma [71]. Accordingly, continuation of omalizumab during pregnancy is recommended for patients already receiving it prior to conception. However, due to the potential risk of anaphylaxis, initiation of omalizumab during pregnancy is not advised [36].A practical challenge associated with omalizumab use in pregnancy is dosing. The medication is administered subcutaneously every 2 or 4 weeks, with dosage based on body weight and total serum IgE levels. Because pregnant individuals may experience rapid weight gain, weight-based titration can become difficult, making accurate dosing more challenging.

5.8 Management of Acute Asthma Exacerbations During Pregnancy

The traditional view of asthma in pregnancy suggests that one-third of patients experience worsening disease control, one-third improve, and the remaining third remain unchanged. A meta-analysis evaluating multiple studies on this topic prospectively followed 366 pregnancies in 330 individuals with asthma and reported worsening in 35%, improvement in 28%, and stability in 33% of cases. The hospitalization rate due to asthma exacerbations during pregnancy was 5.8% (range: 2.4–8.2%) [72, 73].

An asthma exacerbation in pregnancy is defined as a deterioration of symptoms that necessitates an unscheduled hospital or emergency department visit, hospitalization, or use of oral corticosteroids. Exacerbations occur in approximately 20–45% of pregnant patients with asthma. In a prospective study, the risk of a severe exacerbation was 8% in those with mild asthma, 47% in moderate asthma, and 65% in severe asthma [11]. Exacerbations most frequently occur in the late second trimester, peaking around the 25th week of gestation. The most common triggers include viral respiratory infections, poor adherence to ICS therapy, and inadequate overall asthma management [73, 74].

The treatment of asthma exacerbations in pregnant patients generally follows the same approach used in nonpregnant individuals. However, early recognition during pregnancy is especially critical. Symptom worsening, peak expiratory flow (PEF) monitoring, and fetal surveillance provide valuable clinical information. A reduction of more than 50% in PEF indicates a severe exacerbation [50].

Prompt and appropriate treatment is essential. Inhaled salbutamol should be administered at 2.5 mg every 20 min for three doses. If there is inadequate clinical response, therapy should be escalated to include oral or intravenous corticosteroids. When FEV_1 falls below 40% of predicted or when there is no response to SABA, nebulized ipratropium bromide (0.25–0.5 mg every 30 min, up to three doses) may be added. Patients who do not improve with SABA and ICS or whose condition deteriorates should be hospitalized [75].

Oxygen supplementation is necessary to prevent maternal and fetal hypoxia, and systemic corticosteroids should not be delayed when clinically indicated. Continuous maternal and fetal monitoring is required throughout treatment. In the later stages of pregnancy, fetal surveillance should include nonstress testing to assess reactivity of the fetal heart rate, ultrasound evaluation of amniotic fluid volume, and observation of fetal movement, breathing, and heart rate [75]. Treatment response should be reassessed every 30–60 min. Four hours after the initial evaluation, a decision should be made to either discharge the patient or continue inpatient care. If the patient responds adequately and is suitable for discharge, oral prednisone 40–80 mg daily for 5–10 days should be prescribed to prevent recurrence of symptoms [76].

If a patient fails to improve with maximal therapy, clinicians should be prepared to initiate inpatient or intensive care unit (ICU) monitoring. ICU admission should be considered in pregnant individuals with asthma exacerbations when FEV_1 falls below 25% of the predicted value or when post-treatment improvement in FEV_1 is less than 10%. Maternal oxygenation must be assessed promptly, and oxygen saturation should be maintained above 95% to prevent fetal hypoxia [75].

Case reports and series have documented successful use of both noninvasive mechanical ventilation (NIMV) and invasive mechanical ventilation (IMV) in pregnant women with asthma or other indications. IMV is indicated when hypoxemia does not respond to noninvasive oxygen therapy, or in the presence of severe respiratory acidosis, altered mental status, or signs of maternal respiratory fatigue. Ventilatory support should be managed by experienced clinicians using strategies that minimize dynamic hyperinflation and applying low minute ventilation to provide adequate respiratory support [77, 78].

5.9 Labor and Delivery Management

Pre-labor evaluation and multidisciplinary planning are essential components of managing pregnant women with respiratory diseases [46]. In patients with asthma, close coordination between obstetricians and pulmonologists has been shown to decrease the risk of severe respiratory complications [11, 79].

To date, no studies have specifically examined labor management strategies in women with respiratory diseases or evaluated whether cesarean delivery provides any clinical advantage compared with vaginal birth in this population [46]. Although women with moderate to severe asthma are more likely to undergo elective cesarean section than those with mild disease, labor induction is rarely indicated solely on the basis of asthma [79, 80].

During labor and delivery, controller medications—and reliever therapies when needed—should be continued [34, 46]. Owing to endogenous corticosteroid release, approximately 90% of patients do not experience asthma exacerbations during labor. However, labor-associated hyperventilation may trigger bronchoconstriction, which should be treated with short-acting β_2-agonists (SABAs) as needed [34]. In patients taking oral corticosteroids, suppression of the hypothalamic–pituitary–adrenal (HPA) axis may occur. Therefore, administration of hydrocortisone 100 mg every 6–8 h during labor and for 24 h postpartum is recommended [46, 81].

If high doses of SABAs are used during labor, the newborn should be monitored for hypoglycemia during the first 24 h of life. In pregnant individuals with asthma, careful selection of medications for cervical ripening, analgesia, and anesthesia is also important. Oxytocin and prostaglandin E2 are suitable for labor induction. Fentanyl is considered an appropriate analgesic; however, morphine and other opioid analgesics should be avoided due to their potential to induce histamine release and provoke bronchospasm. To minimize respiratory infections and atelectasis, epidural anesthesia is preferred over general anesthesia when there are no contraindications [82].

Asthma in pregnancy represents an important public health issue. Numerous studies have demonstrated that maternal asthma can negatively affect both maternal and fetal health, increasing the risk of multiple complications. Achieving and maintaining optimal asthma control is the most crucial factor in preventing these adverse outcomes. Although concerns about medication use during pregnancy persist, the benefits of maintaining good asthma control and preventing exacerbations outweigh the potential risks of pharmacologic therapy.

Pregnant individuals with asthma should be considered high-risk and require close follow-up by both an obstetrician and a pulmonologist. A stepwise treatment approach should be used with the aim of achieving and sustaining asthma control.

Clinicians should educate and counsel pregnant patients with asthma on trigger avoidance, correct inhaler technique, adherence to prescribed medications, and the importance of seeking medical care promptly if symptoms worsen. Although data on the effects of asthma medications during pregnancy are limited, current evidence largely supports their safety. As with all clinical decisions, the risk–benefit balance should be carefully evaluated, as maternal asthma control has a direct impact on both maternal and fetal outcomes.

References

1. Jolving LR, Nielsen J, Kesmodel US, et al. Prevalence of maternal chronic diseases during pregnancy-a nationwide population based study from 1989 to 2013. Acta Obstet Gynecol Scand. 2016;95:1295–304.
2. Sawicki E, Stewart K, Wong S, et al. Medication use for chronic health conditions by pregnant women attending an Australian maternity hospital. Aust N Z J Obstet Gynaecol. 2011;51:333–8.
3. Kim S, Kim J, Park SY, et al. Effect of pregnancy in asthma on health care use and perinatal outcomes. J Allergy Clin Immunol. 2015;136:1215–23.
4. Murphy VE, Schatz M. Asthma in pregnancy: a hit for two. Eur Respir Rev. 2014;23:64–8.
5. Hodyl NA, Stark MJ, Scheil W, et al. Perinatal outcomes following maternal asthma and cigarette smoking during pregnancy. Eur Respir J. 2014;43:704–16.
6. Kwon HL, Belanger K, Bracken MB. Asthma prevalence among pregnant and childbearing-aged women in the United States: estimates from national health surveys. Ann Epidemiol. 2013;23(4):207–12.
7. Charlton R, Hutchison A, Davis K, De Vries C. Asthma management in pregnancy. PLoS One. 2013;4:8.
8. Clark JM, Hulme E, Devendrakumar V, et al. Effect of maternal asthma on birthweight and neonatal outcome in a British inner-city population. Paediatr Perinat Epidemiol. 2007;21(2):154–62. https://doi.org/10.1111/j.1365-3016.2007.00784.
9. Australian Bureau of Statistics: National Health Survey. First results, 2014–15. 2015. http://www.abs.gov.au/AUSSTATS/abs@.nsf/Lookup/4364.0.55.001Explanatory%20Notes12014-15?OpenDocument.
10. Juniper ENM. Effect of pregnancy on asthma: systematic review and meta-analysis. In: Hn C, Schatz MZR, editors. Asthma and immunological diseases in pregnancy and early infancy. New York: Marcel Dekker; 1993. p. 223–50.
11. Murphy VE, Gibson P, Talbot PI, Clifton VL. Severe asthma exacerbations during pregnancy. Obstet Gynecol. 2005;106:1046–54.
12. Ibrahim WH, Rasul F, Ahmad M, et al. Asthma knowledge, care, and outcome during pregnancy: the QAKCOP study. Chron Respir Dis. 2018;16. https://doi.org/10.1177/1479972318767719.
13. Hodyl NA, Stark MJ, Scheil W, Grzeskowiak LE, Clifton VL. Perinatal outcomes following maternal asthma and cigarette smoking during pregnancy. Eur Respir J. 2014;43(3):704–16. https://doi.org/10.1183/09031936.00054913.
14. Bobrowski RA. Pulmonary physiology in pregnancy. Clin Obstet Gynecol. 2010;53(2):285–300. https://doi.org/10.1097/grf.0b013e3181e04776.
15. Tan EK, Tan EL. Alterations in physiology and anatomy during pregnancy. Best Pract Res Clin Obstet Gynaecol. 2013;27(6):791–802. https://doi.org/10.1016/j.bpobgyn.2013.08.001.
16. Annamraju H, Mackillop L. Respiratory disease in pregnancy. Obstet Gynaecol Reprod Med. 2017;27(4):105–11. https://doi.org/10.1016/j.ogrm.2017.01.011.
17. Mehta N, Chen K, Hardy E, Powrie R. Respiratory disease in pregnancy. Best Pract Res Clin Obstet Gynaecol. 2015;29(5):598–611. https://doi.org/10.1016/j.bpobgyn.2015.04.005.
18. Kourtis AP, Read JS, Jamieson DJ. Pregnancy and infection. N Engl J Med. 2014;370(23):2211–8. https://doi.org/10.1056/nejmra1213566.

19. Clifton V. Maternal asthma during pregnancy and fetal outcomes: potential mechanisms and possible solutions. Curr Opin Allergy Clin Immunol. 2006;6(5):307–11. https://doi.org/10.1097/01.all.0000244788.28789.dd.
20. Robijn AL, Murphy VE, Gibson PG, et al. Asthma in pregnancy. Clin Chest Med. 2011;32:93–110.
21. Tamási L, Horváth I, Bohács A, et al. Asthma in pregnancy immunological changes and clinical management. Respir Med. 2011;105:159–64.
22. Murphy VE, Powell H, Wark PA, et al. A prospective study of respiratory viral infection in pregnant women with and without asthma. Chest. 2013;144:420–7.
23. Schatz M, Harden K, Forsythe A, et al. The course of asthma during pregnancy, post partum, and with successive pregnancies: a prospective analysis. J Allergy Clin Immunol. 1988;81:509–17.
24. Lao TT, Huengsburg M. Labour and delivery in mothers with asthma. Eur J Obstet Gynecol Reprod Biol. 1990;35:183–90.
25. Kircher S, Schatz M, Long L. Variables affecting asthma course during pregnancy. Ann Allergy Asthma Immunol. 2002;8:463–6.
26. Dodds L, Armson BA, Alexander S. Use of asthma drugs is less among women pregnant with boys rather than girls. BMJ. 1999;318:1011.
27. Kwon HL, Belanger K, Holford TR, Bracken MB. Effect of fetal sex on airway lability in pregnant women with asthma. Am J Epidemiol. 2006;16:217–21.
28. Grosso A, Locatelli F, Gini E, et al. The course of asthma during pregnancy in a recent, multicase-control study on respiratory health. Allergy Asthma Clin Immunol. 2018;14:16.
29. Dombrowski MP, Schatz M, Wise R. More asthma during pregnancy. Obstet Gynecol. 2004;103:5–12.
30. Murphy V, et al. A meta-analysis of adverse perinatal outcomes in women with asthma. BJOG. 2011;118:1314–23.
31. Wang G, Murphy VE, Namazy J, et al. The risk of maternal and placental complications in pregnant women with asthma: a systematic review and meta-analysis. J Matern Fetal Neonatal Med. 2014;27:934–42.
32. Morten M, Collison A, Murphy VE, et al. Managing asthma in pregnancy. Breathe (Sheff). 2015;11:258–67.
33. Garne E, Hansen AV, Morris J, et al. Use of asthma medication during preg- nancy and risk of specific congenital anomalies: a European case-mal- formed control study. J Allergy Clin Immunol. 2015;136:1496–502.
34. Global Initiative for Asthma. www.ginasthma.com. 2024.
35. Ali Z, Nilas L, Ulrik CS. Low risk of adverse obstetrical and perinatal outcome in pregnancies complicated by asthma: a case control study. Respir Med. 2016;120:124–30.
36. Kelly W, Massoumi A, Lazarus A. Asthma in pregnancy: physiology, diagnosis, and management. Postgrad Med. 2015;127:349–58.
37. Cooper BG, Cooper BG. An update on contraindications for lung function testing. Thorax. 2011;66:714–23.
38. National Asthma Council Australia. Australian asthma handbook. Melbourne: National Asthma Council Australia; 2023. Website. Available from: http://www.asthmahandbook.org.au.
39. Powell H, Murphy V, Taylor D, Hensley M, McCaffrey K, Giles W, et al. Management of asthma in pregnancy guided by measurement of fraction of exhaled nitric oxide: a double-blind, randomised controlled trial. Lancet. 2011;378:983–90.
40. Bonham CA, Patterson KC, Strek ME. Asthma outcomes and management during pregnancy. Chest. 2017;153:515–27.
41. Bateman E, et al. Global strategy for asthma management and prevention: GINA executive summary. Eur Respir J. 2008;31:143–78.
42. Cusack RP, Whetstone CE, Gauvreau GM. Use of asthma medication during gestation and risk of specific congenital anomalies. Immunol Allergy Clin N Am. 2023;43(1):169–85.

43. Blais L, Forget A. Asthma exacerbations during the first trimester of pregnancy and the risk of congenital malformations among asthmatic women. J Allergy Clin Immunol. 2008;121:1379–84.
44. Dombrowski M, Schatz M. ACOG practice bulletin: clinical management guidelines for obstetrician–gynecologists number 90, February 2008: asthma in pregnancy. Obstet Gynecol. 2008;111:457–64.
45. Lieberman J. Should we encourage allergen immunotherapy during pregnancy? Expert Rev Clin Immunol. 2014;10:317–9.
46. Middleton PG, Gade EJ, Aguilera C, et al. ERS/TSANZ task force statement on the management of reproduction and pregnancy in women with airways diseases. Eur Respir J. 2020;55:1901208.
47. Türk Toraks Derneği Astım Tanı ve Tedavi Rehberi, 2016.
48. Louik C, Schatz M, Hernandez-Diaz S, Werler MM, Mitchell AA. Asthma in pregnancy and its pharmacologic treatment. Ann Allergy Asthma Immunol. 2010;105:110–7.
49. Schatz M, Zeiger R, Harden K, Hoffman CP, Forsythe AB, Chilingar LM, et al. The safety of inhaled beta-agonist bronchodilators during pregnancy. J Allergy Clin Immunol. 1988;82:686–95.
50. Busse WW. NAEPP expert panel report: managing asthma during pregnancy: recommendations for pharmacologic treatment-2004 update. J Allergy Clin Immunol. 2005;115(1):34–46.
51. Delea TE, Hagiwara M, Stempel DA, Stanford RH. Adding salmeterol to fluticasone propionate or increasing the dose of fluticasone propionate in patients with asthma. Allergy Asthma Proc. 2010;31(3):211–8. https://doi.org/10.2500/aap.2010.31.3360.
52. Eltonsy S, Forget A, Beauchesne MF, Blais L. Risk of congenital malformations for asthmatic pregnant women using a long-acting beta(2)-agonist and inhaled corticosteroid combination versus higher-dose inhaled corticosteroid monotherapy. J Allergy Clin Immunol. 2015;135(1):123–30. https://doi.org/10.1016/j.jaci.2014.07.051.
53. Cossette B, Forget A, Beauchesne MF. Impact of maternal use of asthma-controller therapy on perinatal outcomes. Thorax. 2013;68(8):724–30. https://doi.org/10.1136/thoraxjnl-2012-203122.
54. Bay Bjorn AM, Ehrenstein V, Hundborg HH, et al. Use of corticosteroids in early pregnancy is not associated with risk of oral clefts and other congenital malformations in offspring. Am J Ther. 2014;21:73–80.
55. Wendel P, Ramin S, Barnett-Hamm C. Asthma treatment in pregnancy: a randomized controlled study. Am J Obstet Gynecol. 1996;175:150–4.
56. Namazy J, Schatz M, Long L, Lipkowitz M, Lillie MA, Voss M, et al. Use of inhaled steroids by pregnant asthmatic women does not reduce intrauterine growth. J Allergy Clin Immunol. 2004;113:427–32.
57. Kallen B, Rydhstroem H, Aberg A. Congenital malformations after the use of inhaled budesonide in early pregnancy. Obstet Gynecol. 1999;93:392–5.
58. Norjavaara E, De Verdier M. Normal pregnancy outcomes in a population-based study including 2,968 pregnant women exposed to budesonide. J Allergy Clin Immunol. 2003;111:736–42.
59. Williams M, et al. Habitual snoring and asthma comorbidity among pregnancy women. J Asthma. 2011;48:91–7.
60. Park-Wyllie L, Mazzotta P, Pastuszak A, et al. Birth defects after maternal exposure to corticosteroids: prospective cohort study and meta-analysis of epidemiological studies. Teratology. 2000;62:385–92.
61. Kher S, Mota P. Maternal asthma: management strategies. Cleve Clin J Med. 2017;84:296–302.
62. Soler X, Ramsdell J. Anticholinergics/antimuscarinic drugs in asthma. Curr Allergy Asthma Rep. 2014;14:484.
63. Quirce S, Dominguez-Ortega J, Barranco P. Anti-cholinergics for treatment of asthma. J Investig Allergol Clin Immunol. 2015;25:84–5.
64. Castillo JR, Peters SP, Busse WW. Asthma exacerbations: pathogenesis, prevention, and treatment. J Allergy Clin Immunol Pract. 2017;5:918–27.

65. Rocklin RE. Asthma, asthma medications and their effects on maternal/fetal outcomes during pregnancy. Reprod Toxicol. 2011;32:189–97.
66. Tamada T, Ichinose M. Leukotriene receptor antagonists and antiallergy drugs. Handb Exp Pharmacol. 2017;237:153–69.
67. Nelsen LM, Shields KE, Cunningham ML, et al. Congenital malformations among infants born to women receiving montelukast, inhaled corticosteroids, and other asthma medications. J Allergy Clin Immunol. 2012;129:251–4.
68. Kiernan E, Jones KL. Medications that cause fetal anomalies and possible prevention strategies. Clin Perinatol. 2019;46:203–13.
69. Humbert M, Beasley R, Ayres J, Slavin R, Hébert J, Bousquet J, et al. Benefits of omalizumab as add-on therapy in patients with severe persistent asthma who are inadequately controlled despite best available therapy (GINA 2002 step 4 treatment): INNOVATE. Allergy. 2005;60:309–16.
70. Lim A, Stewart K, Konig K, George J. Systematic review of the safety of regular preventive asthma medications during pregnancy. Ann Pharmacother. 2011;45:931–45.
71. Namazy J, Cabana MD, Scheuerle AE, et al. The Xolair Pregnancy Registry (EXPECT): the safety of omalizumab use during pregnancy. J Allergy Clin Immunol. 2015;135:407–12.
72. Gluck JC, Gluck PA. The effect of pregnancy on the course of asthma. Immunol Allergy Clin N Am. 2006;26:63–80.
73. Murphy V, Clifton V, Gibson P. Asthma exacerbations during pregnancy: incidence and association with adverse pregnancy outcomes. Thorax. 2006;61:169–76.
74. Murphy VE, Jensen ME, Gibson PG. Asthma during pregnancy: exacerbations, management, and health outcomes for mother and infant. Semin Respir Crit Care Med. 2017;38:160–73.
75. Schatz M, Dombrowski M. Clinical practice. Asthma in pregnancy. N Engl J Med. 2009;360:1862–9.
76. Maselli DJ, Adams SG, Peters JI, Levine SM. Management of asthma during pregnancy. Ther Adv Respir Dis. 2013;7:87.
77. Allred CC, Matias Esquinas A, Caronia J, et al. Successful use of noninvasive ventilation in pregnancy. Eur Respir Rev. 2014;23:142–4.
78. Dalar L, Caner H, Eryuksel E, Kosar F. Application of non- invasive mechanical ventilation in an asthmatic pregnant woman in respiratory failure: a case report. J Thorac Dis. 2013;5:97–100.
79. Gade EJ, Tidemandsen C, Hansen AV, Ulrik CS, Backer V. Challenges in the successful management of asthma during conception, pregnancy and delivery. Breathe (Sheff) [Internet]. 2022 [cited Dec 24, 2022];18(2):220013.
80. Tinker SC, Broussard CS, Frey MT, Gilboa SM. Prevalence of prescription medication use among non-pregnant women of childbearing age and pregnant women in the United States: NHANES, 1999–2006. Matern Child Health J. 2015;19:1097–106.
81. Vieira AC, Pité H, Morais-Almeida M. Asthma and pregnancy in the 2020 decade: still a matter of concern. J Matern Fetal Neonatal Med. 2022;35(25):6498–504.
82. Wang H, Li N, Huang H. Asthma in pregnancy: pathophysiology, diagnosis, whole-course management, and medication safety. Can Respir J. 2020;9046842:10. https://doi.org/10.1155/2020/9046842.

Chapter 6
Managing Renal Diseases and Nephrolithiasis During Pregnancy

Mustafa Ozan Horsanalı

6.1 Introduction

Urological problems in pregnant patients pose a distinct clinical challenge. Treating these patients can be difficult due to the potential risks related to medications and surgical interventions. Pregnancy involves substantial physiological adaptations, particularly affecting the renal system. While these changes are crucial for fetal development, they also predispose women to various renal disorders. Pregnant patients presenting with urological complaints can often be a challenging population to treat. Recognizing and managing renal diseases during pregnancy is critical, as both maternal and fetal outcomes can be significantly affected if these conditions are left untreated. During pregnancy, various urological issues may develop, such as hydronephrosis, hydroureter, pyelonephritis, and urolithiasis. Symptoms can include flank pain, fever, urinary retention, hematuria, dysuria, and/or a combination of these symptoms [1].

Urolithiasis during pregnancy constitutes a substantial health concern that can influence the well-being of both the mother and the fetus. It is recognized as the predominant cause of urology-related abdominal discomfort among pregnant women [2]. Urolithiasis may be associated with conditions such as ureteral obstruction, upper urinary tract infection, and urosepsis, as well as perinephric abscess, which require urgent hospitalization and intervention, causing significant morbidity to the mother. Furthermore, this condition may initiate preterm labor or interfere with normal labor progression, posing a significant health risk to the fetus [3]. Several physiological and anatomical changes predispose individuals to stone formation during pregnancy, particularly in the upper urinary system. The increase in urinary components and hormonal changes can accelerate stone formation.

M. O. Horsanalı (✉)
Izmir Bakircay University, Faculty of Medicine, Department of Urology, Izmir, Turkey
e-mail: ozan.horsanali@bakircay.edu.tr

© The Author(s), under exclusive license to Springer Nature Switzerland AG 2026

I. Karaca (ed.), *Managing Maternal Chronic Diseases for a Healthy Pregnancy*,
https://doi.org/10.1007/978-3-032-15221-3_6

Physiological changes in pregnancy, such as hypercalciuria and urinary stasis, contribute to stone formation [4].

Sometimes, the diagnosis of urolithiasis during pregnancy may present challenges compared to normal conditions. Diagnosis and treatment can be difficult and highly stressful for the health care providers, given the ineffective use of imaging modalities, anesthesia, and the potential adverse effects on the mother and fetus of radiation exposure through invasive procedures [5]. It may be confused with many clinical conditions in the differential diagnosis, such as appendicitis, placental premature separation, diverticulitis, and ovarian torsion, which can lead to delays in diagnosis [6].

6.2 Changes in the Urinary System During Pregnancy

Several significant physiological changes occur during pregnancy that should be taken into consideration. During pregnancy, the kidneys enlarge by 1–1.5 cm, and their volume can increase by as much as 30% due to increased renal vascular and interstitial pressure volume [7]. Approximately 50–90% of pregnant women in the third trimester may develop physiological hydronephrosis, especially on the right side [3, 8]. Dilatation occurs primarily proximal to the sacroiliac joint, where the ureters cross the pelvic margin, usually in the second and third trimesters [9]. Renal plasma flow increases by 50–80% during pregnancy, peaking in mid-gestation, alongside a 40–50% increase in glomerular filtration rate (GFR), but the total number of nephrons remains constant [10]. Consequently, levels of serum creatinine and blood urea nitrogen decrease. The normal serum creatinine level during pregnancy is in the range of 0.4–0.6 mg/dl. The capacity of the collecting system increases by an estimated 200–300 mL, leading to urinary stasis and hormonal alterations, particularly elevated levels of progesterone, which induce ureteral dilatation and urinary stasis, predisposing individuals to infections and obstructive uropathies. The enlarging uterus exerts mechanical compression while progesterone causes smooth muscle relaxation, leading to physiologic hydronephrosis and urine retention in the collecting system during pregnancy [11].

During a normal pregnancy, urine protein excretion increases, ranging from 60–90 mg/d to 180–250 mg/d, as determined by a 24-h urine collection. Consequently, the threshold for elevated proteinuria in pregnancy has been established at a higher level of 300 mg/d, reflecting this physiological increase in proteinuria. This rise in proteinuria has been ascribed to hyperfiltration, although it may also be attributable to modifications in glomerular permeability [12].

Finally, changes in the innate and adaptive immune systems may affect autoimmune diseases, particularly impairing renal function, especially in young women. Typically, a conversion from a TH1 phenotype to a TH2 phenotype is observed during pregnancy, and humoral-mediated immunity becomes dominant

Table 6.1 Physiological changes occurring during pregnancy

Increased	Decreased
Renal plasma flow (by 50–80%)	Serum creatinine
Glomerular filtration rate (GFR)	Blood urea nitrogen (BUN)
Kidney size and renal length	Ureteral peristaltic activity
Urine volume and frequency	Bladder capacity (in late pregnancy)
Dilation of renal pelvis and ureters (physiologic hydronephrosis)	Urinary osmolality
Sodium and water retention (due to RAAS activation)	Plasma oncotic pressure
Risk of urinary tract infections (due to stasis and hormonal effects)	Concentrating ability of the kidney

over cell-mediated immunity. This change is necessary to establish tolerance to fetal antigens, support trophoblast invasion, and promote placental development. In addition, there is an increase in the number of regulatory T cells (Tregs) that support immune tolerance, thereby contributing further to the establishment of fetal tolerance [13].

Recognizing these regular physiological changes is essential for differentiating them from pathological conditions. Table 6.1 summarizes the physiological alterations during pregnancy [14].

6.3 Epidemiology

Mild physiologic hydronephrosis can manifest as early as 6 weeks into pregnancy due to the effects of progesterone and usually resolves within 4–6 weeks after childbirth; this condition is considered nonpathological. In contrast, moderate to severe hydronephrosis raises concern and is predominantly observed at the beginning of the third trimester [15].

The incidence of urolithiasis during pregnancy is still unclear. Nephrolithiasis impacts as many as 7.1% of women in the general population. At the same time, it is relatively rare during pregnancy; however, it is a significant cause of non-obstetric hospital admissions among this demographic [16]. A recent matched population-based cohort study conducted at a single center reported that the incidence of symptomatic kidney stones during pregnancy is 0.2%. This study also revealed an increased risk of preterm birth, low birth weight, pre-eclampsia, and cesarean section for pregnancies complicated by a symptomatic kidney stone. Approximately one-quarter of pregnant patients admitted for a kidney stone underwent some form of urologic intervention, most commonly a stent or ureterorenoscopy (URS) [17].

6.4 Pathophysiology

Urinary calcium excretion doubles during pregnancy due to an increase in glomerular filtration rate (GFR), resulting in decreased tubular reabsorption. The increased intestinal absorption of calcium, calcium mobilization from the bone driven by the placental formation of 1,25-dihydroxycholecalciferol, and feedback suppression of parathyroid hormone also contribute to absorptive hypercalciuria. This occurs because of the increased GFR during pregnancy and the subsequent rise in net urinary excretion of uric acid, which can also lead to calcium oxalate stone formation [18, 19].

6.5 Clinical Presentation

Pregnant patients experiencing nephrolithiasis usually exhibit typical ureteral colic symptoms. The hallmark symptom is flank pain, which is often sudden, severe, and colicky, occurring in approximately 89% of cases. This pain can radiate toward the groin or labia, akin to nonpregnant individuals, and it may also be accompanied by nausea and vomiting. Hematuria, either gross or microscopic, is quite prevalent, observed in about 95% of cases [20]. Importantly, these findings are linked to physiological changes; for instance, hydronephrosis caused by pregnancy may lead to flank discomfort and microscopic hematuria. Therefore, any unexplained flank pain or hematuria during pregnancy should trigger an assessment for stones.

Less common symptoms include dysuria, urinary urgency, and fever, which may indicate the presence of an infection. In some cases, symptoms may mimic obstetric processes (e.g., preterm labor or appendicitis), so differential diagnosis is broad. Importantly, clinicians should maintain a low threshold for considering nephrolithiasis in any pregnant woman with unilateral or bilateral flank pain, particularly in the second or third trimester [16]. When examining a patient, tenderness in the costovertebral angle (CVA) may be noted. Symptoms of systemic illness, such as fever, tachycardia, and hypotension, indicate a potential superimposed infection and require prompt intervention. It is essential to gather a comprehensive history that includes any previous occurrences of stone disease or relevant risk factors, such as family history and metabolic disorders. Additionally, obstetric considerations, such as gestational age and fetal well-being, should be taken into account during the evaluation.

6.6 Diagnosis

6.6.1 Laboratory Studies

The initial evaluation consists of standard laboratory tests. Urinalysis often reveals hematuria, frequently microscopic, in most cases of stones. The presence of pyuria or positive nitrites may suggest a urinary tract infection, which necessitates immediate treatment. A urine culture should always be performed to identify pathogens. A basic metabolic panel, including serum creatinine, must be assessed; while serum creatinine typically remains normal or slightly decreased during pregnancy, elevated levels could indicate obstructive uropathy or sepsis. Evaluating electrolytes, calcium, and liver enzymes can help rule out conditions that mimic stone disease, such as preeclampsia with hypercalcemia. Inflammatory markers, including a complete blood count (CBC) with differential and C-reactive protein (CRP), are used to assess severity. However, laboratory tests offer limited sensitivity for detecting stones; imaging is usually needed to confirm the diagnosis.

6.6.2 Imagining Studies

Pregnant women face risks from radiation exposure that can lead to both non-stochastic (teratogenic) and stochastic (carcinogenic, mutagenic) effects. Teratogenic impacts accumulate with higher doses and have a threshold below which radiation is deemed safe (<50 mGy), while also being influenced by gestational age; there is minimal risk before the 8th week and after the 23rd week. In contrast, carcinogenic effects can occur even at doses below 10 mGy, and mutations typically require doses between 500 and 1000 mGy, which exceed those typically found in standard radiographic studies. Both carcinogenesis and mutagenesis intensify with increased dosage but do not depend on a dose threshold or the stage of gestation [21]. No imaging technique should be performed routinely on pregnant women. Scientific societies and organizations concur on the safety of diagnostic evaluations when ultrasound, X-ray imaging, and MRI are utilized as necessary [22]. A radiographic procedure should not be denied to a pregnant woman if it is warranted and its omission would impact her medical care. Generally, any investigation that leads to a fetal absorbed dose exceeding 0.5 mGy necessitates justification.

6.6.2.1 Ultrasound

Ultrasound is the primary imaging technique, although its sensitivity for detecting mid-ureteral stones is somewhat limited. Colored Doppler ultrasound enhances stone detection through the twinkling artefact. Renal ultrasound, especially when combined with Doppler, can show hydronephrosis, evaluate ureteral jets, and occasionally identify stones as echogenic foci with shadowing. Transvaginal ultrasound may enhance the detection of distal ureteric stones located near the bladder. A report on a "high-resolution renal ultrasound" should include comments on the renal resistive index as well as the presence of hydronephrosis or ureteral dilation. However, the effectiveness of ultrasonography depends on the operator's skill, which can result in a 30% chance of missing ureteral stones. Additionally, physiological dilation during pregnancy can complicate the interpretation of mild hydronephrosis. Still, ultrasound does not involve ionizing radiation and is safe for both mother and fetus.

6.6.2.2 Magnetic Resonance Imaging (MRI)

If ultrasound results are inconclusive and there are ongoing clinical concerns, such as severe persistent pain or suspected obstruction, magnetic resonance imaging serves as a second-line method for evaluating urinary tract obstruction and visualizing stones as filling defects [23]. The use of gadolinium in pregnancy is typically advised against because of its possible adverse effects on the embryo [23–25]. MRI can detect levels of hydronephrosis and occasionally stones (appearing as signal voids) without using radiation. Recent ACOG guidance highlights that MRI is deemed safe during pregnancy when clinically warranted [24].

6.6.2.3 Low-Dose Computed Tomography (CT)

In detecting urolithiasis among pregnant patients, low-dose CT offers a higher positive predictive value of 95.8%, compared to 80% for MRI and 77% for ultrasound. Nonetheless, CT is typically avoided during pregnancy unless it is essential, such as in cases of life-threatening sepsis with an unknown origin. Guidelines suggest using CT solely as a last resort, employed carefully when ultrasound and MRI fail to provide conclusive results, and the advantages outweigh the radiation risk. According to White et al., low-dose CT improves diagnostic precision, which can help avert unnecessary interventions like ureteroscopy. While low-dose CT protocols are designed to minimize radiation exposure, their application in pregnant women should be reserved solely for critical situations [24]. During CT scans, fetal shielding and low-dose protocols are recommended. According to the Society of Radiologists in Ultrasound and ACOG, doses below approximately 50 mGy are considered non-harmful. Yet, the general guideline is to maintain fetal exposure at "as low as reasonably achievable" levels. In practice, low-dose CT typically leads to fetal exposures of less than 5 mGy, which is significantly below teratogenic thresholds [21].

Crucially, diagnostic imaging must not be delayed if the findings will change management. In emergencies (e.g., fever, hypotension), quick decompression can be lifesaving. During these situations, a collaborative discussion involving a

Table 6.2 Imaging modalities for urolithiasis during pregnancy

Imaging modality	Safety profile	Diagnostic utility	Notes
Ultrasonography	Safe in all trimesters	Moderate sensitivity for stones	First-line imaging; limited for mid-ureteral stones
Color doppler ultrasound	Safe in all trimesters	Improves detection with "twinkling artifact"	Adjunctive to standard ultrasound
MRI (without contrast)	Safe after the first trimester	Good for hydronephrosis and obstruction	No ionizing radiation
Low-dose non-contrast CT	Use only if essential	Highest sensitivity and specificity	Reserved for refractory or unclear cases

Note: Radiation exposure should be minimized whenever possible; MRI is preferred over CT unless diagnosis is critical

radiology consultant informs the imaging decisions. In conclusion, the evaluation process follows this order: ultrasound initially, MRI next, and CT only if necessary [24] (Table 6.2).

6.7 Management

Managing nephrolithiasis during pregnancy necessitates balancing effective treatment with fetal safety. Generally, conservative therapy is the primary approach for most patients, while interventions are reserved for complications or unsuccessful passage. Collaboration among multiple disciplines, including urology, obstetrics, and anesthesia, is essential at every stage. Usually, stones under 5 mm pass on their own.

Management strategies for gestational hydronephrosis depend on existing renal conditions, including stones, pyelonephritis, and intrinsic renal disease. A prior study indicated that double J stent insertion outperformed conservative therapy alone in cases of moderate to severe hydronephrosis [26]. Conservative treatment, which involves hydration and pain relief, is effective in 70–80% of cases.

6.7.1 Conservative Management

Most pregnant patients with kidney stones can typically be managed expectantly. Effective pain control is essential. Acetaminophen (paracetamol) is the recommended first-line analgesic and is deemed safe during all trimesters. For moderate to severe pain, judicious use of short-term opioids, such as morphine or meperidine, may be appropriate. NSAIDS should generally be avoided during late pregnancy due to the risks of miscarriage, renal impairment, and premature closure of the ductus arteriosus [27]. Indeed, NSAID use in pregnancy increases the risk of miscarriage by approximately 80% in some studies. They are contraindicated after

20 weeks according to ACOG guidance. Opiates, though classified as Category C, are often safely used in labor and for renal colic, with monitoring [24].

Adequate oral or intravenous fluids are advised to maintain urine output. Although traditional "bed rest" is no longer routinely recommended, minimizing strenuous activity and lying on one side might help alleviate pain and prevent vena caval compression. Safe antiemetics like ondansetron and intravenous fluids can treat nausea and vomiting during pregnancy. Although smooth muscle relaxants like butylscopolamine are sometimes utilized, evidence supporting their effectiveness is limited.

Alpha-adrenergic blockers (e.g., tamsulosin) and calcium channel blockers (e.g., nifedipine) are widely recognized treatments for facilitating the passage of ureteral stones in nonpregnant adults. During pregnancy, the application of these agents is considered off-label; however, emerging evidence indicates their potential safety for short-term use. A retrospective study revealed that the administration of tamsulosin during the second and third trimesters was not linked to adverse maternal or neonatal outcomes, although it did not result in a statistically significant increase in the stone expulsion rate. Urology specialists suggest that brief courses ($\leq$10 days) of α-blockers may be advisable, particularly for cases involving distal ureteral stones. Any decision regarding the implementation of medical expulsive therapy (MET) should encompass comprehensive counselling concerning the limited existing data. It is essential to note that MET is suitable exclusively within a controlled environment: patients must receive close follow-up, adequate pain management, and exhibit no signs of infection or complete obstruction [16, 28].

Conservative management frequently demonstrates success; aggregated data suggests that around 54% of women ultimately expel stones through mere observation. Pain relief and the process of stone passage should be meticulously monitored. Follow-up ultrasounds or evaluations of symptoms are advisable. Should pain intensify or fail to improve within a timeframe of 48–72 h, or in the event of fever or urinary obstruction, medical intervention is warranted [29].

6.7.2 Interventional Management

Intervention is required in approximately 25–30% of pregnant patients with stones [20]. The goals are relief of obstruction and definitive stone removal, balancing maternal and fetal risk. In certain patients, surgical intervention becomes necessary if conservative therapy is unsuccessful. The absolute indications for surgical intervention are similar to those in nonpregnant patients, encompassing infected or obstructive stones (typically linked with urinary tract infections, fever, and sepsis), an obstructed solitary kidney, or cases of acute renal failure. The most common indication for urological surgery in the pregnant patient is symptomatic urolithiasis [30].

6.7.2.1 Ureteral Stenting

The placement of a double-J ureteral stent is a commonly employed temporizing measure. Stents facilitate the rapid alleviation of obstruction and allow for effective urine drainage. According to recent guidelines, stenting provides more effective relief of symptomatic hydronephrosis than conservative therapy when indicated [31]. Stents are typically positioned under ultrasound guidance or with minimal fluoroscopy, accompanied by appropriate shielding. The primary disadvantages include irritative bladder symptoms and a significant rate of encrustation during pregnancy, attributed to hypercalciuria, which often necessitates stent exchange every 4–6 weeks. Patients with stents should have regular urology follow-up appointments and undergo periodic imaging or stent changes until definitive management is conducted postpartum. It is essential to note that in instances of suspected urosepsis, prompt stent placement is considered safer than percutaneous nephrostomy (PCN), as ureteroscopy or cystoscopy can be performed in a supine position with fetal monitoring, whereas the prone position for PCN is more challenging [32].

6.7.2.2 Percutaneous Nephrostomy (PCN)

A nephrostomy tube might be necessary if retrograde stent placement is unsuccessful or not possible. Percutaneous nephrostomy (PCN) efficiently relieves pressure in the system. Still, it requires the patient to be in a prone position, which can be technically challenging during pregnancy and may pose risks to the fetus. Thus, PCN is typically viewed as a secondary option when cystoscopic stenting isn't practical. In cases of infected, obstructed kidneys, decompression should occur through the fastest method available. Still, the patient's positioning and anesthesia considerations often favor ureteral stenting when it is a viable option [32].

6.7.2.3 Ureteroscopy (URS)

Ureteroscopy with laser lithotripsy has increasingly emerged as the favored definitive treatment option when conservative therapies prove ineffective. The advancement of modern small-caliber ureteroscopes and Holmium:YAG laser lithotripsy enables the fragmentation and extraction of stones without the use of radiation. The European Association of Urology (EAU) and other specialists now advocate for ureteroscopy (URS) as a "reasonable alternative" in the context of pregnancy [33]. In comparison to extended stenting, ureteroscopy (URS) frequently results in expedited stone clearance and a reduction in stent-related symptoms. Published literature demonstrates elevated success rates and minimal complication rates associated with URS in pregnant patients. For instance, a systematic review deduced that with appropriate patient selection and surgical expertise, URS performed during pregnancy correlates with low complication rates and high rates of stone-free status [34].

The pooled systematic analysis indicated stone-free rates ranging from approximately 76–89% for various ureteroscopic techniques, accompanied by complication rates of less than 10%. When performed at experienced medical centers, the outcomes of ureteroscopy (URS) in pregnant women are similar to those observed in the general population. URS is generally performed electively in the second trimester, once fetal organ development is complete, and the uterus has not yet grown excessively large. General or neuraxial anesthesia may be employed, with neuraxial (spinal/epidural) anesthesia frequently preferred to minimize fetal drug exposure [32]. During the third trimester, URS may present a marginally increased risk of preterm labor; consequently, it is advisable to defer the procedure until after delivery if feasible. Should URS be conducted at or beyond 32 weeks of gestation, consultation with the obstetric team regarding administration of steroids for fetal lung maturity and magnesium for neuroprotection is recommended [32].

6.7.2.4 Shock Wave Lithotripsy (SWL)

Extracorporeal shock wave lithotripsy is unequivocally contraindicated during pregnancy. The application of shock waves may compromise fetal tissues and provoke uterine contractions. All established guidelines explicitly prohibit the use of shock wave lithotripsy during pregnancy [35].

6.7.2.5 Percutaneous Nephrolithotomy (PCNL)

Percutaneous nephrolithotomy (PCNL) is infrequently performed during the course of pregnancy. The European Association of Urology (EAU) stipulates that this procedure should only be considered in specialized medical centers and exclusively for selected cases, such as large staghorn calculi. The procedure necessitates the patient to be positioned in a prone posture and administered anesthesia; thus, the associated risks generally outweigh the potential benefits. Typically, the management of large calculi involves staged stenting until the conclusion of the pregnancy [35].

In managing renal stones during pregnancy, there is no notable difference in the rates of adverse pregnancy events between percutaneous nephrostomy (PCN) and ureteral stent placement. Nonetheless, ureteral stent placement is linked with fewer hospital admissions, emergency department visits, exchange procedures, and occurrences of new urinary tract infections (UTIs) or pyelonephritis [36]. Ureteroscopy presents a viable option to prevent the need for prolonged stenting or drainage.

In summary, intervention is indicated for any obstructing stone that causes infection, renal compromise, or uncontrollable pain. The preferred definitive approach is ureteroscopic stone removal. Decompression with stent or PCN is the initial lifesaving therapy in sepsis, with definitive management deferred briefly. All interventions should involve fetal monitoring if the gestational age warrants, and obstetric support.

6.8 Conclusion

During pregnancy, renal diseases and urolithiasis require prompt recognition, careful diagnosis, and individualized management to achieve positive outcomes for both mothers and fetal outcomes. Multidisciplinary collaboration and adherence to evidence-based guidelines are essential in optimizing care for this vulnerable population.

References

1. Lin KL, Shen CJ, Wu MP, Long CY, Wu CH, Wang CL. Comparison of low urinary tract symptoms during pregnancy between primiparous and multiparous women. BioMed Res Int. 2014;2014:303697.
2. Rodriguez PN, Klein AS. Management of urolithiasis during pregnancy. Obstet Gynecol Surv. 1988;43(10):604–5.
3. Pedro RN, Das K, Buchholz N. Urolithiasis in pregnancy. Int J Surg. 2016;36(Pt D):688–92.
4. Stothers L, Lee LM. Renal colic in pregnancy. J Urol. 1992;148(5):1383–7.
5. Swartz MA, Lydon-Rochelle MT, Simon D, Wright JL, Porter MP. Admission for nephrolithiasis in pregnancy and risk of adverse birth outcomes. Obstet Gynecol. 2007;109(5):1099–104.
6. Burgess KL, Gettman MT, Rangel LJ, Krambeck AE. Diagnosis of urolithiasis and rate of spontaneous passage during pregnancy. J Urol. 2011;186(6):2280–4.
7. Bailey RR, Rolleston GL. Kidney length and ureteric dilatation in the puerperium. J Obstet Gynaecol Br Commonw. 1971;78(1):55–61.
8. Grosjean J, Cannie M, de Meyer JM. Physiological hydronephrosis in pregnancy: occurrence and possible causes. An MRI study. Prog Urol. 2017;27(12):603–8.
9. Rasmussen PE, Nielsen FR. Hydronephrosis during pregnancy: a literature survey. Eur J Obstet Gynecol Reprod Biol. 1988;27(3):249–59.
10. Cheung KL, Lafayette RA. Renal physiology of pregnancy. Adv Chronic Kidney Dis. 2013;20(3):209–14.
11. Mandal D, Saha MM, Pal DK. Urological disorders and pregnancy: an overall experience. Urol Ann. 2017;9(1):32–6.
12. Kattah A, Milic N, White W, Garovic V. Spot urine protein measurements in normotensive pregnancies, pregnancies with isolated proteinuria and preeclampsia. Am J Physiol Regul Integr Comp Physiol. 2017;313(4):R418–r24.
13. Aluvihare VR, Kallikourdis M, Betz AG. Regulatory T cells mediate maternal tolerance to the fetus. Nat Immunol. 2004;5(3):266–71.
14. Gonzalez Suarez ML, Kattah A, Grande JP, Garovic V. Renal disorders in pregnancy: core curriculum 2019. Am J Kidney Dis. 2019;73(1):119–30.
15. Au KK, Woo JS, Tang LC, Liang S. Aetiological factors in the genesis of pregnancy hydronephrosis. Aust N Z J Obstet Gynaecol. 1985;25(4):248–51.
16. Wayment RO, Schwartz B. Pregnancy and urolithiasis. Medscape. 2009. http://emedicine.medscape.com/article/455830-overview.
17. Ordon M, Dirk J, Slater J, Kroft J, Dixon S, Welk B. Incidence, treatment, and implications of kidney stones during pregnancy: a matched population-based cohort study. J Endourol. 2020;34(2):215–21.
18. Ringel A, Richter S, Shalev M, Nissenkorn I. Late complications of ureteral stents. Eur Urol. 2000;38(1):41–4.
19. Gertner JM, Coustan DR, Kliger AS, Mallette LE, Ravin N, Broadus AE. Pregnancy as state of physiologic absorptive hypercalciuria. Am J Med. 1986;81(3):451–6.

20. Chan K, Shakir T, El-Taji O, Patel A, Bycroft J, Lim CP, et al. Management of urolithiasis in pregnancy. Curr Urol. 2023;17(1):1–6.
21. Somani BK, Dellis A, Liatsikos E, Skolarikos A. Review on diagnosis and management of urolithiasis in pregnancy: an ESUT practical guide for urologists. World J Urol. 2017;35:1637–49.
22. Asrat T, Roossin MC, Miller EI. Ultrasonographic detection of ureteral jets in normal pregnancy. Am J Obstet Gynecol. 1998;178(6):1194–8.
23. Masselli G, Derme M, Bernieri MG, Polettini E, Casciani E, Monti R, et al. Stone disease in pregnancy: imaging-guided therapy. Insights Imaging. 2014;5:691–6.
24. Jain C. ACOG Committee Opinion No. 723: guidelines for diagnostic imaging during pregnancy and lactation. Obstet Gynecol. 2019;133(1):186.
25. Roy C, Saussine C, Le Bras Y, Delepaul B, Jahn C, Steichen G, et al. Assessment of painful ureterohydronephrosis during pregnancy by MR urography. Eur Radiol. 1996;6:334–8.
26. Tsai YL, Seow KM, Yieh CH, Chong KM, Hwang JL, Lin YH, et al. Comparative study of conservative and surgical management for symptomatic moderate and severe hydronephrosis in pregnancy: a prospective randomized study. Acta Obstet Gynecol Scand. 2007;86(9):1047–50.
27. Li DK, Liu L, Odouli R. Exposure to non-steroidal anti-inflammatory drugs during pregnancy and risk of miscarriage: population based cohort study. BMJ. 2003;327(7411):368.
28. Theriault B, Morin F, Cloutier J. Safety and efficacy of Tamsulosin as medical expulsive therapy in pregnancy. World J Urol. 2020;38(9):2301–6.
29. Salehi-Pourmehr H, Tayebi S, DalirAkbari N, Ghabousian A, Tahmasbi F, Rahmati F, et al. Management of urolithiasis in pregnancy: a systematic review and meta-analysis. Scand J Surg. 2023;112(2):105–16.
30. Giusti G, Proietti S, Peschechera R, Taverna G, Sortino G, Cindolo L, et al. Sky is no limit for ureteroscopy: extending the indications and special circumstances. World J Urol. 2015;33:257–73.
31. Keenan RA, Hegarty NJ, Davis NF. Symptomatic hydronephrosis and ureteral calculi in pregnancy: a narrative review with a proposed management protocol. J Endourol. 2022;36(8):1099–112.
32. Lee MS, Fenstermaker MA, Naoum EE, Chong S, Van de Ven CJ, Bauer ME, et al. Management of nephrolithiasis in pregnancy: multi-disciplinary guidelines from an academic medical center. Front Surg. 2021;8:796876.
33. Teleb M, Ragab A, Dawod T, Elgalaly H, Elsayed E, Sakr A, et al. Definitive ureteroscopy and intracorporeal lithotripsy in treatment of ureteral calculi during pregnancy. Arab J Urol. 2014;12(4):299–303.
34. Semins MJ, Matlaga BR. Ureteroscopy during pregnancy. Indian J Urol. 2009;25(3):291–5.
35. Ramachandra M, Somani BK. Safety and feasibility of percutaneous nephrolithotomy (PCNL) during pregnancy: a review of literature. Turk J Urol. 2020;46(2):89.
36. Mason MM, Nackeeran S, Lokeshwar S, Carino Mason MR, Kohn T, Shah HN, et al. A comparison of adverse pregnancy events between ureteral stents and percutaneous nephrostomy tubes in the treatment of nephrolithiasis during pregnancy: a propensity score-matched analysis of a large multi-institutional research network. World J Urol. 2023;41(7):1721–6.

Chapter 7
Gut Health Through Gestation: Managing Gastrointestinal System Diseases During Pregnancy

Bayram Çolak

7.1 Introduction

Pregnancy has minimal effects on gastrointestinal secretion or absorption; however, it significantly alters the normal physiology of the gastrointestinal (GI) system. The primary changes are related to motility and motor function. Hormonal alterations during pregnancy, along with structural changes such as the enlargement of the uterus, can lead to a range of gastrointestinal disorders.

It is common for pregnant women to experience gastrointestinal symptoms such as nausea, vomiting, constipation, indigestion, and gastroesophageal reflux throughout gestation. In addition, granulomatous changes in the gums (epulis gravidarum), increased salivation, and alterations in taste perception may occur. While the majority of gastrointestinal complaints during pregnancy are mild and improve with dietary and lifestyle modifications, some cases require medical treatment. Furthermore, chronic gastrointestinal diseases that affect women of childbearing age may coexist with pregnancy, and the progression of these diseases and how they are managed can be influenced by the gestational period.

Gastrointestinal disturbances are widespread during pregnancy, although they are usually mild. In fact, most pregnant women experience at least one such disorder during pregnancy. The type and severity of symptoms can vary from person to person, which poses a challenge for healthcare providers. This is particularly true when it comes to evaluating the effects of medications and other interventions on the developing fetus. Although these conditions are rarely life-threatening, they can still cause significant health concerns throughout pregnancy and impair quality of life.

B. Çolak (✉)
Izmir Bakircay University, Faculty of Medicine, Department of General Surgery, Izmir, Turkey
e-mail: bayram.colak@bakircay.edu.tr

© The Author(s), under exclusive license to Springer Nature Switzerland AG 2026

I. Karaca (ed.), *Managing Maternal Chronic Diseases for a Healthy Pregnancy*, https://doi.org/10.1007/978-3-032-15221-3_7

Endoscopy is often used to diagnose and manage gastrointestinal conditions. Esophagogastroduodenoscopy (EGD) is used to evaluate the upper gastrointestinal tract, while colonoscopy is performed to assess the colon and terminal ileum [1]. Among endoscopic procedures, EGD is the most commonly performed during pregnancy [2]. Endoscopic interventions can be safely conducted in pregnant women by experienced specialists [1, 3]. However, such procedures should only be performed after establishing clear indications, preferably during the second trimester, with the use of the least harmful sedative and analgesic agents at the lowest effective doses. They should be carried out as briefly as possible. The patient should be positioned in the left lateral decubitus position, and continuous monitoring of the fetus's well-being should be carried out [4].

7.2 Vomiting, Nausea, and Hyperemesis Gravidarum

Nausea and vomiting are common during pregnancy [5, 6]. Pregnancy is a time when women experience nausea and vomiting, with rates of 50–80% and approximately 50%, respectively [7]. The onset of symptoms is usually around the 4th to 6th week of pregnancy. They typically reach their peak between the 8th and 12th weeks, and usually resolve by the 16th to 20th week [6, 7]. The occurrence of these events can happen at any time of the day, with the length and frequency varying [8]. The Pregnancy-Unique Quantification of Emesis and Nausea (PUQE) scoring system was developed to evaluate the severity of nausea and vomiting symptoms experienced by pregnant women [9].

Hyperemesis gravidarum (HG) is a severe and persistent form of vomiting and nausea experienced during pregnancy [10]. Fortunately, it is relatively uncommon. It occurs in only about 1.2% of pregnancies [3]. There is currently no universally accepted definition or diagnostic criterion for HG. However, widely recognized descriptions include prolonged nausea and vomiting accompanied by weight loss, ketonuria, electrolyte imbalance, dehydration, and/or clinical deterioration requiring hospitalization [11]. HG can have a negative impact on pregnancy outcomes, increasing the risk of preterm delivery, low birth weight, and having an infant who is small for their gestational age [12].

If a woman experiences prolonged and severe nausea and vomiting during pregnancy, any underlying pathological causes must first be ruled out. If laboratory and imaging evaluations are negative, a diagnosis of pregnancy-related nausea and vomiting can be made [10, 13]. Recommended investigations include complete blood count, urinalysis with ketone testing, serum electrolytes, and liver function tests [14]. Some authors also suggest assessing thyroid function and testing for *Helicobacter pylori* [14].

The precise etiology of vomiting and nausea in pregnancy remains unclear, and it is generally considered multifactorial [2]. Contributing factors include human chorionic gonadotropin (hCG), hyperestrogenemia, progesterone, gastric dysrhythmia, vitamin deficiencies, and psychological influences such as anxiety, depression, unwanted pregnancies, and family-related stressors [15]. Progesterone is thought to reduce gastric tone and motility, impairing gastrointestinal transit [16]. Experimental studies demonstrate that progesterone exerts inhibitory effects on both pyloric and small intestinal smooth muscle, leading to decreased contractility [17]. Other studies that compared gastric emptying rates between premenopausal women and men, as well as postmenopausal women, found that the former had slower gastric emptying rates. This supports the hypothesis that delayed gastric emptying is induced by hormones [16].

Consistent literature reports show that women with HG have higher serum hCG levels than controls, with the highest concentrations occurring in the first trimester, when symptoms are most severe. Nevertheless, the exact mechanism by which elevated hCG contributes to HG remains uncertain. One proposed mechanism is that hCG stimulates secretory pathways in the upper gastrointestinal tract [18].

Once alternative physiological causes are excluded, initial management includes dietary and lifestyle modifications. Patients are advised to minimize stress, ensure adequate rest, and maintain hydration. Daily intake of 1–1.5 liters of electrolyte-containing fluids, such as sports drinks or broths rich in sodium, glucose, and potassium, may help prevent dehydration [19]. It is recommended that you eat small, frequent meals and avoid fatty or difficult-to-digest foods. Studies have shown that high-protein liquid supplements can improve gastric rhythm and reduce nausea during the first trimester [19].

Due to concerns regarding teratogenicity, nonpharmacological alternatives have been explored. Thiamine (vitamin B1) and pyridoxine (vitamin B6) have both been shown to reduce nausea and vomiting, and are recommended for patients whose symptoms persist [19, 20]. Pharmacological options include doxylamine (an antihistamine, FDA category B), administered at 10 mg three to four times daily [7]. Second-line agents are dopamine antagonists such as promethazine (FDA category C), prochlorperazine (FDA category C), and metoclopramide (FDA category B) [7, 12]. Ondansetron, a selective serotonin receptor antagonist (FDA category B), is also used for refractory cases [7, 12].

In more severe cases, particularly those with HG, intravenous fluids may be required to correct electrolyte imbalances and dehydration. In patients with persistent symptoms and/or significant weight loss despite appropriate therapy, nasogastric or enteral nutritional support may be considered. For safety reasons, these treatments should only be used in extreme situations where there is a high risk to both mother and fetus [8].

7.3 Constipation

Between 25% and 40% of pregnant women report experiencing abdominal bloating and constipation [21]. Constipation is typically characterized as the number of bowel movements per week should be less than three, passing hard stools, and/or experiencing difficulty defecating [22].

In pregnancy, constipation is attributed to several factors, including altered water absorption, mechanical influences, reduced physical activity, and hormonal changes leading to decreased bowel motility [22]. The reduction in motility is thought to result from increased progesterone levels, enhanced nitric oxide release, and changes in G-protein expression [21]. Iron supplementation may also contribute to constipation during pregnancy [15].

Management of constipation in pregnancy primarily focuses on nonpharmacological measures. These include increasing fluid intake, engaging in regular physical activity, consuming small and frequent meals, and incorporating dietary fiber [21]. Additionally, bowel movements should be encouraged during periods of maximal colonic motility, such as in the morning and after meals [15].

When pharmacological intervention is necessary, the use of laxatives may be considered [21]. Lactulose, glycerin, polyethylene glycol, and sorbitol are generally considered the safest options for treating constipation during pregnancy [21, 22].

7.4 Gastroesophageal Reflux Disease

Gastroesophageal reflux disease (GERD) is a condition involving the involuntary movement of stomach contents back into the esophagus. Clinically, this can present as a simple regurgitation of sour or bitter fluid into the mouth, but in some cases may also lead to pathological changes in the distal esophagus known as esophagitis. Gastroesophageal reflux (GER) is reported in 40–80% of pregnancies [21]. In most cases, reflux symptoms begin in early pregnancy, become more pronounced during the final months of pregnancy, and resolve after delivery [12].

The exact mechanism of GERD in pregnancy is not fully understood. However, it is thought that the primary contributing factors are reduced tone of the lower esophageal sphincter due to progesterone and increased intra-abdominal pressure resulting from uterine enlargement [12]. Symptoms arise from the irritation caused by gastric acid reaching the esophagus. The most common clinical manifestation is retrosternal burning (heartburn), which typically worsens in the supine position [23]. Other frequently reported symptoms include dysphagia, chronic cough, and chest pain [23].

The clinical presentation of gastroesophageal reflux disease in pregnant patients is similar to that in nonpregnant patients, and diagnosis is usually made based solely on symptoms [24]. A barium swallow study should be avoided due to the risk of fetal radiation exposure. Although esophageal manometry and pH monitoring can be performed safely, they are rarely required. For persistent and treatment-resistant GERD symptoms during pregnancy, or in cases of complications, upper gastrointestinal endoscopy is considered the preferred diagnostic method. Such procedures can be performed safely when carried out by experienced specialists, with careful use of sedation, strict blood pressure control, continuous oxygen monitoring, and fetal well-being surveillance [24].

Management of GERD in pregnancy begins with lifestyle modifications. These include raising the head of the bed when lying down, avoiding increased intra-abdominal pressure (e.g., frequent forward bending), eating small and frequent meals, avoiding meals close to bedtime, and eliminating fatty or trigger foods [2, 23]. If pharmacologic therapy becomes necessary, alginic acid and antacids are considered first-line options [2]. Preferably, calcium- and magnesium-based antacids should be used, and bicarbonate-containing preparations should be avoided due to the potential risk of metabolic alkalosis [15]. Sucralfate, an antacid, has also been shown to be safe during pregnancy [15]. H2-receptor antagonists (FDA Category B), such as cimetidine and ranitidine, are recommended as second-line agents [15]. Among proton pump inhibitors, omeprazole (FDA Category C) has not been shown to significantly increase structural anomaly risk, but it should only be used by women with refractory GERD that does not respond to other therapies [15, 25].

7.5 Peptic Ulcer

Peptic ulcer disease is one of the most common gastrointestinal disorders in the general population, and it continues to be a significant cause of morbidity and mortality. It is interesting to note that the severity of symptoms related to peptic ulcers, as well as the frequency of complications, appears to decrease during pregnancy [26].

Several hypotheses have been proposed to explain this phenomenon. Plasma histaminase levels are known to increase during pregnancy due to additional synthesis from the placenta, and these enzymes are thought to metabolize maternal histamine, thereby reducing gastric acid secretion [27]. Moreover, elevated estrogen levels may contribute to hypochlorhydria, while progesterone enhances the secretion of a protective gastric mucus layer, both of which may strengthen defense mechanisms against ulcer formation [28]. In addition, the avoidance of ulcer-causing factors by mothers is crucial such as alcohol, smoking, and the use of nonsteroidal anti-inflammatory drugs (NSAIDs), and reduced psychological stress has been associated with a lower incidence of peptic ulcer disease and related symptoms during pregnancy [29, 30].

NSAIDs carry an increased risk of peptic ulcers because they inhibit cyclooxygenase and have a toxic effect on the gastric mucosa. The typical symptoms of peptic ulcer disease are epigastric pain that worsens after eating and improves when antacids are taken. Patients often report experiencing discomfort that is dull, gnawing, or burning in nature. This discomfort may wake them up at night or in the early morning, before they have eaten.

If you experience back pain alongside abdominal discomfort, it may indicate that the ulcer originates from the posterior wall of the stomach or duodenum, penetrating into the surrounding retroperitoneal structures. Complications of peptic ulcer include perforation—presenting as acute abdomen with rebound tenderness, guarding, and sudden severe abdominal pain—and gastric outlet obstruction, which manifests as prolonged nausea and vomiting. Obstruction typically results from edema and inflammation surrounding a prepyloric or pyloric ulcer.

Initial treatment primarily involves lifestyle and dietary modifications, such as avoiding fatty or acidic foods, caffeine, chocolate, alcohol, and tobacco, as well as minimizing stress and anxiety [12]. The primary pharmacologic therapy is antacids, followed by H2-receptor antagonists and proton pump inhibitors. An upper gastrointestinal endoscopy is rarely necessary and is usually only performed in cases of severe upper gastrointestinal bleeding. Endoscopy is not required solely for diagnosing *Helicobacter pylori* infection during pregnancy [2]. Since eradication therapy requires a multidrug antibiotic regimen (clarithromycin, amoxicillin, and metronidazole), treatment is generally deferred until after delivery [2].

For pharmacologic therapy, antacids are recommended as the first step. Antacids containing magnesium, which are poorly absorbed into the bloodstream, are considered safe during pregnancy. They should be taken in doses of 15–30 ml, 1 h after meals and at bedtime. However, antacids can interfere with iron absorption, and iron deficiency is common during pregnancy. It is recommended that they be administered at different times from iron supplements [31]. Sucralfate, classified as FDA pregnancy category B, is a well-tolerated alternative to antacids. As it is not systemically absorbed and has shown no teratogenic effects in animal studies, it is the preferred option during pregnancy [32].

7.6 Diarrhea

Diarrhea is characterized as having a minimum of three bowel evacuations per day, which is frequently linked to an escalation in faucal output and regularity (in excess of 300 g per day). This is in accordance with the latest medical findings. The only physiological change during pregnancy that is known to contribute to diarrhea is the effect of prostaglandins on smooth muscle. Prostaglandins can induce contractions in the smooth muscle of the intestines, thereby increasing gastrointestinal motility [33].

Diarrhea affects approximately 34% of pregnant women, and the causes are generally the same as for nonpregnant women, with infectious agents being the most common. Viruses are the leading cause, followed by *Salmonella*, *Shigella*, and *Campylobacter* species, *Escherichia coli*, protozoa such as *Entamoeba histolytica, Cryptosporidium*, and *Giardia* [34]. A history of recent antibiotic use should raise suspicion for *Clostridium difficile* infection. Other frequent causes include food poisoning, medication, and irritable bowel syndrome. Additionally, flares of inflammatory bowel disease (IBD) may occur during pregnancy, leading to diarrhea. For this reason, it is emphasized that women with IBD should achieve and maintain clinical remission before, during, and after pregnancy to ensure favorable outcomes [35].

In cases where diarrhea persists for more than 48 h during pregnancy, or when accompanied by excessive watery stools, weight loss, and rectal bleeding, a standard laboratory evaluation should be performed, including stool cultures, parasite analysis, fecal leukocytes, and *Clostridium difficile* testing [35]. If these tests are inconclusive and diarrhea persists, flexible sigmoidoscopy may be performed, as it is considered safe during pregnancy. Importantly, flexible sigmoidoscopy has not been associated with labor induction or congenital malformations [35].

The cornerstone of diarrhea management in pregnancy is conservative treatment [36]. Fluid replacement may be necessary, as may medical therapy. However, commonly used antidiarrheal agents such as diphenoxylate-atropine and bismuth subsalicylate are contraindicated during pregnancy. The use of bismuth subsalicylate is contraindicated due to salicylate absorption [37]. Salicylates are known teratogens that have been linked to prolonged labor, increased perinatal mortality, low birth weight, and bleeding [35, 37]. Diphenoxylate-atropine is teratogenic in humans after the first trimester of pregnancy and should therefore be avoided unless it is absolutely necessary [37].

Most antibiotics used to treat infectious diarrhea are contraindicated at some or all stages of pregnancy. These include quinolones, metronidazole, and tetracyclines. Nonetheless, in cases of severe infectious diarrhea, antibiotic therapy may be warranted, with erythromycin and ampicillin considered safer alternatives due to their more favorable pregnancy profiles [37].

Management should also address the underlying cause when identified. In pregnant women with IBS and diarrhea, a high-fiber diet may be recommended to increase stool bulk. Antidepressants are not advised for IBS-related diarrhea in pregnancy. Anticholinergics and antispasmodics should only be used in refractory cases. Loperamide is often considered when an antidiarrheal agent is required to reduce stool frequency. Previously classified as FDA pregnancy category B, loperamide was reclassified to category C after follow-up studies reported increased risks of hypospadias, cesarean section, placenta previa, and macrosomia in women who used it during early pregnancy [38].

Finally, it is important to remember that diarrhea occurring late in pregnancy or near term may also signal the onset of labor [25].

7.7 Gallstones in Pregnancy

It is not fully understood how gallstones are formed during pregnancy; however, studies have shown that approximately 31% of women develop biliary sludge and around 2% develop new gallstones during pregnancy. The risk is greatest during the second and third trimesters, as well as the postpartum period. Potential contributing factors include increased lithogenicity of bile, impaired gallbladder emptying, and biliary stasis. Pain in the right upper abdomen or epigastric region, fever, vomiting, and jaundice can be symptoms of gallstone disease in pregnant women. Detection of right upper quadrant pain may be more challenging due to uterine enlargement [39].

Conservative management of symptomatic gallstone disease often involves hydration, analgesics, antibiotics, and dietary modifications. In cases complicated by choledocholithiasis, cholangitis, biliary obstruction, or pancreatitis, endoscopic retrograde cholangiopancreatography (ERCP) may be required [37]. For pregnant women needing ERCP, the second trimester is considered the optimal timing compared to other trimesters. However, if delaying ERCP poses a potential threat to maternal–fetal health, its appropriateness should be determined by a multidisciplinary team [37].

Cholecystectomy is indicated in pregnant women with gallbladder disease when symptoms are persistent or recurrent, or when there is significant nutritional compromise or weight loss. After appendectomy, cholecystectomy for gallstone disease is the second most common nonobstetric surgical procedure performed during pregnancy [40, 41]. According to the American Gastroenterological Association (AGA), cholecystectomy is safe during pregnancy, and laparoscopic surgery is considered the standard of care at any stage of pregnancy, although the second trimester is preferred [37].

7.8 Inflammatory Bowel Disease (IBD)

Chronic inflammation of the gastrointestinal tract is a characteristic of inflammatory bowel diseases (IBD), which include Crohn's disease and ulcerative colitis. The most common clinical signs are diarrhea and abdominal pain. Crohn's disease can affect any part of the gastrointestinal tract from the mouth to the anüs with a transmural inflammatory process, whereas ulcerative colitis is typically limited to the mucosal layer and generally confined to the rectum and colon. IBD often affects women of reproductive age, creating challenges in disease management during pregnancy that require close collaboration between obstetricians and gastroenterologists.

The etiology of IBD remains unknown but is considered multifactorial [42]. It is assumed that various infectious agents are pathogenic. A bacterium similar to *Mycobacterium paratuberculosis* has been found in the intestines of patients who have undergone surgery for active Crohn's disease. However, this organism has not been successfully cultured in most patients. Other potential triggers of immune dysregulation include cow's milk proteins, other dietary components, viruses, smoking, and water, though none have been conclusively linked to either disease.

In ulcerative colitis, the inflammation is confined to the colon and affects either the rectum only, the rectum and the left colon, or the entire colon. Crohn's disease, on the other hand, has the potential to affect any part of the gastrointestinal tract. The most common locations are the terminal ileum alone (30%), the colon alone (15–25%), and the ileocolon (40–55%). Diseases of the perianal and perirectal regions are common, presenting as fissures, fistulas, or abscesses.

In ulcerative colitis, mucosal lesions are the most common, while the muscularis propria is rarely affected. Crypt abscesses, characterized by neutrophilic infiltration into the crypt epithelium and lumen, are typical of ulcerative colitis but can also be seen in Crohn's disease. Evidence of chronic inflammation is seen in the form of lymphocytic, plasma cell, and eosinophilic infiltration of the lamina propria. In active ulcerative colitis, edema, hemorrhage, and pseudopolyps are common. Conversely, Crohn's disease is more often associated with transmural inflammation, granulomas, and deep ulcerations extending to the muscularis propria. "Skip lesions" (areas of normal mucosa between inflamed regions) and rectal sparing are characteristic of Crohn's disease.

Patients with either condition may experience abdominal pain, diarrhea, weight loss, fever, and fatigue. These symptoms are often accompanied by extraintestinal manifestations. A serious complication of acute ulcerative colitis is toxic megacolon, which manifests as abdominal distension and may progress to perforation, requiring urgent surgical intervention. Another long-term complication of ulcerative colitis is an increased risk of colorectal cancer after 8–10 years of the disease. This warrants annual colonoscopic surveillance.

In patients presenting with abdominal diarrhea, pain, or rectal bleeding suggestive of IBD, flexible sigmoidoscopy with minimal or no sedation is considered safe during pregnancy [43]. Full colonoscopy, which usually requires deeper sedation, is generally avoided but may be performed with appropriate maternal monitoring if necessary. Radiologic studies involving ionizing radiation should be avoided due to fetal exposure [44].

The risk of disease flare during pregnancy in women with IBD is similar to non-pregnant women, estimated at ~34% per year versus 32%, respectively [45]. For ulcerative colitis, pregnancy does not appear to adversely affect the disease course. Women in remission typically remain stable throughout pregnancy [46, 47]; in contrast, people with active colitis at the time of conception often experience active disease or flares during pregnancy [48]. Women with quiescent Crohn's disease are not at increased risk of disease activation during pregnancy [49, 50]; however, approximately two-thirds of people with active disease continue to experience symptoms or show signs of deterioration [48, 50, 51]. For this reason, women with moderate-to-severe active disease are generally advised to defer conception until remission is achieved.

The impact of IBD on female fertility remains uncertain. Voluntary reduction in pregnancy rates due to fear of disease complications appears more significant than biological infertility [52]. Male fertility may be impaired in patients treated with sulfasalazine due to its direct toxic effect on sperm [52]. The risk of miscarriage is not higher for women with quiescent IBD than for the general population [53]. However, miscarriage risk is increased by up to twofold in women with active disease [47, 53, 54]. IBD has also been linked to an increased risk of giving birth prematurely [52]. Therefore, careful monitoring during the third trimester is recommended. The likelihood of achieving a normal outcome is similar to that in the general population once pregnancy is established, which is encouraging.

To optimize outcomes, patients are advised to conceive during disease remission. It has been shown that it is possible to safely treat women with IBD during pregnancy without this having any negative effects on the mother or fetus. However, drug regimens should be minimized to the lowest effective dose. Studies reporting low birth weight or congenital anomalies have often found it difficult to determine whether disease severity or medication exposure was the main factor.

A multidisciplinary approach involving both gastroenterologists and obstetricians should be adopted for preconception counselling [55]. Women should be encouraged to achieve and maintain remission prior to conception. Medications should be adjusted as needed; those on steroids, methotrexate, or mesalazine should be transitioned to safer alternatives before pregnancy [55]. Both maternal condition and fetal development require close monitoring. Disease activity during pregnancy can be assessed using laboratory markers such as CRP and fecal calprotectin [55, 56]. Fecal calprotectin is a simple and reliable noninvasive tool for monitoring activity throughout gestation.

During pregnancy, continuation of maintenance therapy is recommended to preserve remission. The mode of delivery should be determined by obstetric indications. Cesarean delivery is recommended. This is for women with perineal disease. It is also recommended for women with active rectal involvement [55].

7.9 Irritable Bowel Syndrome (IBS)

Irritable bowel syndrome (IBS) is a chronic functional bowel disorder of unclear etiology. It is characterized by altered bowel habits (constipation and/or diarrhea), abdominal pain, and dyspeptic symptoms such as bloating, flatulence, and belching. This occurs in the absence of any organic pathology [57]. Since there is no specific diagnostic test for IBS and no structural or biochemical markers to confirm the diagnosis, other organic diseases that may present with similar symptoms must be excluded, and the diagnosis relies on a careful evaluation of clinical features [57]. The diagnostic criteria include recurrent abdominal pain for at least 1 day per week over the last 3 months, with symptom onset at least 6 months prior, and fulfillment of at least two of the following three features:

(a) Improvement with defecation
(b) Association with a change in stool frequency
(c) Association with a change in stool form or appearance [58]

Management includes dietary modifications, the use of probiotics and prebiotics, antispasmodics, and, depending on the clinical presentation, either laxatives or antidiarrheal agents. Antidepressants may also be considered in selected cases [2, 57]. IBS does not appear to have a negative impact on either the pregnancy itself or its outcomes [2].

7.10 Hemorrhoids

Hemorrhoids are a common condition. They affect up to 35% of women during pregnancy [59]. They can develop at any stage of pregnancy, but they are more frequently observed during the third trimester and the early postpartum period [2].

Factors contributing to hemorrhoid formation include increased intra-abdominal pressure due to the enlarging uterus, venous compression, constipation, and hormonal changes [12]. The classic clinical feature is painless bright-red rectal bleeding, often noticed on the surface of the stool [2]. Other symptoms include anorectal discomfort, pruritus, prolapse of venous hemorrhoidal cushions, and pain secondary to thrombosis [2]. Around one-third of pregnant women with hemorrhoids experience symptoms, and 10% require treatment [12].

Management during pregnancy and the postpartum period is usually conservative, as symptoms often resolve spontaneously within weeks to months after delivery [2]. Preventing constipation is key to reducing risk. Symptomatic treatment includes dietary adjustments, stool softeners, warm sitz baths, topical analgesics, and anti-inflammatory suppositories [2]. In cases of severely painful thrombosed external hemorrhoids, local anesthesia followed by thrombectomy may be performed safely during pregnancy.

Hemorrhoids are only considered a "disease" when they are symptomatic. They may present as either acute exacerbations or chronic conditions. Pregnancy increases the risk of hemorrhoids because the enlarged uterus puts pressure on the rectal veins, which impairs venous return. Constipation-related straining and hard stools further contribute to their development [60]. Women who have previously experienced hemorrhoids are at an increased risk of experiencing them again during pregnancy [60]. Anal or rectal cancer is a rare differential diagnosis. These should be considered if symptoms do not resolve with conservative management [61].

7.11 Appendicitis

Acute appendicitis is the most common nonobstetric surgical emergency that occurs during pregnancy [62], with an incidence of approximately 1 in 1250–1500 pregnancies [62]. It may occur in any trimester, though it is most frequently diagnosed in the second trimester [2, 63]. The pathogenesis involves obstruction of the appendiceal lumen, leading to distension and initial symptoms of periumbilical pain and anorexia, which later localize to the right lower quadrant, accompanied by acute abdomen signs. Diagnosis during pregnancy is often challenging and can easily be missed if not considered. In early pregnancy, nausea, vomiting, or miscarriage-related symptoms may obscure the diagnosis, while in later stages, the upward displacement of the appendix caused by an enlarged uterus alters clinical presentation and may mimic urinary or obstetric conditions [12, 63]. Physiological leukocytosis and elevated CRP during pregnancy further complicate laboratory diagnosis [63]. The risk of perforation is higher in pregnant women than in nonpregnant women (2.65). Perforated appendicitis can lead to increased maternal and perinatal mortality and morbidity [2, 64]. Reported perinatal mortality is ~1.5% in uncomplicated appendicitis but rises to 10–20% in perforated cases [12, 64].

When it comes to diagnosing issues during pregnancy, ultrasonography and magnetic resonance imaging (MRI) are the go-to tools [2, 65]. Appendectomy is indicated if appendicitis is confirmed by ultrasound [2, 65]. In inconclusive cases, MRI is recommended, with reported sensitivity of 50–95% and specificity of 93–100% [66]. Both laparotomy and laparoscopic appendectomy are acceptable surgical approaches, with the choice left to the surgeon [12, 64]. A meta-analysis showed that there was no significant difference in rates of fetal loss or preterm birth between the two techniques [64]. However, in advanced gestation, laparoscopy should be performed only by experienced surgeons, with careful entry site selection and appropriate technical adjustments.

The risk of preterm labor may be increased by surgical interventions during pregnancy. Thus, appendicitis must be diagnosed with as much certainty as possible while avoiding unnecessary surgeries.

7.12 Pancreatitis

Acute pancreatitis, defined as inflammation of the pancreas, is rare during pregnancy, with an incidence ranging from 1 in 1000 to 1 in 10,000 pregnancies. This usually occurs in the late third trimester or in the early postpartum period [67–69]. Acute pancreatitis poses significant risks for both mother and fetus, including preterm birth, sepsis, shock, and multiple organ dysfunction syndrome. Management is often complex and requires careful maternal and fetal monitoring.

The causes and development of acute pancreatitis in pregnant women are comparable to those in nonpregnant individuals. Gallstones are the most common cause of the condition, accounting for over 70% of cases [70]. The development of gallstones is made more likely by hormonal changes and weight gain during pregnancy [71]. Altered hormone levels may further promote biliary stasis, facilitating stone development. Lodged stones at the ampulla of Vater or stones passing into the duodenum can trigger the premature activation of trypsinogen into trypsin. This can lead to autodigestion and pancreatic injury [72].

Hypertriglyceridemia (serum triglycerides >1000 mg/dL) is the second most common cause, accounting for 4–6% of cases, often associated with familial type I or type V hyperlipoproteinemia [70]. Pregnancy itself elevates triglycerides due to estrogen-driven hepatic synthesis [73], increasing the risk in predisposed women. Alcohol and, rarely, preeclampsia/eclampsia, via microvascular abnormalities, may also cause pancreatitis [70].

Clinical features are similar to nonpregnant patients: acute epigastric pain that radiates to the back, accompanied by nausea and vomiting. Pain worsens in the supine position but may improve in fetal or forward-leaning positions. Jaundice may occur if gallstones obstruct the common bile duct. A diagnosis can be confirmed by elevated serum amylase and/or lipase levels, as these enzymes are not altered by pregnancy [70].

Ultrasound is the first-line investigation, with high accuracy for gallstone detection and no fetal radiation exposure. If common bile duct stones are suspected, endoscopic ultrasound (EUS) or magnetic resonance cholangiopancreatography

(MRCP) is preferred, as both are radiation-free and provide excellent anatomical detail.

Complications include hypovolemia and shock due to third-spacing and persistent vomiting. Preterm delivery is the most common adverse fetal outcome [69], with rates of 15–19% [74], while intrauterine growth restriction and a fetal loss rate of ~4.7% have also been reported [72].

Treatment of uncomplicated cases involves supportive measures: bowel rest, aggressive IV fluid resuscitation, electrolyte correction (particularly hypocalcemia and hypomagnesemia), and analgesia. Opiates may be required; meperidine and fentanyl are considered safe during pregnancy [75]. Prophylactic antibiotics are not recommended unless an infection is present [76]. Importantly, termination of pregnancy does not improve maternal outcomes and is not indicated [77].

7.13 Pregnancy, Microbiota, and Microbiome

Microorganisms within the human body play essential roles in metabolic, immunological, and physiological processes, and maintaining balance in both their numbers and diversity is crucial. The collective community of microorganisms residing in a given habitat is termed the microbiota [78, 79]. The microbiome refers to both the microbiota and its colonized niche, as well as the collective genomes of these microorganisms [78, 79].

Normal pregnancy is accompanied by significant physiological changes in the maternal body, encompassing immunological, metabolic, and hormonal adaptations [80, 81]. Similarly, the gut microbiota undergoes significant shifts. While bacterial load and diversity initially increase during pregnancy, later stages are characterized by slowing expansion but greater compositional changes. An increase in Proteobacteria and a reduction in *Faecalibacterium* have been described. Overall, the maternal gut microbiome during pregnancy shifts toward a pro-inflammatory, pro-diabetogenic state, which is thought to enhance energy storage and support fetal growth [2].

Fungal communities, as an integral component of the gut microbiome, also play critical roles in gut ecology and host health [82, 83]. Recent studies in obese pregnant women and those with gestational diabetes mellitus (GDM) suggest that the maternal gut microbiome may influence host metabolism and contribute to GDM development [84–86]. Although these studies have small sample sizes, they raise the possibility that targeting the maternal gut microbiome may represent a novel intervention to promote healthy pregnancy outcomes.

In light of the well-established impact of maternal nutrition on fetal development and the long-term health of offspring, the intricate relationship between diet and the maternal microbiome must also be taken into account [87]. The microbiome not only produces metabolites that influence fetal programming but is itself modulated by dietary intake. Although there is support from human studies for a correlation between maternal metabolic health and gut microbial composition, there is limited data directly linking maternal diet, microbiome-derived metabolites, and offspring outcomes [88].

Hormonal changes critical for pregnancy maintenance—particularly elevated estrogen and progesterone—also influence the gut environment. These hormones have a direct impact on bacterial metabolism, bacterial growth, and the expression of virulence factors, thereby reshaping the microbiome during gestation [89].

References

1. Friedel D, Stavropoulos S, Iqbal S, et al. Gastrointestinal endoscopy in the pregnant woman. World J Gastrointest Endosc. 2014;6(4):156–67.
2. Bonthala N, Wong MS. Gastrointestinal diseases in pregnancy. In: Landon MB, Galan HL, Jauniaux ERM, Driscoll DA, editors. Gabbe's obstetrics: normal and problem pregnancies. 8th ed. Elsevier; 2021. p. 1019–37.
3. O'Mahony S. Endoscopy in pregnancy. Best Prac Res Clin Gastroenterol. 2007;21:893–9.
4. ASGE Standard of Practice Committee, Shergill AK, Ben-Menachem T, Chandrasekhara V, Chathadi K, Decker GA, Evans JA, Early DS, Fanelli RD, Fisher DA, Foley KQ, Fukami N, Hwang JH, Jain R, Jue TL, Khan KM, Lightdale J, Pasha SF, Sharaf RN, Dominitz JA, Cash BD. Guidelines for endoscopy in pregnant and lactating women. Gastrointest Endosc. 2012;76(1):18–24. https://doi.org/10.1016/j.gie.2012.02.029.
5. van der Minnen LM, Grooten IJ, Dean C, Trovik J, Painter RC. The impact and management of hyperemesis gravidarum: current and future perspectives. Int J Gynaecol Obstet. 2025;171(1):54–62. https://doi.org/10.1002/ijgo.70165.
6. Einarson TR, Piwko C, Koren G. Prevalence of nausea and vomiting of pregnancy in the USA: a meta analysis. J Popul Ther Clin Pharmacol. 2013;20(2):e163–70.
7. ACOG. Practice bulletin number 189, nausea and vomiting of pregnancy. Obstet Gynecol. 2018;131(6):e15.
8. Gazal A, Scarf V, Kay-Smith C, Gidaszewski B, Chua S, Levett K. What are the costs associated with nausea and vomiting in pregnancy and hyperemesis gravidarum? A systematic review. BMC Pregnancy Childbirth. 2025;25(1):807. https://doi.org/10.1186/s12884-025-07921-5.
9. Koot MH, Grooten IJ, van der Post JAM, Bais JMJ, Ris-Stalpers C, Leeflang MMG, Bremer HA, van der Ham DP, Heidema WM, Huisjes A, Kleiverda G, Kuppens SM, van Laar JOEH, Langenveld J, van der Made F, van Pampus MG, Papatsonis D, Pelinck MJ, Pernet PJ, van Rheenen-Flach L, Rijnders RJ, Scheepers HCJ, Vogelvang TE, Mol BW, Roseboom TJ, Painter RC. Determinants of disease course and severity in hyperemesis gravidarum. Eur J Obstet Gynecol Reprod Biol. 2020;245:162–7. https://doi.org/10.1016/j.ejogrb.2019.12.021.
10. Devane D. Interventions for nausea and vomiting in early pregnancy. Pract Midwife. 2010;13(11):38–9.
11. Niemeijer MN, Grooten IJ, Vos N, et al. Diagnostic markers for hyperemesis gravidarum: a systematic review and metaanalysis. Am J Obstet Gynecol. 2014;211(2):150.e1–15.
12. Kelly TF, Savides TJ. Gastrointestinal disease in pregnancy. In: Resnik R, Lockwood, Greene, et al., editors. Creasy and Resnik's maternal-fetal medicine: principles and practice. 8th ed. Elsevier; 2019. p. 1158–72. 95.
13. Liu C, Zhao G, Qiao D, Wang L, He Y, Zhao M, Fan Y, Jiang E. Emerging progress in nausea and vomiting of pregnancy and hyperemesis gravidarum: challenges and opportunities. Front Med. 2022;8:809270. https://doi.org/10.3389/fmed.2021.809270. PMID: 35083256; PMCID: PMC8785858.
14. London V, Grube S, Sherer DM, et al. Hyperemesis gravidarum: a review of recent literature. Pharmacology. 2017;100(3–4):161–71.

15. Gomes CF, Sousa M, Lourenço I, et al. Gastrointestinal diseases during pregnancy: what does the gastroenterologist need to know? Ann Gastroenterol. 2018;31(4):385–94.
16. Richter JE. Heartburn, nausea, and vomiting during pregnancy. In: Pregnancy in gastrointestinal disorders. Bethesda: ACG Monograph American College of Physicians; 2007. p. 18–25. Available at: https://www.acg.gi.org.
17. Verrengia M, Sachdeva P, Gaughan J, et al. Variation of symptoms during the menstrual cycle in female patients with gastroparesis. Neurogastroenterol Motil. 2011;23(7):625–e254.
18. Lowe SA, Steinweg KE. Review article: management of hyperemesis gravidarum and nausea and vomiting in pregnancy. Emerg Med Australas. 2022;34(1):9–15. https://doi.org/10.1111/1742-6723.13909.
19. Jansen LAW, Shaw V, Grooten IJ, Koot MH, Dean CR, Painter RC. Diagnosis and treatment of hyperemesis gravidarum. CMAJ. 2024;196(14):477–85. https://doi.org/10.1503/cmaj.221502.
20. Pope E, Maltepe C, Koren G. Comparing pyridoxine and doxylamine succinate-pyridoxine HCl for nausea and vomiting of pregnancy: a matched, controlled cohort study. J Clin Pharmacol. 2015;55(7):809–14.
21. Keller J, Frederking D, Layer P. The spectrum and treatment of gastrointestinal disorders during pregnancy. Nat Clin Pract Gastroenterol Hepatol. 2008;5(8):430–43.
22. Salari N, Mohamadi S, Hemmati M, Fallahi A, Rasoulpoor S, Zarei H, Shohaimi S, Mohammadi M. Global prevalence of constipation during pregnancy: a systematic review and meta-analysis. BMC Pregnancy Childbirth. 2024;24(1):836. https://doi.org/10.1186/s12884-024-07057-y.
23. Zielinski R, Searing K, Deibel M, et al. Gastrointestinal distress in pregnancy prevalence, assessment, and treatment of 5 common minor discomforts. J Perinat Neonatal Nurs. 2015;29(1):23–31.
24. Dunbar K, Yadlapati R, Konda V. Heartburn, nausea, and vomiting during pregnancy. Am J Gastroenterol. 2022;117(10S):10–5. https://doi.org/10.14309/ajg.0000000000001958.
25. Gill SK, O'Brien L, Einarson TR, Koren G. The safety of proton pump inhibitors (PPIs) in pregnancy: a meta-analysis. Am J Gastroenterol. 2009;104(6):1541–5.
26. Jones PF, McEwan AB, Bernard RM. Hemorrhage and perforation complicating peptic ulcer in pregnancy. Lancet. 1969;2(7616):350–1.
27. Tornqvist A. The effects of exogenous histamine on the forearm blood flow in pregnant and nonpregnant women before and after inhibition of histaminases. Acta Obstet Gynecol Scand. 1968;47(4):391–403.
28. Montoneri C, Drago F. Effects of pregnancy in rats on cysteamine-induced peptic ulcers: role of progesterone. Dig Dis Sci. 1997;42(12):2572–5.
29. Augustin G, Krstulović J, Tavra A, Hrgović Z. Perforated peptic ulcer in pregnancy and puerperium: a systematic review. World J Gastrointest Surg. 2025;17(4):101682. https://doi.org/10.4240/wjgs.v17.i4.101682.
30. Dhamecha R, Pajai S, Bhasin T. Acute abdomen in pregnancy: a comprehensive review of diagnosis and management. Cureus. 2023;15(6):e40679. https://doi.org/10.7759/cureus.40679.
31. Altuwaijri M. Evidence-based treatment recommendations for gastroesophageal reflux disease during pregnancy: a review. Medicine (Baltimore). 2022;101(35):e30487. https://doi.org/10.1097/MD.0000000000030487.
32. Lewis JH, Weingold AB. The use of gastrointestinal drugs during pregnancy and lactation. Am J Gastroenterol. 1985;80(11):912–23.
33. Turawa EB, Musekiwa A, Rohwer AC. Interventions for preventing postpartum constipation. Cochrane Database Syst Rev. 2020;8(8):CD011625. https://doi.org/10.1002/14651858.
34. Menees SB, Lembo A, Charabaty A. Fecal incontinence and diarrhea during pregnancy. Am J Gastroenterol. 2022;117(10S):26–32.
35. Kothari S, Afshar Y, Friedman LS, Ahn J. AGA clinical practice update on pregnancy-related gastrointestinal and liver disease: expert review. Gastroenterology. 2024;167(5):1033–45. https://doi.org/10.1053/j.gastro.2024.06.014.

36. Body C, Christie JA. Gastrointestinal diseases in pregnancy: nausea, vomiting, hyperemesis Gravidarum, gastroesophageal reflux disease, constipation, and diarrhea. Gastroenterol Clin N Am. 2016;45(2):267–83.
37. Bonapace ES Jr, Fisher RS. Constipation and diarrhea in pregnancy. Gastroenterol Clin N Am. 1998;27(1):197–211.
38. Kallen B, Nilsson E, Otterblad OP. Maternal use of loperamide in early pregnancy and delivery outcome. Acta Paediatr. 2008;97(5):541–5.
39. Mądro A. Pancreatitis in pregnancy-comprehensive review. Int J Environ Res Public Health. 2022;19(23):16179. https://doi.org/10.3390/ijerph192316179.
40. Schwulst SJ, Son M. Management of gallstone disease during pregnancy. JAMA Surg. 2020;155(12):1162–3. https://doi.org/10.1001/jamasurg.2020.3683.
41. Ibiebele I, Schnitzler M, Nippita T, Ford JB. Outcomes of gallstone disease during pregnancy: a population-based data linkage study. Paediatr Perinat Epidemiol. 2017;31(6):522–30.
42. Nielsen OH, Gubatan JM, Juhl CB, Streett SE, Maxwell C. Biologics for inflammatory bowel disease and their safety in pregnancy: a systematic review and meta-analysis. Clin Gastroenterol Hepatol. 2022;20(1):74–87.e3. https://doi.org/10.1016/j.cgh.2020.09.021.
43. Nielsen OH, Gubatan JM, Kolho KL, Streett SE, Maxwell C. Updates on the management of inflammatory bowel disease from periconception to pregnancy and lactation. Lancet. 2024;403(10433):1291–303. https://doi.org/10.1016/S0140-6736(24)00052-7.
44. Nielsen OH, Andreasson B, Bondesen S, Jarnum S. Pregnancy in ulcerative colitis. Scand J Gastroenterol. 1983;18(6):735–42.
45. Korelitz BI. Pregnancy, fertility, and inflammatory bowel disease. Am J Gastroenterol. 1985;80(5):365–70.
46. Laube R, Paramsothy S, Leong RW. Review of pregnancy in Crohn's disease and ulcerative colitis. Ther Adv Gastroenterol. 2021;14:17562848211016242. https://doi.org/10.1177/17562848211016242.
47. Mogadam M, Korelitz BI, Ahmed SW, et al. The course of inflammatory bowel disease during pregnancy and postpartum. Am J Gastroenterol. 1981;75(4):265–9.
48. Costa RV, Simões C, Correia L, Pinto L. Inflammatory bowel disease and pregnancy: is it a marker for adverse outcomes? Rev Bras Ginecol Obstet. 2022;44(10):915–24. https://doi.org/10.1055/s-0042-1756149.
49. Miller JP. Inflammatory bowel disease in pregnancy: a review. J R Soc Med. 1986;79(4):221–5.
50. Ali MF, He H, Friedel D. Inflammatory bowel disease and pregnancy: fertility, complications and treatment. Ann Gastroenterol. 2020;33(6):579–90. https://doi.org/10.20524/aog.2020.0536.
51. Lee KS, Kim ES, Song IS, Kim HI, Ahn KH. Association of preterm birth with inflammatory bowel disease and salivary gland disease: machine learning analysis using National Health Insurance Data. Int J Environ Res Public Health. 2022;19(5):3056. https://doi.org/10.3390/ijerph19053056.
52. Forcato S, Aquino ABO, Borges LI, Thomé MLFL, Bilibio JO, Lens HHM, Erthal RP, Guarnier FA, Fernandes GSA, Gerardin DCC. Sulfasalazine exposure during pregnancy and lactation: reproductive outcomes in male rat offspring. Reprod Fertil Dev. 2023;35(8):469–79. https://doi.org/10.1071/RD22240.
53. Nielsen OH, Andreasson B, Bondesen S, et al. Pregnancy in Crohn's disease. Scand J Gastroenterol. 1984;19(5):724–32.
54. Chugh R, Gaidos JKJ. Fertility and pregnancy in Crohn's disease. Gastroenterol Clin N Am. 2022;51(2):381–99. https://doi.org/10.1016/j.gtc.2021.12.012. Epub 2022 Apr 27.
55. Szymanska E, Kisielewski R, Kierkus JJ. Reproduction and pregnancy in inflammatory bowel disease-management and treatment based on current guidelines. J Gynecol Obstet Hum Reprod. 2020;50:101777.
56. Kammerlander H, Nielsen J, Kjeldsen J, et al. Fecal calprotectin during pregnancy in women with moderate-severe inflammatory bowel disease. Inflamm Bowel Dis. 2018;24(4):839–48.

57. Yılmaz B, Akbulut G. İrritabl Bağırsak Sendromuna Güncel Bakış. Bes Diy Derg. 2018;46:276–84.
58. Brandt LJ, Chey WD, Foxx-Orenstein AE, et al. An evidence-based position statement on the management of irritable bowel syndrome. Am J Gastroenterol. 2009;104(suppl 1):S1–S35.
59. Poskus T, Sabonyte-Balsaitiene Z, Jakubauskiene L, Jakubauskas M, Stundiene I, Barkauskaite G, Smigelskaite M, Jasiunas E, Ramasauskaite D, Strupas K, Drasutiene G. Preventing hemorrhoids during pregnancy: a multicenter, randomized clinical trial. BMC Pregnancy Childbirth. 2022;22(1):374. https://doi.org/10.1186/s12884-022-04688-x.
60. Wald A. Constipation, diarrhea and symptomatic hemorrhoids during pregnancy. Gastroenterol Clin N Am. 2003;32(1):309–22.
61. Williams DJ. Physiological changes of normal pregnancy. In: Warrell DA, Cox TM, Firth JD, editors. Oxford textbook of medicine. 5th ed. Oxford University Press; 2014. p. 1069.
62. Kave M, Parooie F, Salarzaei M. Pregnancy and appendicitis: a systematic review and meta-analysis on the clinical use of MRI in diagnosis of appendicitis in pregnant women. World J Emerg Surg. 2019;14:37. https://doi.org/10.1186/s13017-019-0254-1.
63. Tase A, Kamarizan MFA, Swarnkar K. Appendicitis in pregnancy: difficulties in diagnosis and management. Int J Surg Open. 2017;6:5–11.
64. Lee SH, Lee JY, Young YY, et al. Laparoscopic appendectomy versus open appendectomy for suspected appendicitis during pregnancy: a systematic review and updated meta-analysis. BMC Surg. 2019;19:41. https://doi.org/10.1186/s12893-019-0505-9.
65. Moghadam MN, Salarzaei M, Shahraki Z. Diagnostic accuracy of ultrasound in diagnosing acute appendicitis in pregnancy: a systematic review and meta-analysis. Emerg Radiol. 2022;29(3):437–48. https://doi.org/10.1007/s10140-022-02021-9.
66. Yavuz Y, Sentürk M, Gümüş T, Patmano M. Acute appendicitis in pregnancy. Ulus Travma Acil Cerrahi Derg. 2021;27(1):85–8. English. https://doi.org/10.14744/tjtes.2020.22792.
67. ang QY, Hu JW. Prediction of moderately severe and severe acute pancreatitis in pregnancy: several issues. World J Gastroenterol. 2022;28(33):4926–8. https://doi.org/10.3748/wjg.v28.i33.4926.
68. Hughes DL, Hughes A, White PB, Silva MA. Acute pancreatitis in pregnancy: meta-analysis of maternal and fetal outcomes. Br J Surg. 2021;109(1):12–4. https://doi.org/10.1093/bjs/znab221.
69. Alsadery HA, Bamalan OA, Aljubran HJ, Albaish LJ, Al Ghanim BZ. Non-obstetric acute abdomen in pregnancy: a review of literature. Med Arch. 2023;77(4):293–8. https://doi.org/10.5455/medarh.2023.77.293-298.
70. Augustin G, Majerovic M. Non-obstetrical acute abdomen during pregnancy. Eur J Obstet Gynecol Reprod Biol. 2007;131(1):4–12.
71. Olafson SN, Soult AP, Britt RC. The management of gallstones in pregnancy. Adv Surg. 2025;59(1):109–19. https://doi.org/10.1016/j.yasu.2025.05.002.
72. Pitchumoni CS, Yegneswaran B. Acute pancreatitis in pregnancy. World J Gastroenterol. 2009;15(45):5641–6.
73. Lippi G, Albiero A, Montagnana M, et al. Lipid and lipoprotein profile in physiological pregnancy. Clin Lab. 2007;53(3–4):173–7.
74. Zhang T, Wang G, Cao Z, Huang W, Xiao H, Wei H, Lu J, Liu R, Yin C. Acute pancreatitis in pregnancy: a 10-year, multi-center, retrospective study in Beijing. BMC Pregnancy Childbirth. 2022;22(1):414. https://doi.org/10.1186/s12884-022-04742-8.
75. Jain P. Acute pancreatitis in pregnancy: an unresolved issue. World J Gastroenterol. 2010;16(17):2065–6.
76. Haiyan Z, Na P, Yong G, Xiumei B, Jianying B. Impact of acute pancreatitis during pregnancy in Chinese women: a meta-analysis. J Obstet Gynaecol. 2022;42(7):2879–87. https://doi.org/10.1080/01443615.2022.2110462.
77. Benson M, Arena Goncharov D, Jain S. Diagnosis and management of acute pancreatitis in pregnancy. Clin Obstet Gynecol. 2023;66(1):237–49. https://doi.org/10.1097/GRF.0000000000000737.

78. Grech A, Collins CE, Holmes A, Lal R, Duncanson K, Taylor R, Gordon A. Maternal exposures and the infant gut microbiome: a systematic review with meta-analysis. Gut Microbes. 2021;13(1):1–30. https://doi.org/10.1080/19490976.2021.1897210.
79. Gomaa EZ. Human gut microbiota/microbiome in health and diseases: a review. Antonie Van Leeuwenhoek. 2020;113(12):2019–40. https://doi.org/10.1007/s10482-020-01474-7.
80. Newbern D, Freemark M. Placental hormones and the control of maternal metabolism and fetal growth. Curr Opin Endocrinol Diabetes Obes. 2011;18(6):409–16.
81. Hussain T, Murtaza G, Kalhoro DH, Kalhoro MS, Yin Y, Chughtai MI, Tan B, Yaseen A, Rehman ZU. Understanding the immune system in fetal protection and maternal infections during pregnancy. J Immunol Res. 2022;2022:7567708. https://doi.org/10.1155/2022/7567708.
82. Zheng J-S, Wahlqvist M. Regulobiosis: a regulatory and food system-sensitive role for fungal symbionts in human evolution and ecobiology. Asia Pac J Clin Nutr. 2020;29(1):9–15.
83. Shuai M, Fu Y, Zhong H-L, et al. Mapping the human gut mycobiome in middle-aged and elderly adults: multiomics insights and implications for host metabolic health. Gut. 2022;71(9):1812–20.
84. Ferrocino I, Ponzo V, Pellegrini M, et al. Mycobiota composition and changes across pregnancy in patients with gestational diabetes mellitus (GDM). Sci Rep. 2022;12:9192.
85. Vavreckova M, Galanova N, Kostovcik M, et al. Specific gut bacterial and fungal microbiota pattern in the first half of pregnancy is linked to the development of gestational diabetes mellitus in the cohort including obese women. Front Endocrinol (Lausanne). 2022;13:970825.
86. Wu N, Mo H, Mu Q, et al. The gut mycobiome characterization of gestational diabetes mellitus and its association with dietary intervention. Front Microbiol. 2022;13:1–13.
87. Siena M, Laterza L, Matteo MV, et al. Gut and reproductive tract microbiota adaptation during pregnancy: new insights for pregnancy-related complications and therapy. Microorganisms. 2021;9(3):575.
88. Kunasegaran T, Balasubramaniam V, Arasoo VJT, Palanisamy UD, Ramadas A. Diet gut microbiota axis in pregnancy: a systematic review of recent evidence. Curr Nutr Rep. 2023;12(1):203–14.
89. Mulak A, Tache Y, Larauche M. Sex hormones in the modulation of irritable bowel syndrome. World J Gastroenterol. 2014;20(10):2433–48.

Chapter 8
Pregnancy, Pruritus, and Liver: Understanding Cholestasis Challenges

Eyüp Kebabçı

8.1 Introduction

Intrahepatic cholestasis of pregnancy (ICP) is characterized by elevated serum bile acid concentrations and pruritus, typically developing in the late second and/or third trimester and resolving rapidly after delivery.

Among pregnancy-specific hepatic disorders, intrahepatic cholestasis of pregnancy (ICP) is the most frequently encountered condition. Epidemiological data demonstrate substantial regional variability, with prevalence rates reported between 1% and 27.6% worldwide [1–3]. In the United States, ICP affects approximately 0.8% of pregnancies, while in Europe the incidence generally ranges from 0.5% to 1.5% [2, 4]. The highest incidence globally has been documented among the Araucanian Indigenous population in Chile, at 27.6%. The reasons for such marked variation remain unclear, but geographical differences may reflect variations in ethnic susceptibility as well as environmental influences [5, 6].

The incidence of ICP shows seasonal variation, with higher rates reported during winter months in several countries such as Sweden, Finland, and Chile [6, 7]. A previous episode of ICP is a major predictor of recurrence in later pregnancies. Other contributing factors include multiple gestation—documented at 20.9% among twin pregnancies versus 4% in singleton pregnancies in a Chilean cohort, and up to 43% in triplet pregnancies in a Finnish study—as well as chronic hepatitis C infection, a personal or familial history of hepatic cholestasis, and advanced maternal age [7–9].

E. Kebabçı (✉)
Izmir Bakircay University, Faculty of Medicine, Department of General Surgery, Izmir, Turkey
e-mail: eyup.kebabcı@bakircay.edu.tr

© The Author(s), under exclusive license to Springer Nature Switzerland AG 2026

I. Karaca (ed.), *Managing Maternal Chronic Diseases for a Healthy Pregnancy*,
https://doi.org/10.1007/978-3-032-15221-3_8

8.2 Etiology

The etiology of intrahepatic cholestasis of pregnancy (ICP) remains incompletely understood. Current evidence suggests that genetic susceptibility, hormonal influences, environmental exposures, and underlying liver disease all play contributory roles.

8.2.1 *Genetic Susceptibility*

The genetic background of ICP is complex. A high recurrence rate in subsequent pregnancies (60–70%), familial clustering, and increased prevalence among first-degree relatives and specific ethnic groups strongly suggest a hereditary predisposition [10].

Among the implicated genes, mutations in the hepatobiliary transport protein multidrug resistance protein 3 (MDR3), which mediates phospholipid secretion into the bile canalicular membrane, are well recognized [11]. MDR3 gene mutations are identified in approximately 16% of ICP cases and have been linked to more severe clinical manifestations, including total bile acid (TBA) concentrations exceeding 40 μmol/L [12]. Notably, mutations in the MDR3 gene have also been implicated in the development of low-phospholipid–associated gallstone formation and in cholestatic liver injury secondary to drug exposure [13, 14].

MRP2 gene variants have been reported among South American women, but supporting data are still limited [15]. Mutations in the bile salt export pump (BSEP) gene show a stronger association: a large study of 563 ICP cases demonstrated significant correlations with BSEP variants [16]. Rare mutations have also been reported in FIC1 (ATP8B1), encoding a bile canalicular membrane protein, and in FXR (NR1H4), a nuclear receptor regulating bile acid homeostasis [17, 18].

8.2.2 *Hormonal Influences*

Experimental studies suggest that estrogens, progesterone, and their metabolites can impair hepatobiliary transport proteins, reducing bile acid excretion into bile canaliculi [17, 18]. These hormonal effects alter bile composition, increasing hydrophobic bile acids, thereby disrupting maternal–fetal bile acid homeostasis. In uncomplicated pregnancies, the transfer of bile acids occurs from the fetal compartment to the maternal circulation, promoting their metabolic clearance. In contrast, intrahepatic cholestasis of pregnancy (ICP) disrupts this mechanism, causing a reversal of bile acid flow and resulting in elevated concentrations in both the maternal and fetal compartments. High TBA levels contribute to oxidative stress, apoptosis, and hepatocellular injury [19].

Estrogen and progesterone concentrations increase steadily throughout gestation, reaching their highest levels in the third trimester and falling rapidly after delivery—a temporal pattern that mirrors the clinical course of intrahepatic cholestasis of pregnancy (ICP) [20]. The cholestatic effects of 17β-estradiol and sulfated progesterone metabolites have been demonstrated [21]. Several clinical observations support this role: ICP manifests predominantly in the second half of pregnancy, is more frequent in twin gestations, occurs with increased frequency following ovarian hyperstimulation, resolves rapidly postpartum with placental removal, and is more common in women exposed to estrogen–progestin contraceptives [7, 22, 23].

The metabolism of progesterone is also thought to play a significant part in the pathophysiological mechanisms of the disorder. In genetically susceptible women, excessive amounts of sulfated progesterone metabolites are generated, likely as a result of enhanced enzymatic activity of 5α-reductase and 3α-reductase. Saturation of hepatic transport systems may lead to metabolite accumulation [24, 25]. These sulfated metabolites activate TGR5, a G-protein–coupled receptor regulating metabolic processes, and may induce pruritus in a receptor-dependent manner. Reduced sulfotransferase activity in pregnancy further enhances accumulation [26]. Women with ICP exhibit significantly higher levels of progesterone sulfates compared with healthy controls. Although most data are derived from animal studies, the role of these hormones in ICP pathogenesis is strongly supported [27, 28].

The impact of exogenous progesterone on ICP risk remains uncertain. Randomized placebo-controlled trials of progesterone supplementation for preterm birth prevention have not shown a specific increase in ICP incidence. However, hydroxyprogesterone use was reported to increase pruritus rates by ~8% before its market withdrawal [29].

8.2.3 Medications

Thiopurine derivatives such as azathioprine and mercaptopurine have only infrequently been associated with the onset of ICP. In patients receiving these medications—particularly those treated for systemic lupus erythematosus or inflammatory bowel disease—therapy should be promptly discontinued if cholestasis occurs [30].

8.2.4 Environmental Factors

Seasonal and geographical variation in ICP incidence suggests an environmental contribution [3]. Low selenium intake, particularly in regions with selenium-deficient soil, and reduced vitamin D levels have been implicated [9, 31]. Other potential factors include excessive erucic acid intake from rapeseed oil, pesticide exposure, and nutritional deficiencies [32].

8.2.5 *Underlying Liver Disease*

A minority of women with ICP have concurrent chronic liver disease [33–36]. Epidemiological studies link ICP with hepatitis C virus infection and nonalcoholic cirrhosis [34]. Familial forms of recurrent ICP associated with progressive hepatic fibrosis have also been described, as in a report of four sisters with prolonged, recurrent cholestasis during pregnancy [35].

8.3 Clinical Features

The earliest and most characteristic manifestation of ICP is pruritus, which can vary in intensity from mild to severe. Although it may occur throughout the body, it often begins on the palms and soles, where it is typically most pronounced, and tends to intensify during nighttime hours. In some women, pruritus is accompanied by right upper quadrant discomfort, nausea, loss of appetite, sleep disturbance, or fatty stool. Symptoms typically manifest during the late second or third trimester of pregnancy. When pruritus appears transiently in the first trimester, it is most often linked to ovarian hyperstimulation syndrome following in vitro fertilization, whereas spontaneously conceived pregnancies usually demonstrate the characteristic gradual and persistent symptom pattern [23, 37].

8.3.1 *Physical Examination*

Clinical assessment may reveal excoriations, scratch marks, or prurigo nodules that develop secondary to intense itching. Importantly, ICP does not produce any primary skin lesions. Jaundice is observed in approximately 14–25% of patients, usually manifesting 1–4 weeks after the onset of pruritus [38]. The occurrence of jaundice in the absence of itching is unusual and should prompt evaluation for other potential causes.

8.3.2 *Laboratory Findings*

The most characteristic laboratory feature of ICP is an elevated serum total bile acid level, which is found in about 90% of affected pregnancies and may be the earliest or sole detectable abnormality [29, 39, 40]. It is noteworthy that itching typically precedes any biochemical changes [41]. In normal hepatic metabolism, cholic acid and chenodeoxycholic acid, the principal bile acids, are conjugated with either glycine or taurine before they are secreted into the biliary system. In ICP, both acids are elevated, but cholic acid increases disproportionately, producing a markedly higher cholic-to-chenodeoxycholic acid ratio compared with healthy pregnancies (3.4 vs. 1.1) [38, 42, 43]. Most individuals with this altered ratio also exhibit elevated total bile acid concentrations [44]. In contrast, the glycine-to-taurine conjugation ratio is reduced (<1).

8.3.3 *Other Biochemical Abnormalities*

Elevations in serum aminotransferases occur in nearly 60% of ICP cases, most often mild and below twice the upper reference range. In exceptional cases, levels may rise above 1000 U/L, necessitating exclusion of viral hepatitis in the differential diagnosis [29]. Alkaline phosphatase (ALP) can rise up to four times the normal value; however, this is not specific to cholestasis in pregnancy, as placental isoenzyme activity physiologically increases during gestation. Approximately one-quarter of patients demonstrate elevated total and direct bilirubin levels, with total bilirubin seldom exceeding 6 mg/dL. Gamma-glutamyl transpeptidase levels generally remain within normal limits, though mild increases are observed in up to 30% of individuals; marked elevations are atypical and may indicate alternative causes of cholestasis. The prothrombin time is typically normal, and any prolongation is more often attributable to vitamin K deficiency secondary to fat malabsorption—resulting from steatorrhea or bile acid sequestrant therapy (e.g., cholestyramine)—rather than to primary hepatic dysfunction. Steatorrhea is typically mild, and nutritional status is usually preserved.

8.3.4 *Ultrasonography*

Ultrasonographic evaluation in ICP reveals no structural abnormalities. The intrahepatic and extrahepatic bile ducts appear normal in caliber, and the hepatic parenchymal texture remains unremarkable.

8.3.5 *Pathology*

Histopathologic analysis of the liver in ICP demonstrates cholestasis without inflammatory infiltrate [45]. Bile plugs are frequently identified within hepatocytes and bile canaliculi, predominantly in zone 3, whereas the portal tracts are typically preserved. Liver biopsy is seldom required, as diagnosis is clinical and biochemical, and histological confirmation rarely alters management.

8.4 Diagnosis

Intrahepatic cholestasis of pregnancy (ICP) should be suspected in women presenting with generalized pruritus without a rash during the late second or third trimester of pregnancy. The diagnosis is established by detecting elevated total serum bile acids, increased aminotransferase levels, or both, after excluding other potential causes. Because biochemical abnormalities may lag behind pruritus by one or more weeks, repeated laboratory testing is often necessary for confirmation.

Although reference thresholds differ slightly across clinical guidelines, severe disease is generally defined as a sustained serum bile acid concentration above 40 μmol/L, a condition observed in roughly 20% of affected pregnancies. According to a systematic review analyzing 11 studies, application of a 10 μmol/L threshold for diagnosis demonstrated a pooled sensitivity of 0.91 (95% confidence interval [CI], 0.72–0.98) and a specificity of 0.93 (95% CI, 0.81–0.97) in identifying intrahepatic cholestasis of pregnancy [46, 47].

Nevertheless, the diagnostic precision of total bile acid testing remains somewhat uncertain, as most available studies were not prospective and did not include consecutive patient recruitment. Reported cutoff values vary substantially among studies due to differences in analytical methods, fasting conditions, study populations, and gestational age at testing [48]. Moreover, postprandial bile acid levels tend to be higher than fasting concentrations, which can complicate the interpretation of results and limit the assessment of disease severity when samples are obtained in the nonfasting state [49–51].

8.5 Diagnostic Evaluation and Differential Diagnosis

Confirmation of intrahepatic cholestasis of pregnancy and exclusion of other differential diagnoses require a comprehensive clinical evaluation incorporating a detailed patient history, physical examination, and targeted laboratory analyses. The laboratory assessment should include determination of total serum bile acid concentrations (collected in the nonfasting state) together with aminotransferase levels—alanine aminotransferase (ALT) and aspartate aminotransferase (AST) [51].

Pruritus affects approximately 23% of pregnancies; however, only a minority of these cases are caused by intrahepatic cholestasis of pregnancy [52]. Since abnormal liver function tests have multiple potential etiologies, patients must be evaluated comprehensively.

In a retrospective study conducted by Kondrackiene et al., total bile acid (TBA) levels alone were found to lack adequate sensitivity and specificity for the diagnosis of ICP [37]. The investigators identified cholic acid (CA), chenodeoxycholic acid (CDCA) concentrations, and particularly the CA/CDCA ratio as more reliable diagnostic biomarkers [53]. Measuring only total bile acids without bile acid profiling can reduce the positive predictive value by more than 2% [43]. Elevated TBA levels are generally accompanied by increased aminotransferases, particularly ALT. Approximately 60–85% of patients exhibit a 2- to 15-fold increase in ALT activity, sometimes exceeding 1000 IU/L [54].

Differentiating intrahepatic cholestasis of pregnancy (ICP) from other hepatic or dermatologic disorders requires attention to two principal clinical features. The first is the hallmark symptom of generalized pruritus, which distinguishes ICP from other pregnancy-associated diseases with elevated aminotransferase levels. In contrast to ICP, HELLP syndrome, acute fatty liver of pregnancy, and severe preeclampsia tend to present abruptly and are potentially life-threatening. Nevertheless, instances of coexisting or overlapping ICP, preeclampsia, and acute fatty liver of pregnancy have been documented [55, 56]. The second differentiating feature is the absence of primary cutaneous lesions in ICP, aiding in its distinction from pregnancy-specific pruritic dermatoses and unrelated dermatologic disorders characterized by visible eruptions.

8.6 Fetal Effects

8.6.1 Morbidity and Mortality

Maternal bile acids are capable of crossing the placenta. Under normal physiological conditions, a transplacental concentration gradient allows for fetal elimination of bile acids. However, in pregnancies complicated by cholestasis, this gradient becomes reversed, resulting in accumulation of bile acids within the fetus and amniotic fluid, which in turn increases the risk of adverse fetal outcomes [57, 58]. Reported complications include intrauterine fetal demise, meconium-stained amniotic fluid, preterm delivery (occurring in approximately 20–60% of cases), intrauterine hypoxia or asphyxia (up to 44%), and fetal bradycardia or arrhythmias [47, 59, 60].

In a large meta-analysis that included more than 5000 pregnancies, pregnancy outcomes were found to be significantly worse in women with intrahepatic cholestasis of pregnancy (ICP) compared with healthy pregnant women [59]. The study showed higher rates of both medically induced and spontaneous preterm birth, meconium-stained amniotic fluid, admission to the neonatal intensive care unit (NICU), and stillbirth.

The risk of stillbirth increased as total serum bile acid levels rose, especially when concentrations reached or exceeded 100 μmol/L:

- <40 μmol/L: 0.13%
- 40–99 μmol/L: 0.28% (hazard ratio [HR] 2.35; 95% CI 0.52–10.50 vs <40 μmol/L)
- ≥100 μmol/L: 3.44% (HR 30.50; 95% CI 8.83–97.30 vs <40 μmol/L)

Stillbirth risk was also higher with advancing gestational age, particularly after 34–36 weeks [59]. Another systematic review confirmed similar results, showing that higher bile acid concentrations were consistently associated with an increased risk of stillbirth [61].

- <40 μmol/L: 0.4%
- 40–99 μmol/L: 0.3%
- ≥100 μmol/L: 6.8%

Corresponding rates of iatrogenic preterm birth in these categories were 10.8%, 21.6%, and 35.8%, respectively, which may partly explain the relatively lower stillbirth rates observed.

8.6.2 *Pathophysiology of Adverse Pregnancy Outcomes*

The pathophysiological mechanisms underlying fetal morbidity and mortality in ICP remain incompletely understood. Stillbirth may result from fetal arrhythmia induced by elevated bile acid concentrations or from acute vasospasm of the placental chorionic surface vessels [62–64]. The presence of gestational diabetes or preeclampsia may further increase these risks [55, 65]. Bile acids are believed to enhance the expression of oxytocin receptors within the myometrium, a mechanism that may partly explain the higher incidence of preterm and spontaneous preterm labor observed in women with ICP [66, 67]. Moreover, pregnancies that eventually result in spontaneous preterm delivery often exhibit earlier onset of pruritus, supporting a possible pathophysiologic link between bile acid elevation and uterine activity [68].

In addition, there is an inverse relationship between serum bile acid concentrations and birth weight; however, ICP has not been associated with fetal growth restriction or oligohydramnios [29].

8.7 Maternal Management

The management of ICP has two primary objectives:

- To alleviate distressing maternal symptoms
- To reduce the risk of perinatal morbidity and mortality

All patients with clinical symptoms of ICP should be offered therapeutic options. Empirical treatment may be initiated regardless of whether serum bile acid and aminotransferase levels are within normal ranges or elevated. In patients with normal laboratory values, weekly laboratory monitoring is recommended.

8.7.1 Ursodeoxycholic Acid

Ursodeoxycholic acid (UDCA) is the first-line treatment for relieving maternal itching caused by intrahepatic cholestasis of pregnancy (ICP) [69, 70]. It works by replacing harmful, hydrophobic bile acids with safer, hydrophilic ones, which helps protect liver cells and promotes the transfer and elimination of bile acids from the fetal circulation through the placenta. The optimal dosing regimen to achieve clinical efficacy has not been definitively determined. In clinical practice, a commonly employed regimen consists of 300 mg administered three times daily (approximately 15 mg/kg/day) and continued until delivery. Alternatively, 300 mg twice daily (about 10 mg/kg/day) is also acceptable [46]. UDCA is generally well tolerated, although up to one-quarter of patients may report mild gastrointestinal discomfort or dizziness. Most patients experience relief from itching within 1–2 weeks of starting treatment, and liver test results usually return to normal within 3–4 weeks. If pruritus continues after 2 weeks, the UDCA dose can be gradually increased—typically by about 300 mg each week or adjusted based on the patient's response—up to a maximum of 21 mg/kg per day [71–73].

8.7.2 Clinical Evidence for Therapeutic Efficacy

UDCA provides some maternal benefit but has not shown significant advantages for fetal or neonatal outcomes. In a large meta-analysis, UDCA use led to slight improvements in maternal itching scores and liver function tests compared with placebo or other treatments. However, its effects on reducing overall, spontaneous, or medically induced preterm birth showed only a nonsignificant trend [74]. A key limitation of these studies was the uncertainty as to whether the medication had been administered at adequate doses and for sufficient duration [75].

The largest randomized controlled trial to date, which included 605 patients treated with UDCA twice daily versus placebo, demonstrated modest maternal benefits [76]. Although mean maternal bile acid levels were slightly higher in the UDCA group, improvements were noted in itching scores and alanine aminotransferase (ALT) levels. The reduction in pruritus was statistically significant but considered too small to have a meaningful clinical impact for most patients.

Clinical trials have demonstrated no significant difference in fetal or neonatal outcomes between ursodeoxycholic acid (UDCA) and placebo treatment groups. In one large study, the composite endpoint—including perinatal mortality, preterm delivery, or neonatal intensive care unit (NICU) admission—was reported in 27% of pregnancies treated with UDCA compared with 23% of those receiving placebo [75].

8.7.3 Follow-Up Bile Acid Measurements

Management decisions in intrahepatic cholestasis of pregnancy (ICP) should be based on the highest recorded total serum bile acid (TBA) level, evaluated alongside the patient's obstetric history and current clinical presentation. Weekly monitoring of maternal TBA concentrations is advised, as marked elevations are strongly correlated with increased fetal risk. When very high bile acid levels persist, early delivery may be warranted to mitigate the likelihood of stillbirth [59].

If clinical symptoms improve, UDCA dosage does not need to be modified, even in the presence of persistently elevated laboratory values. Similarly, the planned delivery date does not require adjustment. For patients with persistent clinical findings consistent with ICP but normal TBA or aminotransferase levels, laboratory testing should be repeated, as symptoms may precede biochemical abnormalities by several weeks [41]. Unless there is biochemical evidence of ICP, treatment may be deferred; however, in certain cases, empiric UDCA therapy may be initiated for symptom relief. When ursodeoxycholic acid (UDCA) is initiated empirically, subsequent elevations in total bile acids (TBA) or aminotransferases may not be captured or documented, as biochemical abnormalities can normalize rapidly. In cases unresponsive to UDCA, where pruritus remains intense despite maximal dosing, the use of alternative pharmacologic therapies may be warranted.

S-adenosylmethionine (SAMe)
SAMe, a physiologic precursor of glutathione, contributes to maintaining the structural integrity and flexibility of hepatocyte membranes and supports methylation processes that enhance the excretion of hormone metabolites through bile [77, 78].

Cholestyramine
Cholestyramine acts by impairing the reabsorption of bile salts in the ileum, which in turn promotes their increased excretion through the feces. It is initiated at an oral dose of 2–4 g daily in divided doses, titrated as needed for symptom control to a maximum of 16 g/day [79]. However, its antipruritic effect in ICP is limited, and at higher doses (>4 g/day) it can impair the absorption of fat-soluble vitamins (e.g., vitamin K), and cause constipation, abdominal discomfort, and fat malabsorption.

Rifampicin
Rifampicin functions as a potent activator of the pregnane X receptor, a nuclear receptor involved in regulating hepatic detoxification and bile acid transport pathways. In small clinical series reported by Liu et al. and Geenes et al., the drug was used in patients with severe or UDCA-resistant ICP [64, 79]. These reports documented a reduction in pruritus intensity, partial biochemical improvement, and favorable perinatal outcomes, with all neonates delivered healthy between 32 and 37 weeks of gestation.

8.8 Pregnancy Management

8.8.1 Antepartum Fetal Assessment

Pregnancies affected by ICP should undergo twice-weekly monitoring with biophysical profile assessments. However, the effectiveness of antepartum fetal cardiotocography (CTG) in predicting stillbirth risk among these pregnancies remains uncertain. In one study, pregnancies complicated by ICP that ended in stillbirth did not demonstrate an increased frequency of abnormal findings on nonstress testing (NST) [80]. Furthermore, several reports have described cases of stillbirth occurring within days of a reactive NST [81, 82].

Because fetal demise in intrahepatic cholestasis of pregnancy (ICP) is believed to result from an acute, sudden event rather than from chronic placental vascular insufficiency, NST and other tests—such as biophysical profile scoring and daily fetal movement counts—may have limited utility in detecting at-risk fetuses. Evaluation of fetal condition should involve assessment of fetal movements, cardiotocography, and ultrasound examinations [83].

8.8.2 Timing of Delivery

Early delivery is generally favored in order to reduce the risk of stillbirth and initiate resolution of the disease. When the peak total bile acid (TBA) concentration during pregnancy is below 40 μmol/L, delivery is generally advised between 37 0/7 and 38 6/7 weeks of gestation. In the absence of elevated bile acids, early delivery before 37 weeks should be avoided [69].

When the highest TBA concentration is 40–99 μmol/L, delivery is advised between 36 0/7 and 37 0/7 weeks. When the TBA concentration is ≥100 μmol/L, delivery is recommended at 36 0/7 weeks. However, in patients with additional high-risk factors—such as a history of stillbirth related to ICP—earlier delivery may be considered after thorough counseling regarding the associated risks. In such circumstances, administration of antenatal corticosteroids prior to birth is advised to accelerate the developmental maturity of fetal lungs. In patients without elevated TBA levels but with persistent ICP-related symptoms, delivery between the early 37th and late 38th week of gestation may be considered due to the potential for fetal risk in later gestation. If a patient with ICP reaches 39 0/7 weeks with persistent symptoms, induction of labor is appropriate [69].

8.8.3 Delivery

No specific intrapartum modifications are required solely due to ICP. However, given the increased incidence of stillbirth and nonfatal asphyxial events, continuous fetal monitoring during labor is recommended [84, 85]. The Royal College of Obstetricians and Gynaecologists (RCOG) guidelines recommend initiating delivery at 37 + 0 weeks of gestation in ICP pregnancies complicated by significant biochemical abnormalities. In the absence of evidence from randomized trials, the optimal management—particularly when total bile acid levels exceed 40 μmol/L—is to initiate delivery between 36 and 37 weeks of gestation.

When ICP is managed with UDCA, there is no increased risk of postpartum hemorrhage [86]. Therefore, routine pre-delivery coagulation testing or prophylactic vitamin K administration is not necessary. In uncommon instances where symptoms persist despite standard therapy, assessment of prothrombin time is advised, and if prolongation is detected, vitamin K supplementation should be administered [87, 88]. After childbirth, itching generally resolves within several days, accompanied by normalization of serum bile acid levels and improvement in liver function tests [29].

8.8.4 Breastfeeding

Breastfeeding is strongly recommended because of its well-established benefits for both the mother and the newborn. Intrahepatic cholestasis of pregnancy (ICP) does not represent a contraindication to lactation. As ursodeoxycholic acid (UDCA) is discontinued at the onset of labor, only trace amounts, if any, are transferred to the infant, and no adverse effects have been documented in breastfed neonates [89].

In most cases, TBA levels and liver function tests normalize postpartum. If normalization is delayed, further evaluation should be undertaken to rule out other underlying conditions. Referral to a hepatology specialist is recommended when results do not return to normal. Persistent hepatic or biochemical abnormalities following intrahepatic cholestasis of pregnancy (ICP) may later be linked to the development of gallstone disease, hepatitis C infection, hepatic fibrosis, cholangitis, hepatobiliary malignancies, pancreatic disorders, immune-mediated diseases, or cardiovascular conditions [33, 34, 90–92]. Delayed normalization may also be related to comorbidities such as diabetes mellitus, Crohn's disease, and thyroid disorders. Recurrence in subsequent pregnancies occurs in approximately 60–70% of cases, with variable severity; however, episodes are often more severe than in the index pregnancy.

References

1. Geenes V, Williamson C. Intrahepatic cholestasis of pregnancy. World J Gastroenterol. 2009;15(17):2049–66. https://doi.org/10.3748/wjg.15.2049. PMID: 19418576; PMCID: PMC2678574.
2. Riely CA, Bacq Y. Intrahepatic cholestasis of pregnancy. Clin Liver Dis. 2004;8(1):167–76. https://doi.org/10.1016/S1089-3261(03)00131-4. PMID: 15062199.
3. Estin ML, Campbell AIK, Watkins VY, Dotters-Katz SK, Brady CW, Federspiel JJ. Risk of stillbirth in United States patients with diagnosed intrahepatic cholestasis of pregnancy. Am J Obstet Gynecol. 2023;229(4):453.e1–8. https://doi.org/10.1016/j.ajog.2023.06.036.
4. Laifer SA, Stiller RJ, Siddiqui DS, Dunston-Boone G, Whetham JC. Ursodeoxycholic acid for the treatment of intrahepatic cholestasis of pregnancy. J Matern Fetal Med. 2001;10(2):131–5. https://doi.org/10.1080/714052719. PMID: 11392594.
5. Wikström Shemer E, Marschall HU, Ludvigsson JF, Stephansson O. Intrahepatic cholestasis of pregnancy and associated adverse pregnancy and fetal outcomes: a 12-year population-based cohort study. BJOG. 2013;120(6):717–23. https://doi.org/10.1111/1471-0528.12174.
6. Gonzalez MC, Reyes H, Arrese M, Figueroa D, Lorca B, Andresen M, Segovia N, Molina C, Arce S. Intrahepatic cholestasis of pregnancy in twin pregnancies. J Hepatol. 1989;9(1):84–90. https://doi.org/10.1016/0168-8278(89)90079-2.
7. Savander M, Ropponen A, Avela K, Weerasekera N, Cormand B, Hirvioja ML, Riikonen S, Ylikorkala O, Lehesjoki AE, Williamson C, Aittomäki K. Genetic evidence of heterogeneity in intrahepatic cholestasis of pregnancy. Gut. 2003;52(7):1025–9. https://doi.org/10.1136/gut.52.7.1025.
8. Floreani A, Gervasi MT. New insights on intrahepatic cholestasis of pregnancy. Clin Liver Dis. 2016;20(1):177–89. https://doi.org/10.1016/j.cld.2015.08.010.
9. Pataia V, Dixon PH, Williamson C. Pregnancy and bile acid disorders. Am J Physiol Gastrointest Liver Physiol. 2017;313(1):G1–6. https://doi.org/10.1152/ajpgi.00028.2017.
10. Jacquemin E, De Vree JM, Cresteil D, Sokal EM, Sturm E, Dumont M, Scheffer GL, Paul M, Burdelski M, Bosma PJ, Bernard O, Hadchouel M, Elferink RP. The wide spectrum of multidrug resistance 3 deficiency: from neonatal cholestasis to cirrhosis of adulthood. Gastroenterology. 2001;120(6):1448–58. https://doi.org/10.1053/gast.2001.23984.
11. Jacquemin E, Cresteil D, Manouvrier S, Boute O, Hadchouel M. Heterozygous non-sense mutation of the MDR3 gene in familial intrahepatic cholestasis of pregnancy. Lancet. 1999;353:210–1. https://doi.org/10.1016/S0140-6736(05)77221-4.
12. Kawakita T, Parikh LI, Ramsey PS, Huang CC, Zeymo A, Fernandez M, Smith S, Iqbal SN. Predictors of adverse neonatal outcomes in intrahepatic cholestasis of pregnancy. Am J Obstet Gynecol. 2015;213(4):570.e1–8. https://doi.org/10.1016/j.ajog.2015.06.021.
13. Poupon R, Rosmorduc P, Boëlle PY, Chrétien Y, Corpechot C, Chazouillères O, Housset C, Barbu V. Genotype-phenotype relationships in the low-phospholipid-associated cholelithiasis syndrome: a study of 156 consecutive patients. Hepatology. 2013;58:1105–10. https://doi.org/10.1002/hep.26424.
14. Rosmorduc O, Poupon R. Low phospholipid associated cholelithiasis: association with mutation in the MDR3/ABCB4 gene. Orphanet J Rare Dis. 2007;2:29. https://doi.org/10.1186/1750-1172-2-29.
15. Meier Y, Zodan T, Lang C, Zimmermann R, Kullak-Ublick GA, Meier PJ, Stieger B, Pauli-Magnus C. Increased susceptibility for intrahepatic cholestasis of pregnancy and contraceptive-induced cholestasis in carriers of the 1331T>C polymorphism in the bile salt export pump. World J Gastroenterol. 2008;14:38–45. https://doi.org/10.3748/wjg.14.38.
16. Dixon PH, Wadsworth CA, Chambers J, Donnelly J, Cooley S, Buckley R, Mannino R, Jarvis S, Syngelaki A, Geenes V, et al. A comprehensive analysis of common genetic variation around six candidate loci for intrahepatic cholestasis of pregnancy. Am J Gastroenterol. 2014;109:76–84. https://doi.org/10.1038/ajg.2013.406.

17. Müllenbach R, Bennett A, Tetlow N, Patel N, Hamilton G, Cheng F, Chambers J, Howard R, Taylor-Robinson SD, Williamson C. ATP8B1 mutations in British cases with intrahepatic cholestasis of pregnancy. Gut. 2005;54:29–834. https://doi.org/10.1136/gut.2004.058115.
18. Van Mil SW, Milona A, Dixon PH, Mullenbach R, Geenes VL, Chambers J, Shevchuk V, Moore GE, Lammert F, Glantz AG, et al. Functional variants of the central bile acid sensor FXR identified in intrahepatic cholestasis of pregnancy. Gastroenterology. 2007;133:507–16. https://doi.org/10.1053/j.gastro.2007.05.015.
19. McIlvride S, Dixon PH, Williamson C. Bile acids and gestation. Mol Asp Med. 2017;56:90–100. https://doi.org/10.1016/j.mam.2017.05.003.
20. Geier A, Dietrich OG, Gerloff T, Haendly J, Kullak-Ublick GA, Stieger B, Meier PJ, Matern S, Gartung C. Regulation of basolateral organic anion transporters in ethinylestradiol-induced cholestasis in the rat. Biochim Biophys Acta. 2003;1609:87–94. https://doi.org/10.1016/S0005-2736(02)00657-0.
21. Barth A, Klinger G, Rost M. Influence of ethinyloestradiolpropanolsulphonate on serum bile acids in healthy volunteers. Exp Toxicol Pathol. 2003;54:381–6. https://doi.org/10.1078/0940-2993-00274.
22. Mutlu MF, Aslan K, Guler I, Mutlu I, Erdem M, Bozkurt N, Erdem A. Two cases of first onset intrahepatic cholestasis of pregnancy associated with moderate ovarian hyperstimulation syndrome after IVF treatment and review of the literature. J Obstet Gynaecol. 2017;37(5):547–9. https://doi.org/10.1080/01443615.2017.1286302.
23. Meng LJ, Reyes H, Palma J, Hernandez I, Ribalta J, Sjövall J. Effects of ursodeoxycholic acid on conjugated bile acids and progesterone metabolites in serum and urine of patients with intrahepatic cholestasis of pregnancy. J Hepatol. 1997;27(6):1029–40. https://doi.org/10.1016/s0168-8278(97)80147-x.
24. Abu-Hayyeh S, Ovadia C, Lieu T, et al. Prognostic and mechanistic potential of progesterone sulfates in intrahepatic cholestasis of pregnancy and pruritus gravidarum. Hepatology. 2016;63(4):1287–98. https://doi.org/10.1002/hep.28265.
25. Davies MH, Ngong JM, Yucesoy M, et al. The adverse influence of pregnancy upon sulphation: a clue to the pathogenesis of intrahepatic cholestasis of pregnancy? J Hepatol. 1994;21:1127.
26. Bacq Y, Sapey T, Bréchot MC, Pierre F, Fignon A, Dubois F. Intrahepatic cholestasis of pregnancy: a French prospective study. Hepatology. 1997;26(2):358–64. https://doi.org/10.1002/hep.510260216.
27. Abu-Hayyeh S, Papacleovoulou G, Lövgren-Sandblom A, et al. Intrahepatic cholestasis of pregnancy levels of sulfated progesterone metabolites inhibit farnesoid X receptor resulting in a cholestatic phenotype. Hepatology. 2013;57:716–26. https://doi.org/10.1002/hep.26055.
28. Abu-Hayyeh S, Williamson C. Progesterone metabolites as farnesoid X receptor inhibitors. Hepatology. 2014;60:1815–7. https://doi.org/10.1159/000371565.
29. FDA alerts health care professionals of pregnancy problems associated with thiopurines. Federal Drug Administration. https://www.fda.gov/drugs/drug-safety-and-availability/fda-alerts-health-care-professionals-pregnancy-problems associated-thiopurines. Accessed 25 June 2024.
30. Paffzek A, Duskova M, Vftek L, et al. The role of steroid hormones in the development of intrahepatic cholestasis of pregnancy. Physiol Res. 2015;64(Suppl 2):S203–9. https://doi.org/10.33549/physiolres.933117.
31. Marschall HU, Wikström Shemer E, Ludvigsson JF, Stephansson O. Intrahepatic cholestasis of pregnancy and associated hepatobiliary disease: a population-based cohort study. Hepatology. 2013;58(4):1385–91. https://doi.org/10.1002/hep.26444.
32. Dixon PH, Williamson C. The pathophysiology of intrahepatic cholestasis of pregnancy. Clin Res Hepatol Gastroenterol. 2016;40:141–53. https://doi.org/10.1016/j.clinre.2015.12.008.
33. Ropponen A, Sund R, Riikonen S, Ylikorkala O, Aittomäki K. Intrahepatic cholestasis of pregnancy as an indicator of liver and biliary diseases: a population-based study. Hepatology. 2006;43(4):723–8. https://doi.org/10.1002/hep.21111.

34. Leevy CB, Koneru B, Klein KM. Recurrent familial prolonged intrahepatic cholestasis of pregnancy associated with chronic liver disease. Gastroenterology. 1997;113(3):966–72. https://doi.org/10.1016/s0016-5085(97)70193-8.
35. Turunen K, Mölsa A, Helander K, et al. Health history after intrahepatic cholestasis of pregnancy. Acta Obstet Gynecol Scand. 2012;91(6):679–85. https://doi.org/10.1111/j.1600-0412.2012.01403.x.
36. Hubschmann AG, Orzechowski KM, Berghella V. Severe first trimester recurrent intrahepatic cholestasis of pregnancy: a case report and literature review. AJP Rep. 2016;6(1):e38–41. https://doi.org/10.1055/s-0035-1565922.
37. Kondrackiene J, Kupcinskas L. Intrahepatic cholestasis of pregnancy-current achievements and unsolved problems. World J Gastroenterol. 2008;14(38):5781–8. https://doi.org/10.3748/wjg.14.5781.
38. Heikkinen J, Maentausta O, Ylöstalo P, Janne O. Changes in serum bile acid concentrations during normal pregnancy, in patients with intrahepatic cholestasis of pregnancy and in pregnant women with itching. Br J Obstet Gynaecol. 1981;88(3):240–5.
39. Lunzer M, Barnes P, Byth K, O'Halloran M. Serum bile acid concentrations during pregnancy and their relationship to obstetric cholestasis. Gastroenterology. 1986;91(4):825–9. https://doi.org/10.1016/0016-5085(86)90682-7.
40. Kenyon AP, Piercy CN, Girling J, et al. Obstetric cholestasis, outcome with active management: a series of 70 cases. BJOG. 2002;109(3):282–8. https://doi.org/10.1111/j.1471-0528.2002.01368.x.
41. Brites D, Rodrigues CM, Oliveira N, et al. Correction of maternal serum bile acid profile during ursodeoxycholic acid therapy in cholestasis of pregnancy. J Hepatol. 1998;28(1):91–8. https://doi.org/10.1016/s0168-8278(98)80207-9.
42. Diken Z, Usta IM, Nassar AH. A clinical approach to intrahepatic cholestasis of pregnancy. Am J Perinatol. 2014;31(1):1–8. https://doi.org/10.1055/s-0033-1333673.
43. Huang WM, Gowda M, Donnelly JG. Bile acid ratio in diagnosis of intrahepatic cholestasis of pregnancy. Am J Perinatol. 2009;26(4):291–4. https://doi.org/10.1055/s-0028-1103158.
44. Rolfes DB, Ishak KG. Liver disease in pregnancy. Histopathology. 1986;10(6):555–70. https://doi.org/10.1111/j.1365-2559.1986.tb02510.x.
45. Bicocca MJ, Sperling JD. Chauhan SP intrahepatic cholestasis of pregnancy: review of six national and regional guidelines. Eur J Obstet Gynecol Reprod Biol. 2018;231:180–7. https://doi.org/10.1016/j.ejogrb.2018.10.041.
46. Manzotti C, Casazza G, Stimac T, et al. Total serum bile acids or serum bile acid profile, or both, for the diagnosis of intrahepatic cholestasis of pregnancy. Cochrane Database Syst Rev. 2019;7(7):CD012546. https://doi.org/10.1002/14651858.
47. Ovadia C, Seed PT, Sklavounos A, Geenes V, et al. Association of adverse perinatal outcomes of intrahepatic cholestasis of pregnancy with biochemical markers: results of aggregate and individual patient data meta-analyses. Lancet. 2019;393(10174):899–909. https://doi.org/10.1016/S0140-6736(18)31877-4. Epub 2019 Feb 14. Erratum in: Lancet. 2019 Mar 16;393(10176):1100. https://doi.org/10.1016/S0140-6736(19)30504-5.
48. Engelking LR, Dasher CA, Hirschowitz BI. Within-day fluctuations in serum bile-acid concentrations among normal control subjects and patients with hepatic disease. Am J Clin Pathol. 1980;73(2):196–201. https://doi.org/10.1093/ajcp/73.2.196.
49. Smith DD, Kiefer MK, Lee AJ, et al. Effect of fasting on total bile acid levels in pregnancy. Obstet Gynecol. 2020;136(6):1204–10. https://doi.org/10.1097/AOG.0000000000004160.
50. Mitchell AL, Ovadia C, Syngelaki A, et al. Re-evaluating diagnostic thresholds for intrahepatic cholestasis of pregnancy: case-control and cohort study. BJOG. 2021;128(10):1635–44. https://doi.org/10.1111/1471-0528.16669.
51. Kenyon AP, Tribe RM, Nelson-Piercy C, et al. Pruritus in pregnancy: a study of anatomical distribution and prevalence in relation to the development of obstetric cholestasis. Obstet Med. 2010;3(1):25–9. https://doi.org/10.1258/om.2010.090055.

52. Arafa A, Dong JY. Association between intrahepatic cholestasis of pregnancy and risk of gestational diabetes and preeclampsia: a systematic review and meta-analysis. Hypertens Pregnancy. 2020;39(3):354–60. https://doi.org/10.1080/10641955.2020.1758939.
53. Sentilhes L, Verspyck E, Roman H, Marpeau L. Intrahepatic cholestasis of pregnancy and bile acid levels. Hepatology. 2005;42(3):737–8.
54. Prati D, Taioli E, Zanella A, Della Torre E, Butelli S, Del Vecchio E, Vianello L, Zanuso F, Mozzi F, Milani S, et al. Updated definitions of healthy ranges for serum alanine aminotransferase levels. Ann Intern Med. 2002;137(1):1–10. https://doi.org/10.7326/0003-4819-137-1-200207020-00006.
55. Vanjak D, Moreau R, Roche-Sicot J, et al. Intrahepatic cholestasis of pregnancy and acute fatty liver of pregnancy. An unusual but favorable association? Gastroenterology. 1991;100(4):1123–5. https://doi.org/10.1016/0016-5085(91)90292-s.
56. Rioseco AJ, Ivankovic MB, Manzur A, et al. Intrahepatic cholestasis of pregnancy: a retrospective case-control study of perinatal outcome. Am J Obstet Gynecol. 1994;170(3):890–5. https://doi.org/10.1016/s0002-9378(94)70304-3.
57. Geenes V, Lövgren-Sandblom A, Benthin L, et al. The reversed feto-maternal bile acid gradient in intrahepatic cholestasis of pregnancy is corrected by ursodeoxycholic acid. PLoS One. 2014;9(1):e83828. https://doi.org/10.1371/journal.pone.0083828.
58. Zecca E, De Luca D, Baroni S, et al. Bile acid-induced lung injury in newborn infants: a bronchoalveolar lavage fluid study. Pediatrics. 2008;121(1):e146–9. https://doi.org/10.1542/peds.2007-1220.
59. Di Mascio D, Quist-Nelson J, Riegel M, et al. Perinatal death by bile acid levels in intrahepatic cholestasis of pregnancy: a systematic review. J Matern Fetal Neonatal Med. 2021;34(21):3614–22. https://doi.org/10.1080/14767058.2019.1685965.
60. Castaño G, Lucangioli S, Sookoian S, et al. Bile acid profiles by capillary electrophoresis in intrahepatic cholestasis of pregnancy. Clin Sci (Lond). 2006;110(4):459–65. https://doi.org/10.1042/CS20050302.
61. Williamson C, Miragoli M, Sheikh Abdul Kadir S, et al. Bile acid signaling in fetal tissues: implications for intrahepatic cholestasis of pregnancy. Dig Dis. 2011;29(1):58–61. https://doi.org/10.1159/000324130.
62. Zhan Y, Xu T, Chen T, et al. Intrahepatic cholestasis of pregnancy and fetal cardiac dysfunction: a systematic review and meta-analysis. Am J Obstet Gynecol MFM. 2023;5(8):100952. https://doi.org/10.1016/j.ajogmf.2023.100952.
63. Sepulveda WH, Gonzalez C, Cruz MA, Rudolph MI. Vasoconstrictive effect of bile acids on isolated human placental chorionic veins. Eur J Obstet Gynecol Reprod Biol. 1991;42(3):211–5. https://doi.org/10.1016/0028-2243(91)90222-7.
64. Geenes V, Chappell LC, Seed PT, et al. Association of severe intrahepatic cholestasis of pregnancy with adverse pregnancy outcomes: a prospective population-based case-control study. Hepatology. 2014;59(4):1482–91. https://doi.org/10.1002/hep.26617.
65. Germain AM, Kato S, Carvajal JA, et al. Bile acids increase response and expression of human myometrial oxytocin receptor. Am J Obstet Gynecol. 2003;189(2):577–82. https://doi.org/10.1067/s0002-9378(03)00545-3.
66. Israel EJ, Guzman ML, Campos GA. Maximal response to oxytocin of the isolated myometrium from pregnant patients with intrahepatic cholestasis. Acta Obstet Gynecol Scand. 1986;65(6):581–2. https://doi.org/10.3109/00016348609158391.
67. Williamson C, Hems LM, Goulis DG, et al. Clinical outcome in a series of cases of obstetric cholestasis identified via a patient support group. BJOG. 2004;111(7):676–81. https://doi.org/10.1111/j.1471-0528.2004.00167.x.
68. Uyar I, Gülhan I, Öztekin D, et al. Intrahepatic cholestasis of pregnancy may lead to low birth weight. Turk J Med Sci. 2015;45(3):723–8. https://doi.org/10.3906/sag-1403-7.
69. Society for Maternal-Fetal Medicine (SMFM). Electronic address: pubs@smfm.org, Lee RH, Mara Greenberg, Metz TD, Pettker CM. Society for maternal-fetal medicine consult series

#53: intrahepatic cholestasis of pregnancy: replaces consult #13, April 2011. Am J Obstet Gynecol. 2021;224(2):B2–9. https://doi.org/10.1016/j.ajog.2020.11.002.
70. Williamson C, Geenes V. Intrahepatic cholestasis of pregnancy. Obstet Gynecol. 2014;124(1):120–33. https://doi.org/10.1097/AOG.0000000000000346.
71. Pusl T, Beuers U. Intrahepatic cholestasis of pregnancy. Orphanet J Rare Dis. 2007;2:26. https://doi.org/10.1186/1750-1172-2-26.
72. Bacq Y, le Besco M, Lecuyer AI, et al. Ursodeoxycholic acid therapy in intrahepatic cholestasis of pregnancy: results in real-world conditions and factors predictive of response to treatment. Dig Liver Dis. 2017;49(1):63–9. https://doi.org/10.1016/j.dld.2016.10.006.
73. Walker KF, Chappell LC, Hague WM, et al. Pharmacological interventions for treating intrahepatic cholestasis of pregnancy. Cochrane Database Syst Rev. 2020;7(7):CD000493. https://doi.org/10.1002/14651858.CD000493.
74. Haslinger C. The problem of uncertain adherence to study interventions: what can we conclude? BJOG. 2021;128(6):1076. https://doi.org/10.1111/1471-0528.16613.
75. Chappell LC, Bell JL, Smith A, et al. Ursodeoxycholic acid versus placebo in women with intrahepatic cholestasis of pregnancy (PITCHES): a randomised controlled trial. Lancet. 2019;394(10201):849–60. https://doi.org/10.1016/S0140-6736(19)31270-X.
76. Ozkan S, Ceylan Y, Ozkan OV, Yildirim S. Review of a challenging clinical issue: intrahepatic cholestasis of pregnancy. World J Gastroenterol. 2015;21(23):7134–41. https://doi.org/10.3748/wjg.v21.i23.7134.
77. Zhang Y, Lu L, Victor DW, et al. Ursodeoxycholic acid and S-adenosylmethionine for the treatment of intrahepatic cholestasis of pregnancy: a meta-analysis. Hepat Mon. 2016;16(8):e38558. https://doi.org/10.5812/hepatmon.38558.
78. Coltorti M, Bortolini M, Di Padova C. A review of the studies on the clinical use of S-adenosylmethionine (SAMe) for the symptomatic treatment of intrahepatic cholestasis. Methods Find Exp Clin Pharmacol. 1990;12(1):69–78.
79. Liu J, Murray AM, Mankus EB, et al. Adjuvant use of rifampin for refractory intrahepatic cholestasis of pregnancy. Obstet Gynecol. 2018;132(3):678–81. https://doi.org/10.1097/AOG.0000000000002794.
80. Alsulyman OM, Ouzounian JG, Ames-Castro M, Goodwin TM. Intrahepatic cholestasis of pregnancy: perinatal outcome associated with expectant management. Am J Obstet Gynecol. 1996;175(4 Pt 1):957–60. https://doi.org/10.1016/s0002-9378(96)80031-7.
81. Laatikainen T, Tulenheimo A. Maternal serum bile acid levels and fetal distress in cholestasis of pregnancy. Int J Gynaecol Obstet. 1984;22(2):91–4. https://doi.org/10.1016/0020-7292(84)90019-5.
82. Girling J, Knight CL, Chappell L, Royal College of Obstetricians and Gynaecologists. Intrahepatic cholestasis of pregnancy: green-top guideline no. 43 June 2022. BJOG. 2022;129(13):e95–114. https://doi.org/10.1111/1471-0528.17206.
83. Ozyuncu O, Orgul G, Ozten G, Yurdakok M, Beksac MS. Outpatient versus inpatient follow-up for intrahepatic cholestasis of pregnancy. Clin Exp Hepatol. 2019;5(4):289–93. https://doi.org/10.5114/ceh.2019.88616.
84. Oztekin D, Aydal I, Oztekin O, et al. Predicting fetal asphyxia in intrahepatic cholestasis of pregnancy. Arch Gynecol Obstet. 2009;280(6):975–9. https://doi.org/10.1007/s00404-009-1052-x.
85. Furrer R, Winter K, Schaffer L, et al. Postpartum blood loss in women treated for intrahepatic cholestasis of pregnancy. Obstet Gynecol. 2016;128(5):1048–52. https://doi.org/10.1097/AOG.0000000000001693.
86. Maldonado M, Alhousseini A, Awadalla M, et al. Intrahepatic cholestasis of pregnancy leading to severe vitamin K deficiency and coagulopathy. Case Rep Obstet Gynecol. 2017;2017:5646247. https://doi.org/10.1155/2017/5646247.
87. DeLeon A, De Oliveira GS, Kalayil M, et al. The incidence of coagulopathy in pregnant patients with intrahepatic cholestasis: should we delay or avoid neuraxial analgesia? J Clin Anesth. 2014;26(8):623–7. https://doi.org/10.1016/j.jclinane.2014.04.013.

88. Cemortan M, Sagaidac I, Cernetchi O. Comparative analysis of vitamin K levels in women with intrahepatic cholestasis of pregnancy. BMC Pregnancy Childbirth. 2025;25(1):405. https://doi.org/10.1186/s12884-025-07515-1.
89. Hirvioja ML, Kivinen S. Inheritance of intrahepatic cholestasis of pregnancy in one kindred. Clin Genet. 1993;43(6):315–7. https://doi.org/10.1111/j.1399-0004.1993.tb03826.x.
90. Wikström Shemer EA, Stephansson O, Thuresson M, et al. Intrahepatic cholestasis of pregnancy and cancer, immune-mediated and cardiovascular diseases: a population-based cohort study. J Hepatol. 2015;63(2):456–61. https://doi.org/10.1016/j.jhep.2015.03.010.
91. Hamalainen ST, Turunen K, Mattila KJ, et al. Intrahepatic cholestasis of pregnancy and comorbidity: a 44-year follow-up study. Acta Obstet Gynecol Scand. 2019;98(12):1534–9. https://doi.org/10.1111/aogs.13695.
92. Curtis KM, Tepper NK, Jatlaoui TC, et al. U.S. medical eligibility criteria for contraceptive use, 2016. MMWR Recomm Rep. 2016;65(3):1–103. https://doi.org/10.15585/mmwr.rr6503a1.

Chapter 9
Navigating Anemia Challenges During Pregnancy and Hematologic Disorders

Onur Yavuz

9.1 Introduction

Anemia is the most common hematologic complication in pregnancy, affecting approximately one-third of pregnant women worldwide [1]. The World Health Organization (WHO) defines anemia in pregnancy as a hemoglobin concentration below 11.0 g/dL in the first and third trimesters and below 10.5 g/dL in the second trimester [2]. While mild cases may be asymptomatic, moderate to severe anemia can lead to substantial risks, including maternal fatigue, reduced work capacity, cardiac stress, and increased risk of maternal mortality [3].

The burden of anemia is most profound in resource-limited settings due to a combination of dietary insufficiency, high rates of parasitic infections, and inadequate antenatal care [4]. Nevertheless, even in high-income countries, iron deficiency and underrecognized hemoglobinopathies remain common and can lead to adverse pregnancy outcomes if unaddressed.

The etiologies of anemia during pregnancy are multifactorial. Iron-deficiency anemia accounts for the majority of cases, resulting from increased maternal iron requirements coupled with insufficient intake or absorption. Other contributors include folate and vitamin B12 deficiencies, hemoglobinopathies such as sickle cell disease and thalassemia, chronic inflammation, and bone marrow failure syndromes. Each type has distinct pathophysiological mechanisms, diagnostic features, and treatment approaches.

Untreated anemia is associated with poor obstetric outcomes. Maternal complications include fatigue, immune dysfunction, postpartum hemorrhage, and an increased need for transfusions. Fetal complications may include prematurity, low

O. Yavuz (✉)
Dokuz Eylul University, Faculty of Medicine, Department of Obstetrics and Gynecology, Izmir, Turkey
e-mail: onur.yavuz@deu.edu.tr

© The Author(s), under exclusive license to Springer Nature Switzerland AG 2026

I. Karaca (ed.), *Managing Maternal Chronic Diseases for a Healthy Pregnancy*,
https://doi.org/10.1007/978-3-032-15221-3_9

birth weight, and impaired neurodevelopment [5]. Identifying and correcting anemia early in pregnancy improves outcomes and is a priority in global maternal health strategies [6].

Effective management begins with an understanding of the physiologic hematologic changes that occur during pregnancy, which influence both laboratory interpretation and clinical thresholds for intervention.

9.2 Hematological Adaptations During Pregnancy

Pregnancy induces a complex series of hematologic and cardiovascular adaptations that are essential to support fetal growth and maternal survival during childbirth. These physiological changes begin early in gestation and continue to evolve throughout the pregnancy, significantly affecting the interpretation of laboratory results and the thresholds for diagnosing hematologic disorders.

One of the most significant adaptations is the expansion of plasma volume, which can increase by 40–50% by the third trimester [7]. In contrast, red blood cell (RBC) mass increases by only 20–30%. This mismatch creates a dilutional effect, reducing the concentration of hemoglobin and hematocrit—a condition referred to as physiologic anemia of pregnancy [8]. Though hemoglobin values may appear low, this is often a normal finding in healthy pregnancies and should be interpreted in context.

In addition to plasma expansion, leukocyte counts typically rise during pregnancy. The white blood cell (WBC) count can reach 12,000–16,000/μL in the absence of infection, predominantly due to neutrophilia [9]. This physiologic leukocytosis is considered benign but may be misinterpreted as a sign of infection if the clinical context is not considered.

Another common change is a mild decrease in platelet count, termed gestational thrombocytopenia, which affects approximately 5–10% of pregnancies [10]. In most cases, platelet levels remain above 100,000/μL, and the condition resolves spontaneously postpartum without intervention. Unlike immune thrombocytopenic purpura (ITP) or preeclampsia-associated thrombocytopenia, gestational thrombocytopenia is not associated with bleeding or adverse fetal outcomes.

Cardiovascular changes also play a role in hematologic adaptation. Systemic vascular resistance decreases, while cardiac output increases by as much as 30–50%, leading to enhanced perfusion of maternal organs and the uterus [11]. These hemodynamic shifts may contribute to symptoms such as fatigue, palpitations, and lightheadedness, which can sometimes mimic or mask the clinical features of anemia.

Iron metabolism undergoes a significant transformation during pregnancy. As fetal demands increase, maternal iron absorption rises to compensate. This process is regulated by hepcidin, a key hormone in iron homeostasis. Normally, hepcidin is suppressed during pregnancy to enhance iron uptake from the diet. However, in states of infection or inflammation, elevated hepcidin can block intestinal iron absorption, leading to functional iron deficiency, even when total body iron stores are adequate [12].

Recognizing these physiological changes is essential to avoid misdiagnosing normal adaptations as pathology or, conversely, to avoid missing true anemia due to inappropriate thresholds. Clinical judgment, supported by trimester-specific reference ranges, is necessary for accurate diagnosis and appropriate management.

9.3 Iron-Deficiency Anemia (IDA)

9.3.1 Pathophysiology

Iron-deficiency anemia (IDA) is the most common cause of anemia in pregnancy, accounting for up to 70% of all cases worldwide [13]. During pregnancy, iron demand increases significantly due to several physiological needs: expanding maternal red blood cell mass, development of the fetus and placenta, and preparation for blood loss during delivery. The total iron requirement in a singleton pregnancy is estimated to be approximately 1000–1200 mg [14].

Iron is essential for hemoglobin synthesis, cellular respiration, and enzymatic functions. To meet gestational demands, intestinal iron absorption increases, regulated by hepcidin, a key peptide hormone produced by the liver. Hepcidin controls systemic iron levels by binding to ferroportin, the iron exporter on enterocytes, causing its degradation. When hepcidin is suppressed—as occurs physiologically in pregnancy—iron absorption from the intestine increases [15]. However, in conditions of chronic inflammation, infections, or obesity, hepcidin levels can remain elevated, limiting iron bioavailability even in the presence of adequate dietary intake—a phenomenon known as functional iron deficiency [16].

The depletion of iron progresses through three stages: first, storage iron (reflected by serum ferritin) is reduced; second, circulating iron becomes insufficient, affecting transferrin saturation; finally, hemoglobin synthesis becomes impaired, leading to microcytic, hypochromic anemia. Erythrocytes become smaller (low mean corpuscular volume, MCV) and paler (low mean corpuscular hemoglobin concentration, MCHC), which can be detected on a peripheral blood smear.

9.3.2 Clinical Features

The clinical presentation of IDA during pregnancy can vary depending on the severity and the woman's baseline health. In mild cases, symptoms may be absent or misattributed to the pregnancy itself. As anemia worsens, typical symptoms begin to manifest, including:

- Fatigue and generalized weakness
- Shortness of breath on exertion

- Palpitations or tachycardia
- Dizziness or faintness
- Headache
- Pale skin, mucous membranes, or nail beds

In more advanced cases, pregnant individuals may develop pica, a craving for non-nutritive substances such as ice, clay, or starch. Restless leg syndrome has also been associated with iron deficiency. Severe or untreated IDA increases the risk of complications such as:

- Intrauterine growth restriction (IUGR)
- Preterm birth
- Low birth weight
- Postpartum hemorrhage
- Increased maternal susceptibility to infection
- Maternal cardiac decompensation in extreme cases [17]

On physical examination, signs may include pale conjunctiva, systolic flow murmurs, and koilonychia (spoon-shaped nails), although these are less frequently observed in well-nourished populations. It is essential to assess both symptoms and laboratory markers to confirm the diagnosis and determine the need for intervention.

9.3.3 Diagnosis

Diagnosing iron-deficiency anemia (IDA) in pregnancy requires careful interpretation of laboratory data within the context of pregnancy-induced hematologic changes. Physiologic hemodilution complicates the use of hemoglobin and hematocrit as sole diagnostic criteria. Therefore, a combination of hematologic and biochemical markers is essential for accurate diagnosis.

The World Health Organization defines anemia in pregnancy as a hemoglobin concentration below 11.0 g/dL in the first and third trimesters, and below 10.5 g/dL in the second trimester [2]. However, these thresholds may vary slightly across clinical guidelines and institutions.

Serum ferritin is the most widely accepted marker of iron stores. In pregnant women, a ferritin level below 30 ng/mL is generally considered diagnostic of iron deficiency, even in the absence of anemia [18]. Ferritin is also an acute-phase reactant and may be falsely elevated in inflammatory states. Therefore, concurrent measurement of C-reactive protein (CRP) is useful to distinguish between pure IDA and anemia of chronic disease.

Other supportive laboratory findings in IDA include:

- Low serum iron
- Elevated total iron-binding capacity (TIBC)
- Low transferrin saturation (<20%)

- Increased soluble transferrin receptor (sTfR)
- Low reticulocyte hemoglobin content (CHr)

Peripheral blood smear may show microcytosis, hypochromia, and anisopoikilocytosis. Red cell distribution width (RDW) is often elevated, reflecting a heterogeneous erythrocyte population.

In early pregnancy, anemia may be asymptomatic and only detected during routine first-trimester labs. Therefore, universal screening for anemia is recommended at the first prenatal visit and again in the late second or early third trimester, especially in high-risk populations [19].

A diagnostic algorithm for anemia in pregnancy typically involves:

1. CBC (complete blood count) with differential
2. Ferritin and transferrin saturation
3. Reticulocyte count
4. CRP (if ferritin borderline or elevated)
5. Additional tests as needed: B12, folate, hemoglobin electrophoresis

It is critical not to assume iron deficiency in all anemic pregnancies. Misdiagnosis can lead to unnecessary iron therapy, delayed identification of other etiologies (e.g., thalassemia trait, vitamin deficiencies), and failure to address the underlying cause.

9.3.4 *Management of Iron-Deficiency Anemia in Pregnancy*

The management of iron-deficiency anemia (IDA) during pregnancy depends on the severity of anemia, gestational age, patient tolerance to therapy, and urgency of correction. Early identification and prompt treatment are essential to minimize complications for both mother and fetus.

9.3.4.1 Oral Iron Therapy

First-line treatment for mild to moderate IDA in pregnancy is oral iron supplementation. Ferrous salts such as ferrous sulfate, ferrous fumarate, and ferrous gluconate are commonly used, with ferrous sulfate being the most widely prescribed. These preparations typically provide 60–120 mg of elemental iron daily [20].

For best absorption, iron should be taken:

- On an empty stomach
- With vitamin C (ascorbic acid), which enhances absorption
- At least 1–2 h apart from calcium-rich foods or supplements, antacids, and tea/coffee

However, gastrointestinal side effects such as nausea, constipation, metallic taste, and epigastric discomfort are common and lead to poor adherence in up to

30–50% of patients [21]. Slow-release or enteric-coated formulations may reduce side effects but also decrease iron absorption.

Clinical response to oral iron therapy is usually observed within 2–3 weeks, with a hemoglobin rise of 10.0 g/dL or more over 2–4 weeks being a positive sign. If there is no response, reasons such as poor adherence, malabsorption (e.g., celiac disease), continued bleeding, or incorrect diagnosis must be considered.

9.3.4.2 Intravenous Iron Therapy

IV iron is indicated in the following situations:

- Moderate to severe anemia (Hb <9.0 g/dL) diagnosed in the late second or third trimester
- Intolerance or noncompliance with oral iron
- Functional iron deficiency (e.g., high hepcidin, inflammation)
- Imminent delivery when rapid correction is needed
- Iron-refractory iron-deficiency anemia

Commonly used intravenous iron formulations include:

- *Ferric carboxymaltose:*
- This formulation allows for the administration of up to 1000 mg per session. It is generally well tolerated and enables correction of iron deficiency with fewer infusions due to the possibility of a single high-dose administration.
- *Iron sucrose:*
- The maximum dose per infusion is limited to 200 mg, necessitating multiple sessions to achieve total iron repletion. While effective, this may increase the treatment burden for patients.
- *Iron isomaltoside (ferric derisomaltose):*
- This agent permits flexible dosing up to 20 mg/kg per session. It is associated with a lower incidence of anaphylactic reactions and may be preferable in patients with a history of hypersensitivity.

Intravenous iron is generally considered safe in pregnancy, especially after the first trimester. Anaphylaxis is extremely rare with newer preparations, although all infusions should be administered in monitored settings.

9.3.4.3 Monitoring and Follow-Up

After initiating treatment:

- Re-check hemoglobin after 2–4 weeks
- If oral iron is used, monitor ferritin after 4–6 weeks

- Continue supplementation for 3 months after anemia correction and at least 6 weeks postpartum to replenish iron stores [22]

It is important to tailor the iron regimen based on patient tolerance, anemia severity, gestational age, and expected delivery timing. In women at high risk for recurrent IDA (e.g., multiple pregnancies, low dietary intake), routine prophylactic iron may be extended through lactation.

9.4 Folate and Vitamin B12 Deficiency Anemias

9.4.1 Folate Deficiency

Folate (vitamin B9) plays a vital role in DNA synthesis, cellular replication, and erythropoiesis. During pregnancy, the demand for folate significantly increases to support rapid fetal growth and placental development. Inadequate folate intake or increased requirements can lead to megaloblastic anemia, characterized by the presence of large, immature red blood cells.

Daily folate requirements rise from 400 mcg in nonpregnant women to at least 600 mcg in pregnancy, and up to 4 mg/day is recommended in high-risk cases (e.g., prior neural tube defects, antiepileptic drug use) [23].

Folate deficiency in pregnancy is associated with:

- Neural tube defects (NTDs) such as spina bifida and anencephaly
- Preterm birth
- Abruptio placentae
- Low birth weight
- Maternal anemia and elevated homocysteine levels, increasing vascular risk [24]

Clinical signs of folate deficiency anemia may include fatigue, glossitis (smooth, red tongue), pallor, and irritability. Laboratory findings show:

- Macrocytic anemia (MCV >100 fL)
- Hypersegmented neutrophils on blood smear
- Low serum folate
- Elevated homocysteine (specific to folate and B12 deficiency)

Diagnosis is confirmed via serum or red blood cell folate levels. Since folate stores are relatively limited in the body, deficiency can develop within weeks of poor intake. Treatment involves oral folic acid supplementation, usually 1–5 mg/day until hematologic recovery, followed by standard prenatal supplementation.

9.4.2 *Vitamin B12 Deficiency*

Vitamin B12 (cobalamin) is essential for DNA synthesis, neurological function, and myelin formation. It is absorbed in the ileum via intrinsic factor-mediated transport. B12 deficiency in pregnancy is less common than folate deficiency but has serious consequences if unrecognized.

Common causes include:

- Malabsorption (e.g., pernicious anemia, Crohn's disease, gastric surgery)
- Inadequate intake (e.g., strict vegan diet)
- Use of metformin or proton pump inhibitors

Clinical manifestations are broader than folate deficiency and may include:

- Fatigue, pallor
- Glossitis
- Neurologic symptoms: paresthesia, numbness, impaired proprioception, memory changes
- Gait disturbances and mood disorders in severe cases

Lab findings include:

- Macrocytic anemia (often more severe than folate-related)
- Hypersegmented neutrophils
- Low serum B12 (<200 pg/mL)
- Elevated methylmalonic acid (MMA) and homocysteine

Untreated B12 deficiency can lead to irreversible neurologic damage, especially in the fetus, including developmental delay and hypotonia. Therefore, early detection is critical.

Treatment requires parenteral therapy, typically 1000 mcg intramuscularly weekly for 4 weeks, followed by monthly maintenance. Oral high-dose B12 (1000–2000 mcg/day) may be used for non-neurologic cases but is less reliable in malabsorptive conditions [25].

Combined folate and B12 deficiencies can coexist. Supplementing folate alone in B12-deficient individuals can correct anemia but worsen neurologic symptoms, so both should be checked in macrocytic anemia.

9.5 Hemoglobinopathies in Pregnancy

Hemoglobinopathies are inherited disorders of hemoglobin structure or production that can significantly complicate pregnancy. The two most clinically important types are sickle cell disease (SCD) and thalassemias, both of which are more common in certain geographic and ethnic populations. These disorders require specialized management during pregnancy to minimize maternal and fetal risks.

9.5.1 Sickle Cell Disease (SCD)

SCD is caused by a point mutation in the β-globin gene, leading to the production of hemoglobin S (HbS). Under deoxygenated conditions, HbS polymerizes, causing red blood cells to become rigid and sickle-shaped. These abnormally shaped cells occlude small blood vessels, resulting in vaso-occlusive crises, chronic hemolysis, and multiorgan damage [26].

Pregnancy in women with SCD is considered high-risk due to the increased metabolic demands and prothrombotic state. Common complications include:

- Increased frequency of vaso-occlusive crises
- Acute chest syndrome (a leading cause of maternal morbidity)
- Preeclampsia and eclampsia
- Urinary tract infections and pyelonephritis
- Intrauterine growth restriction (IUGR)
- Preterm delivery
- Stillbirth and perinatal death [27]

Management of SCD in pregnancy includes:

- Multidisciplinary care with obstetricians and hematologists
- Close antenatal surveillance (serial growth scans, Doppler)
- Folic acid 4 mg/day due to high erythropoietic demand
- Avoidance of hydroxyurea, which is teratogenic
- Prophylactic transfusions in selected cases (e.g., history of severe disease, frequent crises)
- Prompt treatment of infections and pain control (e.g., acetaminophen, opioids when needed)

Delivery planning is individualized. Cesarean section is reserved for obstetric indications. Epidural analgesia is preferred during labor to reduce pain-induced hypoxia.

9.5.2 Thalassemia Syndromes

Thalassemias are inherited disorders caused by reduced or absent synthesis of α- or β-globin chains. The clinical spectrum ranges from asymptomatic carriers to transfusion-dependent anemia.

- β-thalassemia trait (minor) is typically asymptomatic. Women may present with mild microcytic anemia but should not be treated with iron unless iron deficiency is confirmed.
- β-thalassemia intermedia may require occasional transfusions during pregnancy.
- β-thalassemia major often leads to infertility due to iron-induced hypogonadism; however, with improved care, pregnancy is becoming more feasible.

Complications in thalassemia pregnancies include:

- Cardiac decompensation due to iron overload
- Endocrine abnormalities (e.g., diabetes, hypothyroidism)
- Hepatic dysfunction
- Increased risk of thromboembolic events [28]

Management strategies include:

- Preconception counseling and genetic testing of both partners
- Hemoglobin electrophoresis for diagnosis and risk assessment of fetal inheritance
- Monitoring iron overload via serum ferritin and MRI (if applicable)
- Regular transfusions to maintain Hb >10.0 g/dL if needed
- Chelation therapy (e.g., deferoxamine) avoided during pregnancy unless absolutely necessary

Prenatal diagnosis (chorionic villus sampling or amniocentesis) is offered if both parents are carriers, especially for β-thalassemia major or hemoglobin Bart's hydrops fetalis.

9.6 Bone Marrow Failure and Thrombocytopenic Disorders in Pregnancy

9.6.1 Aplastic Anemia and Myelodysplastic Syndromes

Aplastic anemia is a rare but potentially life-threatening condition during pregnancy, characterized by pancytopenia and hypocellular bone marrow without infiltration or fibrosis. It can be idiopathic or secondary to autoimmune diseases, drugs, viral infections, or environmental toxins [29]. The condition may be present before pregnancy or emerge de novo during gestation.

Clinical manifestations include:

- Fatigue and pallor (due to anemia)
- Frequent infections (due to neutropenia)
- Easy bruising or bleeding (due to thrombocytopenia)

Diagnosis is confirmed by bone marrow biopsy, which reveals a markedly hypocellular marrow with fatty replacement. CBC shows low counts in all three cell lines.

Management is challenging:

- Supportive care with transfusions is the mainstay.
- Immunosuppressive therapy (e.g., antithymocyte globulin + cyclosporine) may be used after weighing fetal risks.
- Hematopoietic stem cell transplantation is generally deferred until postpartum unless the condition is life-threatening.

Pregnancy is often discouraged in women with a history of severe aplastic anemia unless remission is achieved. In diagnosed cases, multidisciplinary care and individual risk assessment are essential.

Myelodysplastic syndromes (MDS) are exceedingly rare in pregnancy and typically occur in older women. These clonal disorders involve ineffective hematopoiesis, cytopenias, and a risk of transformation to acute leukemia. In pregnancy, management is usually conservative unless transformation occurs. Fetal growth and maternal counts must be monitored closely [30].

9.6.2 Thrombocytopenia and Hypercoagulability in Pregnancy

Pregnancy is a naturally hypercoagulable state, an adaptive mechanism to prevent postpartum hemorrhage. However, this state increases the risk of thromboembolic events and complicates the evaluation of platelet disorders.

Gestational thrombocytopenia is the most common cause of low platelet count in pregnancy, accounting for ~75% of cases. It usually occurs in the third trimester, with platelet counts remaining above 70,000/μL. It is benign, asymptomatic, and does not require treatment [31].

Immune thrombocytopenic purpura (ITP) is an autoimmune condition in which antibodies destroy platelets. It may predate pregnancy or be newly diagnosed. Platelet levels may fall below 50,000/μL, increasing bleeding risk during labor or surgery.

Treatment options include:

- Corticosteroids (prednisone 1 mg/kg/day)
- Intravenous immunoglobulin (IVIG) for refractory or urgent cases
- Splenectomy in severe, chronic cases (preferably in the second trimester)

Delivery planning depends on platelet count:

- Vaginal delivery: ≥50,000/μL
- Cesarean or regional anesthesia: ≥75,000–80,000/μL

Antiphospholipid syndrome (APS) is a prothrombotic autoimmune condition associated with recurrent miscarriage, pre-eclampsia, fetal growth restriction, and thrombosis. Diagnosis requires clinical criteria and persistently positive antiphospholipid antibodies.

Management includes:

- Low-dose aspirin (81 mg daily)
- Prophylactic or therapeutic low molecular weight heparin (e.g., enoxaparin)

Women with known thrombophilias or a history of thromboembolism may also require anticoagulation during pregnancy and the postpartum period.

9.7 Public Health Implications and Global Perspectives

Anemia during pregnancy is not only a clinical issue but also a major public health concern, especially in low- and middle-income countries (LMICs). Its high prevalence is driven by multiple, interrelated factors:

- Nutritional deficiencies (iron, folate, B12)
- High rates of parasitic infections (e.g., hookworm, malaria)
- Limited access to prenatal care and diagnostic services
- Frequent and closely spaced pregnancies
- Socioeconomic inequities and gender-based disparities

The World Health Organization (WHO) estimates that more than 40% of pregnant women in LMICs are anemic [1]. This has significant implications for maternal mortality, neonatal outcomes, and long-term child development.

Evidence-based public health strategies for reducing anemia include:

- Universal iron-folic acid supplementation during pregnancy
- Food fortification (e.g., wheat flour with iron and folic acid)
- Deworming in endemic regions
- Malaria prophylaxis and treatment
- Micronutrient education and behavioral change campaigns

National policies that promote early antenatal care, integrate nutrition with reproductive health services, and expand access to diagnostics are essential. Community-based interventions, especially in rural areas, are crucial to address systemic barriers.

Moreover, data collection and monitoring systems are needed to evaluate progress. Reducing anemia prevalence in pregnancy is a key step toward achieving Sustainable Development Goals (SDGs) related to maternal and child health.

Anemia and hematologic disorders during pregnancy represent a diverse and complex group of conditions with far-reaching consequences for both mother and fetus. While iron-deficiency anemia remains the most common cause, clinicians must remain vigilant for other etiologies such as folate and vitamin B12 deficiency, hemoglobinopathies, and bone marrow failure syndromes.

Pregnancy introduces unique physiological changes that affect hematologic parameters and can mask or mimic disease. Effective diagnosis and management depend on a combination of clinical judgment, targeted laboratory testing, and evidence-based interventions.

A multidisciplinary approach—involving obstetricians, hematologists, dietitians, and public health professionals—is essential for optimal care. Prevention strategies, especially in high-burden regions, must be scaled through health policy and community engagement.

Ultimately, reducing the burden of maternal anemia is not only a medical goal but a global health priority with lasting benefits for generations to come.

References

1. Kassebaum NJ, Jasrasaria R, Naghavi M, Wulf SK, Johns N, Lozano R, et al. A systematic analysis of global anemia burden from 1990 to 2010. Blood. 2014;123(5):615–24.
2. World Health Organization. Haemoglobin concentrations for the diagnosis of anaemia and assessment of severity. Geneva: WHO; 2011.
3. Stevens GA, Finucane MM, De-Regil LM, Paciorek CJ, Flaxman SR, Branca F, et al. Global, regional, and national trends in hemoglobin concentration. Lancet Glob Health. 2013;1(1):e16–25.
4. Aguayo VM, Paintal K. Determinants of anemia among women in India. Matern Child Nutr. 2016;12(Suppl 1):69–82.
5. Daru J, Zamora J, Fernández-Félix BM, Vogel J, Oladapo OT, Tunçalp Ö, et al. Risk of maternal mortality in women with severe anemia. Lancet Glob Health. 2018;6(5):e548–54.
6. Balarajan Y, Ramakrishnan U, Özaltin E, Shankar AH, Subramanian SV. Anaemia in low-income and middle-income countries. Lancet. 2011;378(9809):2123–35.
7. Cunningham FG, Leveno KJ, Bloom SL, Dashe JS, Hoffman BL, Casey BM, et al. Williams obstetrics. 25th ed. New York: McGraw-Hill; 2018.
8. Milman N. Iron and pregnancy—a delicate balance. Ann Hematol. 2006;85(9):559–65.
9. Abbassi-Ghanavati M, Greer LG, Cunningham FG. Pregnancy and laboratory studies: a reference table. Obstet Gynecol. 2009;114(6):1326–31.
10. Reese JA, Peck JD, Deschamps DR, McIntosh JJ, Owings CL, Bougie DW, et al. Platelet counts during pregnancy. Am J Hematol. 2013;88(11):1034–9.
11. Ueland K, Hansen JM. Maternal cardiovascular dynamics. Am J Obstet Gynecol. 1969;104(6):856–64.
12. Sangkhae V, Nemeth E. Regulation of the iron homeostatic hormone hepcidin. Adv Nutr. 2017;8(1):126–36.
13. Pavord S, Daru J, Prasannan N, Robinson S, Stanworth S, Girling J. UK guidelines on the management of iron deficiency in pregnancy. Br J Haematol. 2020;188(6):819–30.
14. Bothwell TH. Iron requirements in pregnancy and strategies to meet them. Am J Clin Nutr. 2000;72(1):257S–64S.
15. Zimmermann MB, Hurrell RF. Nutritional iron deficiency. Lancet. 2007;370(9586):511–20.
16. Young MF, Oaks BM, Tandon S, Martorell R, Dewey KG, Wendt AS. Maternal hepcidin and iron absorption during pregnancy. J Nutr. 2022;152(2):319–27.
17. Lone FW, Qureshi RN, Emmanuel F. Maternal anemia and its impact on perinatal outcome in a tertiary care hospital in Pakistan. East Mediterr Health J. 2004;10(6):801–7.
18. De Benoist B, McLean E, Egli I, Cogswell M. Worldwide prevalence of anaemia 1993–2005. Geneva: WHO; 2008.
19. Centers for Disease Control and Prevention. Recommendations to prevent and control iron deficiency in the United States. MMWR Recomm Rep. 1998;47(RR-3):1–29.
20. Peña-Rosas JP, De-Regil LM, Garcia-Casal MN, Dowswell T. Daily oral iron supplementation during pregnancy. Cochrane Database Syst Rev. 2015;7:CD004736.
21. Tolkien Z, Stecher L, Mander AP, Pereira DI, Powell JJ. Ferrous sulfate supplementation causes significant gastrointestinal side-effects. PLoS One. 2015;10(2):e0117383.
22. National Institute for Health and Care Excellence. Antenatal care for uncomplicated pregnancies. NICE guideline CG62. London: NICE; 2019.
23. De-Regil LM, Fernández-Gaxiola AC, Dowswell T, Peña-Rosas JP. Folic acid supplementation for preventing neural tube defects. Cochrane Database Syst Rev. 2015;10:CD007950.
24. Scholl TO. Maternal iron and folate status and pregnancy outcome. J Nutr. 2005;135(9):1961–5.
25. O'Leary F, Samman S. Vitamin B12 in health and disease. Nutrients. 2010;2(3):299–316.
26. Oteng-Ntim E, Meeks D, Seed PT, Webster L, Howard J, Doyle P, et al. Adverse pregnancy outcomes in women with sickle cell disease. BJOG. 2015;122(4):480–8.
27. Villers MS, Jamison MG, De Castro LM, James AH. Morbidity associated with sickle cell disease in pregnancy. Am J Obstet Gynecol. 2008;199(2):125.e1–5.

28. Taher AT, Musallam KM, Cappellini MD. Thalassemias. Hematology Am Soc Hematol Educ Program. 2021;2021(1):256–66.
29. Desai PC, Aranoff GM, Petrucci R. Aplastic anemia in pregnancy. Hematol Oncol Clin North Am. 2011;25(2):293–310.
30. Della Porta MG, Tuechler H, Malcovati L, Schanz J, Savic A, Valent P, et al. Myelodysplastic syndromes: diagnostic and prognostic considerations. Lancet. 2022;400(10352):2233–47.
31. Gernsheimer T. Thrombocytopenia in pregnancy: evaluation and management. Hematology Am Soc Hematol Educ Program. 2012;2012(1):421–6.

Chapter 10
Thyroid and Parathyroid Disease During Pregnancy

İlker Kızıloğlu

10.1 Introduction

Thyroid disease represents one of the most prevalent endocrine diseases encountered during pregnancy, exerting profound effects on maternal health and fetal development. Pregnancy induces complex physiological changes, including increased human chorionic gonadotropin (hCG) and estrogen levels, which modulate thyroid hormone synthesis, binding, and metabolism. These alterations are vital for accommodating gestational metabolic demands and supporting early fetal neurodevelopment, yet they may obscure or simulate thyroid pathology, complicating clinical assessment.

Hypothyroidism, especially in its subclinical form, is frequently underdiagnosed but associated with significant obstetric complications such as miscarriage, preeclampsia, placental abruption, low birth weight, and neurodevelopmental impairments. Levothyroxine continues to be the mainstay of treatment, especially for overt cases of hypothyroidism and selectively for subclinical hypothyroidism when thyroid autoimmunity is present. In contrast, hyperthyroidism—most commonly due to Graves' disease—is less prevalent but associated with maternal thyrotoxic crisis, gestational hypertension, and fetal risks including intrauterine restriction of fetal growth and/or the possibility of preterm delivery. Treatment necessitates trimester-specific use of antithyroid medications, with propylthiouracil favored in early pregnancy due to teratogenic concerns.

Autoimmune thyroiditis, particularly Hashimoto's disease, often manifests as isolated thyroid antibody positivity in euthyroid women and has been implicated in adverse reproductive outcomes. While the use of levothyroxine therapy in these

İ. Kızıloğlu (✉)
Izmir Bakircay University, Faculty of Medicine, Department of General Surgery, Izmir, Turkey
e-mail: ilker.kiziloglu@bakircay.edu.tr

© The Author(s), under exclusive license to Springer Nature Switzerland AG 2026

I. Karaca (ed.), *Managing Maternal Chronic Diseases for a Healthy Pregnancy*,
https://doi.org/10.1007/978-3-032-15221-3_10

cases is still debated, there is evidence to suggest it may provide a selective benefit. Current screening practices for thyroid dysfunction during pregnancy are debated; while targeted screening is widely endorsed, the potential benefits of universal screening for subclinical disease remain under investigation.

Benign thyroid nodules and differentiated thyroid carcinoma identified during gestation are typically indolent and can often be managed conservatively. Surgery, when indicated, is optimally performed during the second trimester. Overall, the management of thyroid disorders in pregnancy necessitates individualized, multidisciplinary care tailored to gestational physiology, disease severity, and evolving clinical guidelines to optimize maternal and fetal outcomes.

Parathyroid diseases during pregnancy represent a rare but clinically significant group of disorders that can profoundly affect maternal and fetal outcomes. These conditions include primary hyperparathyroidism (PHPT), hypoparathyroidism, pseudohypoparathyroidism, and secondary hyperparathyroidism. Physiological adaptations in calcium metabolism during pregnancy, such as induced absorption of intestinal calcium and elevated levels of 1,25-dihydroxyvitamin D, are essential for fetal skeletal development, particularly in the third trimester. Disruption of this finely tuned system, as seen in parathyroid disorders, may lead to complications including nephrolithiasis, preeclampsia, pancreatitis, and life-threatening maternal or neonatal hypocalcemia.

Primary hyperparathyroidism, though rare, is the most common parathyroid disorder encountered during pregnancy. This condition is frequently asymptomatic but can manifest with symptoms related to hypercalcemia and lead to adverse outcomes, including growth restriction of the fetus, neonatal hypocalcemia, and preterm delivery. For moderate to severe cases, surgical intervention in the second trimester is the preferred treatment approach. In contrast, hypoparathyroidism, which is marked by low serum calcium levels and suppressed parathyroid hormone levels, necessitates careful biochemical monitoring along with treatment using calcium and active vitamin D analogs. Pseudohypoparathyroidism and secondary hyperparathyroidism present further diagnostic and therapeutic challenges.

Screening for parathyroid dysfunction should be recommended for pregnant women with risk factors, such previous history of endocrine disorders, nephrolithiasis, or previous fetal loss. Management strategies during pregnancy and lactation must balance maternal biochemical stability with fetal safety, emphasizing individualized care. Emerging evidence also highlights the role of vitamin D status in modulating disease severity and outcomes. Prompt diagnosis and interdisciplinary management are essential for optimizing both maternal and perinatal health.

10.2 Thyroid Disease During Pregnancy

10.2.1 Thyroid Physiology During Pregnancy

Pregnancy induces complex endocrine adaptations involving the hypothalamic–pituitary–thyroid (HPT) axis to support fetal development and maternal metabolic demands. The maternal thyroid gland undergoes both functional and structural changes throughout gestation, mediated by placental hormones, increased estrogen levels, and alterations in iodine homeostasis. Understanding these physiological modifications is crucial for accurate interpretation of thyroid function tests and optimal clinical management of thyroid disorders during pregnancy [1–5].

During normal pregnancy, the maternal thyroid gland enlarges by approximately 10–40%, particularly in iodine-deficient regions, primarily due to glandular hyperplasia and increased vascularity stimulated by elevated thyroid-stimulating hormones or their analogs. During pregnancy, the secretion of thyroxine (T4) and triiodothyronine (T3) rises by about 50% compared to nonpregnant levels. This physiological increase is essential to meet the elevated maternal metabolic requirements and to ensure optimal fetal neurodevelopment, particularly during the first trimester when the fetal thyroid gland remains functionally immature [1–7].

Estrogen plays a key role in modifying thyroid physiology by stimulating hepatic synthesis of thyroxine-binding globulin (TBG), leading to a two- to threefold increase in TBG concentrations during pregnancy. The increased binding capacity elevates total serum T4 and T3 levels, though free hormone levels often remain stable if measured accurately. TBG levels rise within the first few weeks of pregnancy, plateau around midgestation, and remain elevated until delivery [1–3, 8, 9]. During pregnancy, physiological changes alter thyroid hormone dynamics, necessitating the recalibration of reference intervals for laboratory assessment. To prevent diagnostic errors in identifying thyroid dysfunction, both the American Thyroid Association (ATA) and the Endocrine Society advocate the use of population-specific and trimester-adjusted reference ranges for thyroid-stimulating hormone (TSH) and free thyroxine (fT4) [1, 2, 10].

Human chorionic gonadotropin (hCG), synthesized by the placenta, also significantly impacts thyroid function. hCG shares structural homology with TSH, particularly at the β-subunit and receptor-binding regions, allowing it to weakly stimulate the TSH receptor. hCG levels peak between 10 and 12 weeks of gestation, coinciding with a transient suppression of TSH and mild increases in fT4 and free T3 (fT3). This physiological response may mimic subclinical thyrotoxicosis and should not be misinterpreted as pathological, especially during the first trimester [2, 9, 11]. As hCG concentrations decline in mid to late gestation, TSH levels gradually increase, often normalizing to pre-pregnancy levels [11, 12].

Early in gestation, maternal renal clearance of iodine increases as a result of a heightened glomerular filtration rate, leading to decreased circulating iodine levels. In addition, the placenta metabolizes maternal thyroid hormones and actively transports iodine to the fetus, further depleting maternal iodine stores [13]. Consequently, the daily iodine requirement increases from 150 to 250 μg during pregnancy. Failure to meet these demands can lead to maternal hypothyroxinemia and potential neurodevelopmental impairments in the fetus. Therefore, both the ATA and the Royal College of Obstetricians and Gynaecologists recommend iodine supplementation (typically 150 μg/day via prenatal vitamins) for all women (pregnant, lactating, or planning pregnancy), especially in regions with marginal iodine intake [1, 4].

By the 10th–12th week of pregnancy, the fetal thyroid gland acquires the capacity to concentrate iodine, and autonomous synthesis and secretion of thyroid hormones commence between the 18th and 22nd weeks. Nevertheless, maternal thyroxine (T4) remains a pivotal source of fetal thyroid hormone throughout pregnancy—constituting up to 30–50% of the total fetal T4 pool during the first trimester. The maternal-to-fetal transfer of T4 plays a fundamental role in neurodevelopmental processes such as neuronal proliferation, cortical migration, and myelination. Notably, even transient reductions in maternal T4 concentrations have been correlated with impaired neurocognitive outcomes in later life, underscoring the necessity of maintaining euthyroidism during early gestation [1, 2, 14].

Interpreting thyroid function tests during pregnancy is complex and requires consideration of assay limitations and physiological changes. Although total T4 and T3 concentrations increase due to thyroid-binding globulin (TBG), free hormone levels may vary depending on the assay methodology used. The direct measurement of free T4 (fT4) through equilibrium dialysis combined with liquid chromatography–tandem mass spectrometry (LC-MS/MS) is agreed as the gold standard, though it is not commonly accessible in routine clinical practice. Immunoassays, though commonly used, may yield lower fT4 values during pregnancy due to interference by elevated TBG and free fatty acids [15, 16]. In such cases, calculating the free T4 index (FTI) may provide a more reliable estimation of thyroid hormone status. In summary, pregnancy is a physiological state that alters thyroid hormone synthesis, metabolism, and transport. These adaptations are essential for ensuring adequate thyroid hormone supply to both mother and fetus. Recognizing and appropriately adjusting for these physiological changes is crucial in the clinical assessment and management of thyroid function in pregnancy.

10.2.2 Hypothyroidism in Pregnancy

Hypothyroidism constitutes one of the most frequent endocrine abnormalities in pregnancy and poses considerable risks to maternal and fetal health when timely diagnosis and appropriate management are not achieved. It is defined by insufficient production or action of thyroid hormones and classified into overt and subclinical hypothyroidism based on laboratory findings. Overt hypothyroidism is characterized by elevated thyroid-stimulating hormone (TSH) and decreased free thyroxine (FT4) levels, whereas subclinical hypothyroidism is defined by elevated TSH with normal FT4 levels [1, 2, 4, 17]. The main causes of hypothyroidism during pregnancy encompass autoimmune thyroiditis (Hashimoto's thyroiditis), iodine deficiency, thyroidectomy or radioiodine ablation, and, more rarely, central hypothyroidism. In iodine-sufficient populations, Hashimoto's thyroiditis remains the foremost etiology, typically marked by the presence of circulating anti-thyroid peroxidase (anti-TPO) and anti-thyroglobulin (anti-Tg) antibodies. Iatrogenic etiologies, including prior surgical or ablative interventions, further contribute to the burden of hypothyroidism, especially among women with known thyroid disease prior to conception [18]. Pregnancy exerts profound influences on thyroid physiology through several mechanisms, including increased estrogen levels leading to elevated thyroxine-binding globulin (TBG) concentrations, augmented renal iodine clearance, and stimulation of the thyroid gland by human chorionic gonadotropin (hCG). These adaptations necessitate the establishment of trimester-specific reference intervals for thyroid hormone assessment. The accepted reference ranges for TSH are approximately 0.1–2.5 mIU/L during the first trimester, 0.2–3.0 mIU/L during the second, and 0.3–3.5 mIU/L during the third [19, 20]. Because free T4 (fT4) and free T3 (fT3) levels exhibit physiological variability, their interpretation should rely on local laboratory-specific, method-dependent pregnancy reference intervals.

The diagnosis of hypothyroidism during pregnancy is established through the assessment of serum thyroid-stimulating hormone (TSH) and free thyroxine (fT4) concentrations. Present clinical guidelines discourage universal screening for thyroid dysfunction in pregnancy, favoring a targeted approach restricted to women exhibiting specific risk factors. These include a personal or familial history of thyroid disease, palpable goiter, concurrent autoimmune disorders, or a history of infertility or recurrent pregnancy loss. Nonetheless, considerable controversy remains regarding the potential advantages of universal screening, given the association between undiagnosed subclinical hypothyroidism and unfavorable maternal and perinatal outcomes [18, 21].

Maternal hypothyroidism that remains untreated during pregnancy confers significant maternal and fetal risks. Maternal complications include miscarriage, gestational hypertension, preeclampsia, placental abruption, preterm delivery, and postpartum hemorrhage. In the fetus, hypothyroidism is linked to intrauterine growth restriction, decreased birth weight, impaired neurodevelopment, and lower intelligence quotient (IQ), with severe cases potentially resulting in cretinism. Notably, the risk of neurocognitive impairment is most pronounced when overt hypothyroidism develops during the first trimester, a period critical for central nervous system maturation [17, 22, 23]. Levothyroxine (LT4) remains the choice of treatment. In overt hypothyroidism, LT4 therapy should be initiated immediately to maintain TSH within trimester-specific reference ranges. For women already on LT4 therapy preconception, the dose typically requires an increase of approximately 30–50% early in pregnancy. Subsequent monitoring every 4–6 weeks is advised. For subclinical hypothyroidism, treatment is recommended if TSH exceeds 4.0 mIU/L or in the presence of positive TPO antibodies [24, 25]. Dose adjustments should be made based on weight, etiology, and gestational age, with careful monitoring to avoid both under- and overtreatment. Hypothyroidism during pregnancy is a common but treatable condition. Timely diagnosis and adequate LT4 replacement can mitigate the maternal and fetal risks. Adherence to guideline-recommended TSH targets, early intervention, and close monitoring throughout gestation are critical components of optimal care.

10.2.3 Hyperthyroidism in Pregnancy

Hyperthyroidism, a condition characterized by excessive production of thyroid hormones, occurs in approximately 0.1–0.4% of pregnancies and is most commonly caused by Graves' disease. Other etiologies include gestational transient thyrotoxicosis (GTT), toxic multinodular goiter, toxic adenoma, and, rarely, thyroiditis or trophoblastic disease [26]. Graves' disease, an autoimmune disorder marked by thyroid-stimulating immunoglobulins (TSIs), remains the primary cause of hyperthyroidism in pregnancy. TSIs stimulate the TSH receptor, leading to excessive thyroid hormone secretion. GTT, on the other hand, is typically self-limiting and related to elevated human chorionic gonadotropin (hCG) levels, which stimulate the TSH receptor due to structural similarity. Unlike Graves' disease, GTT lacks TSIs and does not require antithyroid drug therapy [4, 27, 28]. Hyperthyroidism during pregnancy is diagnosed primarily by suppressed serum TSH in conjunction with elevated free or total thyroxine (T4). Accurate interpretation of thyroid function tests during pregnancy necessitates consideration of the physiological adaptations that occur throughout gestation, including elevated thyroxine-binding globulin (TBG) concentrations and transient suppression of thyroid-stimulating hormone (TSH) mediated by human chorionic gonadotropin (hCG). Applying trimester-specific reference ranges is essential, as TSH levels typically fall to around 0.1 mIU/L in the first trimester, while free thyroxine (fT4) concentrations often exceed those observed in nonpregnant individuals [29]. Distinguishing between Graves' disease and gestational transient thyrotoxicosis (GTT) is essential for guiding treatment decisions. Clinical findings such as persistent symptoms beyond the first trimester, a history of autoimmune thyroid disease, ophthalmopathy, and detectable TSIs favor Graves' disease [30]. The 2018 European Thyroid Association (ETA) guideline provides a comprehensive and evidence-based algorithm for the diagnosis and management of Graves' hyperthyroidism (GH), emphasizing both general care and special conditions such as pregnancy, pediatrics, and comorbidities. In areas with sufficient iodine intake, Graves' disease (GD) represents the predominant etiology of hyperthyroidism. It is defined by the presence of circulating thyroid-stimulating hormone receptor antibodies (TRAb), which drive the overproduction of thyroid hormones [31].

Inadequately managed hyperthyroidism is linked to various adverse outcomes, including miscarriage, preeclampsia, heart failure, preterm delivery, and low birth weight. Fetal complications may include fetal tachycardia, intrauterine growth restriction (IUGR), hydrops fetalis, and fetal or neonatal thyrotoxicosis resulting from the transplacental transfer of thyroid-stimulating immunoglobulins (TSIs) [31, 32]. Treatment aims to sustain maternal free thyroxine (fT4) concentrations at the upper limit of normal or mildly above, ensuring adequate fetal thyroid hormone availability and avoiding fetal hypothyroidism. Treatment aims to sustain maternal free thyroxine (fT4) concentrations at the upper limit of normal or mildly above, ensuring adequate fetal thyroid hormone availability and avoiding fetal hypothyroidism. Antithyroid drugs (ATDs) are the cornerstone of therapy. During pregnancy, propylthiouracil (PTU) is recommended in the first trimester owing to its comparatively lower teratogenic risk, while methimazole (MMI) is advised in the second and third trimesters because of its more favorable hepatic safety profile. Minimal effective doses are used to avoid fetal thyroid suppression [26, 33]. During the pregnancy, the guideline provides specific recommendations regarding the differential diagnosis of gestational thyrotoxicosis versus GH, careful titration of PTU or MMI to the lowest effective dose, and the importance of TRAb measurement during each trimester to predict neonatal thyrotoxicosis. For patients undergoing definitive therapy, RAI is contraindicated during pregnancy and lactation. Thyroidectomy is considered in patients intolerant or unresponsive to ATDs or when malignancy is suspected. Preoperative preparation, including euthyroidism and beta-blocker use (propranolol), is recommended to reduce perioperative risk [31]. Fetal monitoring includes serial ultrasound for fetal growth, heart rate, and goiter. TSIs should be measured in the second trimester; high levels may warrant closer fetal surveillance [34]. Graves' disease may worsen postpartum, necessitating re-evaluation of ATD therapy. Breastfeeding is generally considered safe with low-dose MMI or PTU. Neonatal thyroid function should be examined, especially in babies of mothers with active Graves' disease or elevated TSIs [35].

10.2.4 Inflammatory and Autoimmune Diseases of the Thyroid Gland in Pregnancy

Autoimmune and inflammatory thyroid diseases represent a substantial portion of thyroid dysfunctions encountered in pregnancy, with Hashimoto's thyroiditis predominating as the cause of hypothyroidism in regions with adequate iodine intake. Immunological modulation during gestation plays an essential role in determining both the expression and progression of these disorders [36, 37]. Pregnancy is characterized by a complex interplay between immune tolerance and activation to support fetal development. This dynamic immune adaptation results in the modulation of autoimmune activity, often leading to remission or amelioration of symptoms in certain autoimmune thyroid diseases during gestation, followed by exacerbation in the postpartum period [38].

Hashimoto's thyroiditis is defined by the presence of anti-thyroid peroxidase (anti-TPO >35 IU/mL) and anti-thyroglobulin (anti-Tg >40 IU/mL) antibodies. These antibodies can be found in 10–20% of pregnant women, although not all demonstrate overt thyroid dysfunction. Thyroid autoimmunity (TAI), even among women with normal thyroid function, confers an elevated risk of adverse obstetric events, including miscarriage, preterm labor, placental abruption, and postpartum thyroiditis. Recent meta-analyses provide robust evidence reinforcing the causal association between TAI and unfavorable maternal and fetal outcomes [38–40]. Antigen-presenting cells, particularly dendritic cells, play a pivotal role in initiating the autoimmune cascade by activating autoreactive CD4+ T cells. These T helper cells (Th1 and Th17 subsets) contribute to inflammation via the production of cytokines such as IFN-γ and IL-17, which recruit cytotoxic T lymphocytes and macrophages to the thyroid tissue. Regulatory T cells (Tregs), which normally suppress autoimmunity, are often dysfunctional or decreased in HT, exacerbating the disease course [41].

Postpartum thyroiditis (PPT), typically a self-limited condition, occurs in approximately 5–10% of women within the first year postpartum and is often seen in those with preexisting anti-thyroid antibodies. The clinical course of postpartum thyroiditis (PPT) may involve an initial transient thyrotoxic phase, which is then followed by hypothyroidism. This condition can ultimately resolve or progress to permanent hypothyroidism [39, 42].

Management of autoimmune disease of the thyroid gland during pregnancy primarily involves vigilant monitoring of maternal thyroid function. Levothyroxine therapy is indicated for women presenting with subclinical or overt hypothyroidism in the presence of thyroid autoantibodies, in order to optimize maternal euthyroidism and minimize adverse obstetric and fetal outcomes. Moreover, euthyroid women with TAI may benefit from levothyroxine supplementation, particularly in cases of recurrent pregnancy loss or assisted reproductive techniques, although the evidence remains inconclusive [43]. Adjuvant therapies such as selenium supplementation (60–200 μg/day) have been shown to reduce TPO antibody titers and the risk of PPT in some trials. Similarly, vitamin D deficiency, prevalent in autoimmune thyroiditis, may influence immunological responses. Limited studies have evaluated the role of cholecalciferol in reducing antibody levels and improving thyroid autoimmunity, although further research is warranted [44, 45]. Overall, close monitoring of TSH and free T4 levels throughout pregnancy, especially in women with known TAI, is essential. Evaluation every 4–6 weeks is recommended, and levothyroxine doses should be adjusted accordingly to maintain trimester-specific TSH targets.

10.2.5 Thyroid Nodule in Pregnancy

Thyroid nodules (TN) are a common finding during pregnancy, with prevalence estimates ranging from 3% to 30%. These nodules may develop de novo or enlarge secondary to pregnancy-associated physiological alterations. Elevated human chorionic gonadotropin (hCG), estrogen-induced increases in thyroxine-binding globulin (TBG), and the accompanying rise in thyroid hormone synthesis collectively drive thyroid hyperplasia and nodular transformation, reflecting the gland's adaptive response to gestational demands [2, 46]. The pathogenesis of TN in pregnancy includes hormonal stimulation by hCG and insulin-like growth factors, alongside predisposing factors such as iodine deficiency, multiparity, advanced maternal age, and the presence of uterine fibroids, which may elevate the risk of goiter and nodules through hormonal interplay [46–48]. An increased prevalence of TN has also been observed in iodine-sufficient populations, where excess iodine intake may paradoxically induce nodular development [49].

The diagnostic approach to TN during pregnancy aligns with standard nonpregnant protocols, beginning with clinical evaluation, history of rapid growth, compressive symptoms, or family history of thyroid disease. Thyroid ultrasonography remains the cornerstone imaging modality due to its safety and sensitivity [1, 12, 50]. Fine-needle aspiration cytology (FNAC) is generally deferred to postpartum unless sonographic features strongly suggest malignancy. In high-risk cases, particularly Bethesda category IV or higher, FNAC may be considered in the second trimester [1, 3, 50–52]. Management of benign nodules typically involves surveillance with periodic ultrasonography and thyroid function monitoring. TSH suppression therapy with levothyroxine may be cautiously employed in selected cases with large or growing nodules, although evidence supporting this is limited [51, 52]. Surgical management is indicated for patients presenting with rapid nodule enlargement or symptomatic compression, with thyroidectomy preferentially performed during the second trimester to mitigate fetal risk [2, 46, 51]. Iodine status is a critical determinant in the development of nodular thyroid disease, as both iodine deficiency and excess have been implicated in promoting thyroid nodule formation. Recent evidence suggests that thyroglobulin may serve as a useful biomarker reflecting iodine insufficiency and the presence of nodular changes during pregnancy, although this association requires further validation through prospective studies [6, 49]. Thyroid nodules in pregnancy require a balanced approach integrating risk stratification, judicious use of diagnostics, and avoidance of unnecessary interventions. While most TN are benign and nonprogressive, individualized care based on sonographic findings, maternal–fetal risks, and biochemical markers remains paramount.

10.2.6 Thyroid Cancer in Pregnancy

Thyroid cancer is the second most frequently diagnosed endocrine malignancy among women of reproductive age and is increasingly identified during pregnancy, thanks to routine prenatal imaging and the trend of delayed childbearing. The majority of thyroid cancers detected in pregnancy are differentiated thyroid carcinomas (DTC), most commonly papillary thyroid carcinoma (PTC), which is approximately 80–85% of cases, followed by follicular thyroid carcinoma (FTC). Other rare histological types, such as medullary thyroid carcinoma and anaplastic thyroid carcinoma, are exceedingly rare in pregnancy [2, 4, 53]. Pregnancy-associated hormonal changes, particularly elevated human chorionic gonadotropin (hCG), can suppress TSH, complicating the biochemical evaluation of thyroid nodules. Thyroid ultrasonography remains the cornerstone for nodule assessment, facilitating identification of features predictive of malignancy, including hypoechogenicity, microcalcifications, irregular margins, and increased vascularity. Fine-needle aspiration cytology (FNAC) is indicated for nodules ≥1 cm with suspicious sonographic characteristics or for smaller nodules in high-risk patients, and should ideally be performed during the second trimester to minimize fetal risk [2, 10, 52, 54]. The most frequent histologic subtype is papillary thyroid carcinoma (PTC), which generally follows an indolent course. FTC is less common but may exhibit hematogenous spread. Medullary thyroid carcinoma (MTC), derived from parafollicular C-cells, constitutes a clinically challenging entity owing to its potential for early metastatic spread and its growth that is independent of thyroid-stimulating hormone (TSH), necessitating specialized diagnostic and therapeutic strategies. Anaplastic thyroid carcinoma (ATC), while rare in pregnancy, is highly aggressive and typically associated with poor prognosis [2, 10, 52–55]. Studies have shown that pregnancy does not significantly worsen the prognosis of DTC. Tumor progression during gestation is rare, and overall outcomes are comparable to nonpregnant women when appropriately managed [2, 56–58]. The management of thyroid cancer in pregnant women must balance optimal maternal treatment and fetal safety. In cases of confirmed DTC without aggressive features, surgery may be deferred until the postpartum period. However, thyroidectomy may be considered during the second trimester in cases of rapid tumor growth, compressive symptoms, or cytologic findings suggestive of aggressive histology [52, 53, 55, 59]. When surgery is postponed, levothyroxine therapy is administered to maintain TSH suppression, aiming for a TSH level below 0.1–0.5 mIU/L to mitigate potential tumor stimulation. Radioiodine therapy is contraindicated during pregnancy and should be postponed until after delivery and cessation of breastfeeding [52–54, 59]. Postpartum follow-up includes a comprehensive re-evaluation, including neck ultrasonography, serum thyroglobulin levels, and consideration for radioactive iodine ablation when appropriate [2, 52, 60]. Thyroid cancer during pregnancy, predominantly PTC, generally has a favorable prognosis. Management decisions should be individualized, emphasizing multidisciplinary coordination and gestational age. Timely diagnosis, selective surgical intervention, and suppression therapy allow for safe maternal and fetal outcomes.

10.2.7 Thyroid Surgery During Pregnancy

Surgical or interventional treatment of thyroid disease in pregnancy is indicated in select cases where conservative management is insufficient or inappropriate. While most thyroid conditions in pregnancy are managed medically, specific clinical scenarios—such as suspected or confirmed malignancy, compressive goiter, or refractory hyperthyroidism—may necessitate timely surgical consideration. The approach requires a multidisciplinary framework balancing maternal health and fetal safety [2, 54].

The main indications for surgical intervention during pregnancy include:

- Rapidly growing or compressive goiters causing dysphagia, dyspnea, or vascular compromise.
- Nodules with cytology suggestive of malignancy (Bethesda V or VI) or high-risk ultrasound features.
- Confirmed thyroid cancer with aggressive features (e.g., local invasion, nodal metastasis).
- Hyperthyroidism unresponsive or intolerant to antithyroid drug therapy (e.g., methimazole or propylthiouracil) [61–64].

The timing of surgery is critical. The second trimester (14–28 weeks of gestation) is considered optimal, as teratogenic risk has declined, and uterine size is still amenable to safe anesthesia and positioning. Surgery in the first trimester carries a higher risk of miscarriage, while third-trimester procedures pose risks of preterm labor and increased anesthetic complications [2, 3, 54, 59]. Surgical planning during pregnancy requires coordination with obstetricians, anesthesiologists, and endocrinologists [63]. Preoperative evaluation includes high-resolution ultrasonography and, when necessary, fine-needle aspiration cytology. Vocal cord assessment is recommended to minimize the risk of unrecognized recurrent laryngeal nerve palsy [61]. Total thyroidectomy is preferred over lobectomy when malignancy is known or strongly suspected [61–64]. Fetal heart rate monitoring and intraoperative uterine tone monitoring are necessary during procedures performed after viability (typically >24 weeks). Postoperative complications can include transient or permanent hypocalcemia, hemorrhage, and injury to the recurrent laryngeal nerve. Hypocalcemia is particularly prevalent following total thyroidectomy and should be managed proactively [3]. Radioactive iodine (RAI) is strictly contraindicated during pregnancy. It crosses the placenta and can affect the fetal thyroid as early as 12 weeks of gestation, leading to congenital hypothyroidism. Radioactive iodine (RAI) therapy should be postponed until after the postpartum period, and lactating women should stop breastfeeding well before undergoing treatment [1–3, 31, 48, 65]. Novel interventional procedures, including radiofrequency ablation (RFA) and ethanol injection for benign nodules, are currently not recommended during pregnancy due to a lack of safety data and procedural risks. These should be reserved for postpartum periods when appropriate [48, 51, 52]. Surgery may be indicated for Graves' disease in pregnant women, who are intolerant or resistant to antithyroid medications. Thyroidectomy is a safe and definitive treatment option in the second trimester. In patients requiring surgery for hyperthyroidism, preoperative preparation includes beta-blockade (e.g., propranolol) and antithyroid therapy to achieve euthyroid state and prevent thyroid storm [62, 63]. Post-thyroidectomy, levothyroxine therapy is initiated promptly to maintain euthyroidism and support pregnancy outcomes. Dose adjustments are guided by trimester-specific TSH reference ranges. Regular monitoring every 4–6 weeks is essential to ensure optimal hormonal balance [2, 62–64]. Surgical and interventional management of thyroid diseases in pregnancy is reserved for select indications where maternal or fetal well-being is at risk. The second trimester is the safest window for thyroidectomy. Radioiodine therapy and thermal ablation are contraindicated during pregnancy. Careful perioperative management, maternal–fetal monitoring, and postoperative hormonal replacement are critical for favorable outcomes.

10.2.8 Screening of Thyroid Disease in Pregnancy

Thyroid function screening during pregnancy remains a subject of ongoing debate, particularly regarding the comparative merits of universal versus risk-based approaches. Maternal thyroid dysfunction, including subclinical hypothyroidism and thyroid autoimmunity, has been consistently associated with adverse outcomes such as miscarriage, preterm birth, gestational hypertension, and impaired neurocognitive development in offspring [1, 2, 4, 26]. Current professional guidelines differ in their recommendations; the American Thyroid Association (ATA) and the

Endocrine Society advocate for selective, risk-based screening, targeting women with identifiable maternal risk factors, including prior thyroid disease, clinical manifestations of thyroid dysfunction, type 1 diabetes, coexisting autoimmune conditions, previous head or neck irradiation, and a history of infertility or recurrent miscarriage [1, 2]. However, this strategy may miss up to 30%–55% of women with thyroid dysfunction, prompting a growing interest in universal screening [5, 66–68]. Universal screening entails measuring serum TSH levels in all pregnant women, usually during the initial prenatal visit or within the first trimester. Supporters of this approach argue that early detection and treatment of subclinical hypothyroidism with levothyroxine can enhance pregnancy outcomes and is cost-effective in many contexts [68, 69]. A study from Denmark revealed significant variation in clinical practice and emphasized the importance of establishing consistent national protocols [67]. In contrast, opponents highlight the potential for overdiagnosis and overtreatment, especially in women with marginally elevated TSH or transient changes due to hCG-related thyroid stimulation [70]. The dynamic physiological changes during early pregnancy necessitate the use of gestation-specific and population-specific TSH reference ranges to reduce misclassification [71, 72]. Thyroid autoantibodies, especially thyroid peroxidase antibodies (TPOAb), are increasingly recognized as a marker of autoimmune thyroid disease and a predictor of future hypothyroidism. Their role in risk stratification and treatment decisions remains under investigation [21]. In a meta-analysis encompassing 19 prospective cohort studies with 47,045 participants, Korevaar et al. reported that subclinical hypothyroidism (OR 1.29), isolated hypothyroxinemia (OR 1.46), and positivity for thyroid peroxidase antibodies (OR 1.33) were independently linked to a heightened risk of preterm delivery [73]. In conclusion, while targeted screening remains the current standard in many countries, growing evidence supports the potential utility of universal thyroid screening in early pregnancy. The development of dynamic, evidence-based guidelines that integrate risk assessment, local epidemiology, and resource availability is essential to optimize maternal and fetal outcomes.

10.2.9 Perinatal Outcomes of Thyroid Disease

Thyroid dysfunction in pregnancy, whether overt or subclinical, has been consistently linked to unfavorable maternal and perinatal outcomes. Maternal thyroid hormones play an essential role in fetal growth and neurological development, particularly during the first trimester, when the fetus relies entirely on the transplacental transfer of maternal thyroxine to sustain normal brain maturation and metabolic regulation [1–4]. Overt maternal hypothyroidism has been consistently linked to heightened risks of spontaneous miscarriage, preterm delivery, low birth weight, and preeclampsia, emphasizing the critical importance of early detection and management. Moreover, insufficient maternal thyroid hormone availability during gestation may result in irreversible neurocognitive deficits in the offspring due to disrupted fetal brain development [21, 69, 73]. Subclinical hypothyroidism, although less well-defined in its consequences, has been linked in several studies to elevated risks of pregnancy loss, gestational hypertension, and placental abruption, particularly when TSH levels exceed pregnancy-specific reference ranges [1, 73, 74]. Uncontrolled maternal hyperthyroidism, most commonly resulting from Graves' disease, is associated with serious maternal and fetal outcomes, including spontaneous miscarriage, intrauterine growth restriction, stillbirth, preterm delivery, and, in severe cases, maternal heart failure [30, 31]. In addition, transplacental transfer of thyroid-stimulating hormone receptor antibodies (TRAb) may induce fetal or neonatal thyrotoxicosis, which can manifest as tachycardia, intrauterine growth restriction, and advanced bone maturation. Therefore, meticulous maternal–fetal monitoring and individualized adjustment of antithyroid drug therapy are essential to balance maternal euthyroidism while minimizing fetal exposure and potential adverse effects [24, 28]. Thyroid hormones are critical for fetal brain development. Several cohort studies have linked maternal hypothyroxinemia and overt hypothyroidism to reduced IQ and altered psychomotor development in children. Although universal screening remains debated, early identification and treatment of thyroid dysfunction may reduce the risk of long-term neurodevelopmental impairment [1, 6, 33, 74, 75]. Thyroid disease during pregnancy can significantly impact both maternal and perinatal outcomes. Careful screening, diagnosis, and management—particularly during the first trimester—are essential to minimize risks. Individualized care guided by updated guidelines and gestation-specific reference ranges is recommended to ensure favorable outcomes for both mother and child.

10.3 Parathyroid Disease During Pregnancy

10.3.1 Parathyroid Gland Physiology During Pregnancy

The regulation of calcium homeostasis during pregnancy is a complex process involving adaptive changes in the maternal endocrine system, particularly the parathyroid glands. These adaptations aim to meet the increased fetal demand for calcium, especially during the third trimester when fetal skeletal mineralization peaks [76–78]. During pregnancy, the fetal requirement for calcium reaches approximately 25–30 g, primarily in the third trimester, necessitating substantial changes in maternal calcium metabolism to sustain this demand without depleting maternal skeletal stores [76–78]. Maternal physiology accommodates this by increasing intestinal calcium absorption rather than relying on bone resorption, which becomes more prominent during lactation [76–79].

The augmentation of maternal calcium absorption is largely driven by increased concentrations of 1,25-dihydroxyvitamin D [$1,25(OH)_2D$], the hormonally active vitamin D metabolite. Both placental and renal synthesis of $1,25(OH)_2D$ are markedly upregulated, reflecting increased 1α-hydroxylase activity induced by placental lactogen, estrogen, and parathyroid hormone-related protein (PTHrP) [76, 78, 80]. As a result, circulating $1,25(OH)_2D$ levels double by the third trimester [79, 81].

Parathyroid hormone (PTH) levels follow a distinct trajectory across gestation. In early pregnancy, PTH concentrations are often suppressed into the low-normal or subnormal range due to elevated 1,25$(OH)_2$D and elevated calcium absorption. However, as gestation advances, PTH levels gradually rise, reaching mid-normal levels by the third trimester to sustain calcium homeostasis amid the increasing fetal calcium demand [79, 81–83].

The role of PTHrP is especially critical. Synthesized by placental, fetal, and maternal tissues, PTHrP facilitates active calcium transfer across the placenta, modulates renal calcium handling, and contributes to skeletal metabolism. While it shares structural homology and receptor pathways with PTH, its functions in pregnancy are physiologically distinct. The placental–fetal calcium gradient (maternal: fetal = 1:1.4) allows efficient fetal mineralization without compromising maternal bone integrity [76, 78, 84]. Despite a reduction in total serum calcium due to hemodilution and hypoalbuminemia, ionized calcium levels—the biologically active fraction—remain stable throughout pregnancy. This distinction is clinically important, as reliance on total serum calcium may underestimate true calcium status in pregnant women [80, 82, 85]. Disruption of these finely tuned mechanisms by parathyroid disorders, such as primary hyperparathyroidism (PHPT) or hypoparathyroidism, may pose significant risks for both maternal and fetal health. In such cases, the altered calcium–PTH–vitamin D axis necessitates vigilant monitoring and management [82, 83, 86].

Moreover, determinants such as maternal vitamin D status, dietary calcium intake, geographic latitude, seasonality, and parity influence PTH dynamics in pregnancy, further underlining the complex interplay of endocrine and environmental factors in gestational calcium regulation [87].

10.3.2 Hypoparathyroidism in Pregnancy

Hypoparathyroidism during pregnancy is an uncommon but clinically significant disorder that presents unique diagnostic and therapeutic challenges. It may be due to surgical removal of the parathyroid glands, autoimmune destruction, genetic syndromes (e.g., DiGeorge syndrome), or infiltrative diseases. The physiological adaptations of calcium homeostasis in pregnancy further complicate its management [82, 88]. The most common etiology is postsurgical hypoparathyroidism following thyroidectomy or parathyroidectomy. Idiopathic and autoimmune hypoparathyroidism are rarer but possible causes. During pregnancy, the physiological increase in intestinal calcium absorption mediated by elevated calcitriol levels reduces maternal parathyroid hormone (PTH) secretion. However, in women with hypoparathyroidism, endogenous PTH is absent or deficient, making calcium homeostasis dependent on exogenous calcium and vitamin D supplementation [88, 89]. Symptoms during pregnancy may be subtle or nonspecific, including paresthesia, muscle cramps, fatigue, or more severe complications such as tetany and seizures. Inadequate treatment can result in hypocalcemia, with potential risks for fetal outcomes such as intrauterine restriction of fetal growth, preterm, or low-weight birth. Neonatal hypocalcemia may also occur due to chronic suppression of fetal parathyroid glands from maternal calcium supplementation [90, 91].

Therapeutic management aims to sustain serum calcium concentrations within the low-normal range—total calcium 8.0–8.5 mg/dL and ionized calcium 1.0–1.15 mmol/L—to minimize clinical symptoms and reduce the risk of hypercalciuria. Active vitamin D analogs (e.g., calcitriol) and calcium supplements are the mainstays of therapy. Regular monitoring of serum calcium, phosphate, creatinine, and 24-hour urinary calcium excretion is recommended every 3–4 weeks [78, 82, 92].

Lactation presents additional complexity, as mammary PTHrP production increases and promotes skeletal calcium resorption, potentially improving serum calcium in hypoparathyroid women. This may necessitate dose reduction or discontinuation of calcitriol and calcium during breastfeeding. Monitoring must be individualized due to interpatient variability. In pseudohypoparathyroidism, characterized by the resistance of end-organs to PTH, PTH levels are elevated but ineffective, and management remains similar to that of classical hypoparathyroidism [77, 82, 93, 94]. Hypoparathyroidism in pregnancy requires individualized care guided by physiological adaptations of calcium metabolism. Interdisciplinary management involving endocrinology and obstetrics is vital to optimize maternal and neonatal outcomes.

10.3.3 Pseudohypoparathyroidism in Pregnancy

Pseudohypoparathyroidism (PHP) represents a group of rare endocrine disorders caused by impaired target organ responsiveness to parathyroid hormone (PTH). Despite normal or increased circulating PTH concentrations, resistance at the renal and skeletal level results in biochemical features resembling hypoparathyroidism, including hypocalcemia and hyperphosphatemia. It results in hypocalcemia and hyperphosphatemia due to impaired cyclic AMP generation following PTH receptor activation. PHP is primarily caused by inactivating mutations in the GNAS gene, and its subtypes (e.g., PHP1A, PHP1B, and PPHP) display varying degrees of hormone resistance and phenotypic features such as Albright's hereditary osteodystrophy (AHO) [91, 95]. Pregnancy poses both diagnostic and therapeutic challenges in PHP. Physiological adaptations in gestation, including increased 1,25-dihydroxyvitamin D production and enhanced placental calcium transfer, may attenuate the biochemical severity of hypocalcemia in PHP patients. However, symptoms such as muscle cramps, tetany, paresthesia, or seizures may occur, particularly in the first trimester or postpartum period when calcium demands and hormonal fluctuations are high [91, 95, 96]. According to a recent case series, well-managed pregnancies in women with PHP—using adjusted doses of active vitamin D (e.g., calcitriol) and calcium supplementation—are usually uneventful, with good maternal and fetal outcomes [91]. Nonetheless, the postpartum period is critical, as the abrupt cessation of transplacental calcium flow and the rise in PTH-related peptide (PTHrP) from lactating breast tissue can lead to significant hypocalcemic episodes, requiring careful monitoring and dose adjustments [97]. Management of pseudohypoparathyroidism (PHP) during pregnancy should focus on maintaining maternal serum calcium concentrations within the low-normal range (total calcium: 8.0–8.5 mg/dL; ionized calcium: 1.0–1.15 mmol/L) to minimize both maternal symptomatology and fetal complications. Close biochemical surveillance is essential, with serial measurements of serum calcium, phosphate, magnesium, and creatinine, along with 24-hour urinary calcium excretion, recommended every 2–4 weeks throughout gestation. Adjustment of calcium and active vitamin D supplementation should be guided by these values to avoid hypocalcemic or hypercalcemic episodes. Furthermore, genetic counseling is advised due to the autosomal dominant inheritance pattern observed in several PHP subtypes, particularly those involving GNAS mutations [97].

10.3.4 Primary Hyperparathyroidism in Pregnancy

Primary hyperparathyroidism (PHPT) is defined as autonomous PTH secretion, mostly due to a single parathyroid adenoma (80–85%), with less frequent causes including multiglandular hyperplasia and rarely parathyroid carcinoma [76, 85]. Hereditary syndromes such as MEN1 and MEN2A or familial isolated hyperparathyroidism may also be implicated in younger women. PHPT is diagnosed during pregnancy at an estimated rate of 0.03–0.05%, although underdiagnosis is common due to the physiological suppression of total calcium levels by hypoalbuminemia during gestation [98]. In pregnancy, the usual calcium-lowering effect of increased $1,25(OH)_2D$ and PTH-related peptide (PTHrP) may mask hypercalcemia, delaying diagnosis. PTH remains inappropriately normal or elevated despite hypercalcemia. Normocalcemic PHPT (elevated PTH with normal calcium) may also occur and has implications for bone health and fetal development [76, 78].

Undiagnosed or untreated PHPT during pregnancy carries a substantial risk. Maternal complications include nephrolithiasis, pancreatitis, hyperemesis gravidarum, hypertension, preeclampsia, and hypercalcemic crises, particularly in the postpartum period when PTHrP-driven skeletal resorption abruptly declines [99, 100]. Fetal risks are even more pronounced: due to maternal hypercalcemia suppressing fetal parathyroid gland development in utero, neonates are prone to severe postnatal hypocalcemia, tetany, seizures, and apnea, typically manifesting within 48–72 hours postpartum [76, 87, 101]. Additionally, studies report increased rates of miscarriage, limitation of intrauterine growth (IUGR), low birth weight, and stillbirth in untreated maternal PHPT [76, 77, 87, 101].

Diagnosis is based on elevated serum calcium (corrected for albumin or ionized calcium) and inappropriately normal or high PTH levels. Because total calcium may fall in pregnancy, measuring ionized calcium is preferred. A 24-hour urinary calcium excretion test is useful for distinguishing PHPT from familial hypocalciuric hypercalcemia (FHH). Serum phosphate is often low, and alkaline phosphatase is unreliable due to placental isoenzyme elevation [76, 78, 85]. Neck ultrasound is the preferred imaging modality during pregnancy; sestamibi scans and CT are contraindicated due to fetal radiation exposure [78, 82].

Management is stratified based on symptom severity and biochemical parameters:

A. Asymptomatic/Mild Cases (Ca <11 mg/dL): Conservative management includes adequate hydration, oral phosphate supplementation (if tolerated), and frequent calcium monitoring. Dietary calcium should not be restricted excessively to avoid rebound bone resorption [78, 82, 98].
B. Symptomatic or Severe Hypercalcemia (Ca >11 mg/dL): Parathyroidectomy is the treatment of choice, ideally performed in the second trimester to minimize teratogenic risks and preterm labor. Surgery reduces maternal–fetal complications and neonatal hypocalcemia [76, 78, 98].
C. First/Third Trimester or Nonsurgical Candidates: Aggressive hydration, limited use of loop diuretics, and possibly calcitonin may be considered. Calcitonin does not cross the placenta and is relatively safe but may cause tachyphylaxis. Cinacalcet is off-label and generally avoided due to insufficient safety data [82, 98, 99].

After delivery, PTHrP-driven bone resorption and renal calcium conservation are augmented by lactation, potentially lowering serum calcium. However, PHPT-related hypercalcemia may paradoxically worsen in the early postpartum period due to abrupt withdrawal of placental calcium transfer and decreased maternal $1,25(OH)_2D$ levels [76, 87, 99]. Breastfeeding may be continued in most cases, but calcium levels must be closely monitored. In some cases, postpartum parathyroidectomy is planned electively after weaning [78, 85]. The use of calcimimetics and bisphosphonates is discouraged during lactation due to potential transmission into breast milk and effects on neonatal bone metabolism [76, 98, 102].

10.3.5 Secondary Hyperparathyroidism in Pregnancy

Secondary hyperparathyroidism (SHPT) arises as a physiological adaptation to chronic hypocalcemia or vitamin D deficiency, leading to compensatory PTH elevation. In pregnancy, SHPT may be caused by Vitamin D deficiency—particularly common in high-latitude regions or in women with limited sun exposure, skin covering, or poor dietary intake—as well as by chronic kidney disease (CKD), due to impaired phosphate excretion and 1α-hydroxylation of vitamin D. Malabsorption syndromes, e.g., celiac disease or conditions following bariatric surgery [76, 79, 82, 89], may also contribute. PTH elevations are typically modest, and serum calcium is low or normal. Unlike PHPT, SHPT does not cause fetal hypercalcemia, but maternal bone loss and increased risk of postpartum osteoporosis or fracture may occur [82, 87, 103]. Management focuses on correcting the underlying cause. Cholecalciferol (vitamin D3) supplementation is first-line, aiming for 25(OH) D levels ≥30 ng/mL. If the calcium level is low, oral calcium supplementation is added. Vitamin D analogs (e.g., calcitriol) may be cautiously used in CKD, with attention to serum calcium and phosphate levels. Parathyroidectomy is not indicated in SHPT during pregnancy [76, 82, 98].

10.3.6 Inflammatory, Autoimmune, Genetic, and Neoplastic Parathyroid Disorders and Surgery in Pregnancy

Autoimmune and inflammatory disorders of the parathyroid glands are exceptionally rare during gestation but can present within the framework of autoimmune polyendocrine syndromes. Autoimmune Polyglandular Syndrome Type 1 (APS1), associated with AIRE gene mutations, characteristically includes autoimmune hypoparathyroidism as a defining clinical feature, underscoring the importance of recognizing these syndromes in pregnant patients [104–106]. Recent evidence indicates the presence of autoantibodies targeting the calcium-sensing receptor (CaSR) on parathyroid cells in individuals with autoimmune hypoparathyroidism. In certain cases, these anti-CaSR antibodies have been shown to exert functional agonist activity on the receptor, leading to suppression of parathyroid hormone secretion and contributing directly to the pathogenesis of hypocalcemia [105]. Pregnant women with APS1 may present with hypocalcemia, which, if not adequately treated, can result in fetal complications such as secondary hyperparathyroidism, fetal skeletal demineralization, and intrauterine growth restriction [107].

No pregnancy-specific cases of IgG4-related parathyroiditis have been reported in the literature. However, autoimmune destruction of the parathyroid gland has been described histologically in chronic hypoparathyroidism, often with lymphocytic infiltration [108]. Differentiation of hypocalcemia from other diseases, such as pseudohypoparathyroidism and vitamin D deficiency, is essential, particularly in pregnant women with neuromuscular symptoms [87, 96].

Parathyroid adenomas are the leading cause of primary hyperparathyroidism (PHPT) in pregnancy, representing up to 85% of cases [109–111]. Clinically significant PHPT during gestation is associated with hypercalcemia, fatigue, nausea, vomiting, and nephrolithiasis. In a systematic review of 75 cases of parathyroid adenoma diagnosed during pregnancy, maternal complications included preeclampsia (6.7%), nephrolithiasis (5.3%), and pancreatitis (4%), while fetal complications included preterm labor (7%) and intrauterine growth restriction (5.3%) [109]. Ultrasound is the imaging modality of choice, while scintigraphy and CT are generally avoided during gestation due to ionizing radiation risks [87, 96, 99].

Several hereditary syndromes associated with parathyroid pathology have important implications for pregnancy, both in terms of maternal and fetal outcomes and in preconception planning. Among these, Multiple Endocrine Neoplasia Type 1 (MEN1) is characterized with germline mutations in the MEN1 gene, leading to multiglandular parathyroid hyperplasia as well as tumors of the pituitary and pancreas. Women with MEN1 have an increased risk of recurrent or persistent primary hyperparathyroidism (PHPT), which may worsen during pregnancy due to the physiological changes in calcium homeostasis. For this reason, subtotal parathyroidectomy is often recommended prior to conception in known mutation carriers to mitigate maternal and fetal complications associated with hypercalcemia [112].

MEN2A is an inherited autosomal dominant syndrome resulting from activating mutations in the RET proto-oncogene, located on chromosome 10q11.2. The classic clinical phenotype includes medullary thyroid carcinoma (MTC), pheochromocytoma, and parathyroid hyperplasia or adenoma. The penetrance and temporal pattern of tumor emergence are mutation-dependent, underscoring the critical role of genetic counseling and individualized mutation-specific surveillance protocols. In pregnant women with MEN2A, early identification and appropriate surgical management of associated tumors are critical, particularly because undiagnosed pheochromocytoma may lead to hypertensive crises and severe obstetric complications. Biochemical screening and multidisciplinary planning are essential in patients with known RET mutations or a family history of MEN2A [113].

Hyperparathyroidism–Jaw Tumor Syndrome (HPT-JT) is a rare autosomal dominant disorder attributable to germline mutations in the CDC73 gene, which encodes the tumor suppressor parafibromin. The syndrome is clinically distinguished by a substantially increased risk of parathyroid carcinoma, in addition to ossifying fibromas of the mandible or maxilla and, less commonly, renal and uterine neoplasms. Given the aggressive behavior of parathyroid lesions in HPT-JT, women of reproductive age should undergo detailed preconception genetic counseling and a comprehensive endocrine evaluation to guide risk mitigation and reproductive planning. In many cases, early or pre-pregnancy parathyroidectomy is advisable to mitigate the risks of hypercalcemia-related maternal and fetal complications during gestation. Given the 50% inheritance risk, prenatal genetic counseling and possible cascade screening of family members are recommended [114, 115]. In all of these syndromes, pregnancy planning should include individualized risk assessment, early biochemical and genetic screening, and a multidisciplinary approach to management. The timing of surgical intervention—either prior to pregnancy or during the second trimester—should be based on the severity of hypercalcemia, tumor behavior, and maternal–fetal risks [78, 87].

Parathyroid carcinoma, though rare, must be considered when PTH levels are significantly elevated (>two–threefold), calcium levels exceed 3.0 mmol/L, or when ultrasound reveals a large, irregular, or invasive lesion. A case report by Dematapitiya et al. detailed a parathyroid carcinoma diagnosed during the second trimester of pregnancy, with histopathology confirming vascular and capsular invasion, and molecular analysis revealing a novel frameshift mutation in the CDC73 gene [116]. CDC73 mutations are characteristic of Hyperparathyroidism-Jaw Tumor Syndrome (HPT-JT), a rare autosomal dominant condition predisposing to parathyroid carcinoma, as well as ossifying fibromas of the jaw, and renal neoplasms [114]. In the context of pregnancy, CDC73 mutation testing is indicated in young women with recurrent PHPT, multiglandular disease, or a family history of parathyroid neoplasia. Early genetic diagnosis enables appropriate surgical planning and postpartum surveillance [115].

Surgical management is considered for PHPT in pregnancy when total serum calcium is persistently >2.75 mmol/L (11 mg/dL), or when maternal complications such as nephrolithiasis, pancreatitis, or severe neuropsychiatric symptoms occur [117]. Consensus guidelines recommend that parathyroidectomy be performed during the second trimester, ideally between 13 and 24 weeks of pregnancy, to minimize the complications of miscarriage and preterm delivery [118]. In a review by Pothiwala and Levine, second-trimester surgery was associated with better maternal–fetal outcomes than conservative therapy in cases of severe hypercalcemia [119]. Ultrasound-guided fine-needle aspiration with PTH washout may be used to confirm parathyroid tissue prior to surgery, although this method is contraindicated in suspected parathyroid carcinoma due to the risk of needle tract seeding [119, 120]. Intraoperative PTH monitoring is useful to confirm adequate excision. Surgery is typically performed under general anesthesia, with preoperative planning coordinated among endocrinology, obstetrics, and anesthesiology teams [78, 120, 121].

10.3.7 Screening of Parathyroid Function in Pregnancy and Perinatal Outcomes of Parathyroid Disease

Maternal calcium and phosphate homeostasis undergo significant adaptations during pregnancy to support fetal skeletal development, particularly in the third trimester. These adaptations include increased intestinal calcium absorption, changes in parathyroid hormone (PTH) dynamics, and high circulating levels of 1,25-dihydroxyvitamin D [84, 89]. Disruptions in these processes due to primary hyperparathyroidism (PHPT), hypoparathyroidism, pseudohypoparathyroidism, or secondary hyperparathyroidism cause adverse maternal and fetal results, underscoring the importance of screening for parathyroid dysfunction during pregnancy [76, 81, 83, 122].

Routine screening of parathyroid function is not currently recommended for all pregnant individuals. However, targeted evaluation is necessary in women with nephrolithiasis, osteoporosis, recurrent miscarriage, unexplained intrauterine fetal demise, low fetal birth weight, or familial syndromes such as MEN1, MEN2A, or HPT-JT [86, 96]. Initial evaluation should include measurements of serum total and ionized calcium, phosphorus, albumin, PTH, and 25(OH) vitamin D levels. Measurement of ionized calcium is particularly significant in pregnancy due to the hemodilutional reduction in total serum calcium [76, 83, 123].

Hypercalcemia in pregnancy may be misattributed to physiological changes; hence, careful interpretation of laboratory findings is critical. PHPT is typically characterized by elevated serum calcium with suppressed or inappropriately normal PTH levels, whereas hypoparathyroidism presents with low calcium and low or undetectable PTH. Pseudohypoparathyroidism may be suggested by high PTH in the context of hypocalcemia and hyperphosphatemia [76, 82, 95].

Undiagnosed or poorly managed parathyroid disorders are related to significant maternal and fetal comorbidity. Maternal pathologies include nephrolithiasis, hyperemesis, pancreatitis, preeclampsia, and cardiac arrhythmias [82, 87, 95]. Hypercalcemia may exacerbate volume depletion and lead to hypertensive crises [80, 85]. Hypoparathyroidism, on the other hand, may present with seizures or tetany due to hypocalcemia and poses additional risks if vitamin D supplementation is inadequate [96].

Fetal complications of maternal PHPT include intrauterine growth retardation (IUGR), preterm birth, and neonatal hypocalcemia or tetany due to suppressed fetal parathyroid function. The abrupt withdrawal of maternal calcium following delivery leads to transient neonatal hypocalcemia, particularly in cases where maternal hypercalcemia was not corrected [88, 95]. In contrast, poorly controlled hypoparathyroidism in pregnancy may impair fetal skeletal mineralization and contribute to low birth weight and seizures in the newborn [82, 95, 96].

Recent studies have demonstrated that maternal vitamin D deficiency may amplify the adverse effects of both hyperparathyroidism and hypoparathyroidism. Inadequate vitamin D impairs calcium absorption and contributes to secondary hyperparathyroidism, complicating maternal management and increasing fetal risk [79, 82, 98].

For hypoparathyroidism, the therapeutic goal during pregnancy is to preserve serum total calcium in the low-to-mid normal range (8.0–9.0 mg/dL or 2.0–2.25 mmol/L) and ionized calcium within the normal range. Treatment includes oral calcium supplementation at doses of 1000–2000 mg/day divided into 2–3 doses, and calcitriol (1,25-dihydroxyvitamin D3) starting at 0.25 μg/day and titrated up to 2.0 μg/day depending on calcium levels [80, 85, 95]. Vitamin D3 (cholecalciferol) at 1000–2000 IU/day is also commonly added if 25(OH)D is <30 ng/mL [82, 87]. During lactation, calcitriol requirements often decrease due to increased bone resorption mediated by PTH-related peptide (PTHrP), necessitating frequent calcium monitoring and dose adjustment [87, 124].

In pseudohypoparathyroidism, a similar regimen is used as PTH resistance results in hypocalcemia and hyperphosphatemia. Calcium supplementation and active vitamin D analogs remain the mainstay, with careful phosphate control [96, 97].

For primary hyperparathyroidism (PHPT), asymptomatic patients with mild hypercalcemia (<11 mg/dL) can often be managed conservatively with hydration. In symptomatic or moderate-to-severe cases, parathyroidectomy is preferred during the second trimester [80, 118, 125]. Short-term treatment with hydration and furosemide (used cautiously) may help manage acute hypercalcemia. Calcitonin, at 100–200 IU subcutaneously every 6–12 hours, is considered safe in pregnancy and can be used as bridging therapy [76, 85, 96]. Cinacalcet is not recommended due to a lack of safety data [85, 100, 101].

Following delivery, newborns of mothers with untreated or severe PHPT should be monitored closely for hypocalcemia. Likewise, in hypoparathyroidism and pseudohypoparathyroidism, both maternal and neonatal calcium levels should be evaluated in the postpartum period [76, 78, 87, 91, 96].

References

1. De Groot L, Abalovich M, Alexander EK, Amino N, Barbour L, Cobin RH, et al. Management of thyroid dysfunction during pregnancy and postpartum: an endocrine society clinical practice guideline. J Clin Endocrinol Metab. 2012;97(8):2543–65.
2. Alexander EK, Pearce EN, Brent GA, Brown RS, Chen H, Dosiou C, et al. 2017 Guidelines of the American Thyroid Association for the diagnosis and management of thyroid disease during pregnancy and the postpartum. Thyroid. 2017;27(3):315–89.
3. Thyroid disease in pregnancy: ACOG Practice Bulletin, Number 223. Obstet Gynecol. 2020;135(6):e261–74. https://doi.org/10.1097/AOG.0000000000003893. PMID: 32443080.
4. Chan SY, Marsh MS, Gilbert J, Boelaert K, Evans C, Dhillon-Smith R. Management of thyroid disorders in pregnancy. BJOG Int J Obstet Gynaecol. 2025;132(8):e130–61.
5. Dickens LT, Cifu AS, Cohen RN. Diagnosis and management of thyroid disease during pregnancy and the postpartum period. JAMA – J Am Med Assoc. 2019;321(19):1928–9.
6. Harding KB, Peña-Rosas JP, Webster AC, Yap CMY, Payne BA, Ota E, et al. Iodine supplementation for women during the preconception, pregnancy and postpartum period. Cochrane Database Syst Rev. 2017;2017(3):CD011761.
7. Taylor PN, Vaidya B. Iodine supplementation in pregnancy – is it time? Clin Endocrinol (Oxf). 2016;85(1):10–4.
8. Nathan N, Sullivan SD. Thyroid disorders during pregnancy. Endocrinol Metab Clin N Am. 2014;43(2):573–97.
9. Yap YW, Onyekwelu E, Alam U. Thyroid disease in pregnancy. Clin Med J R Coll Physicians Lond. 2023;23(2):125–8.
10. Rotondi M, Capelli V, Chiovato L, Nappi RE. 2017 ATA guidelines on the management of thyroid dysfunctions in pregnancy: what do OB/GYNs need to know? Gynecol Endocrinol [Internet]. 2019;35(4):276–9. Available from: https://doi.org/10.1080/09513590.2018.1532496.
11. Vandana KA, Khatuja R, Mehta S. Thyroid dysfunction during pregnancy and in postpartum period: treatment and latest recommendations. Arch Gynecol Obstet. 2014;289(5):1137–44.
12. Velasco I, Vila L, Goya M, Oleaga A, de la Calle M, Santamaria FJ. Executive summary of the SEEN (Sociedad Española de Endocrinología y Nutrición [Spanish Society of Endocrinology and Nutrition])-SEGO (Sociedad Española deGinecología y Obstetricia [Spanish Society of Gynaecology and Obstetrics]) consensus document on the management of thyroid dysfunction during pregnancy. Endocrinol Diabetes Nutr (English Ed). 2023;70:38–50.
13. Osinga JAJ, Liu Y, Männistö T, Vafeiadi M, Tao FB, Vaidya B, et al. Risk factors for thyroid dysfunction in pregnancy: an individual participant data meta-analysis. Thyroid. 2024;34(5):646–58.
14. Aktaş A, Pekkolay Z. Thyroid diseases and treatment in pregnancy. J Clin Exp Investig. 2016;7(1):119–23.
15. Patton PE, Samuels MH, Trinidad R, Caughey AB. Controversies in the management of hypothyroidism during pregnancy. Obstet Gynecol Surv. 2014;69(6):346–58. https://doi.org/10.1097/OGX.0000000000000075. PMID: 25101844.
16. Nowak A, Podlewski J, Hubalewska-Dydejczyk A, Trofimiuk-Müldner M. The impact of insulin resistance on thyroid function and the prevalence of thyroid follicular nodular disease in pregnant women. Eur Thyroid J. 2025;14(2):e240317.
17. Fang Y, Yao L, Sun J, Zhang J, Li Y, Yang R, Yang K, Tian L. Appraisal of clinical practice guidelines on the management of hypothyroidism in pregnancy using the appraisal of guidelines for research and evaluation II instrument. Endocrine. 2018;60(1):4–14. https://doi.org/10.1007/s12020-018-1535-2. Epub 2018 Feb 14. PMID: 29445919.
18. Azizi F, Amouzegar A, Mehran L, Alamdari S, Subekti I. Screening and management of hypothyroidism. Endocr J. 2014;61(7):697–704.
19. Dorizzi RM, Spiazzi G, Rolli N, Maltoni P, Mingolla L, Sgarzani C, et al. Trimester-specific reference intervals for thyroid function parameters in pregnant Caucasian women using

Roche platforms: a prospective study. J Endocrinol Invest [Internet]. 2023;46(12):2459–69. Available from: https://doi.org/10.1007/s40618-023-02098-0.

20. Ollero MD, Toni M, Pineda JJ, Martínez JP, Espada M, Anda E. Thyroid function reference values in healthy iodine-sufficient pregnant women and influence of thyroid nodules on thyrotropin and free thyroxine values. Thyroid. 2019;29(3):421–9.
21. Spencer L, Bubner T, Bain E, Middleton P. Screening and subsequent management for thyroid dysfunction pre-pregnancy and during pregnancy for improving maternal and infant health. Cochrane Database Syst Rev. 2015;2015(9):CD011263.
22. Liu J, Xie X, García-Patterson A, Asla Q, Sardà H, Chico A, et al. Association between inadequate weight gain according to the institute of medicine 2009 guidelines and pregnancy outcomes in women with thyroid disorders. Arch Gynecol Obstet [Internet]. 2024;310(2):961–9. Available from: https://doi.org/10.1007/s00404-023-07279-z.
23. Özon A, Tekin N, Şıklar Z, Gülcan H, Kara C, Taştekin A, et al. Neonatal effects of thyroid diseases in pregnancy and approach to the infant with increased TSH: Turkish Neonatal and Pediatric Endocrinology and Diabetes Societies consensus report. Turk Pediatr Ars. 2018;53:S209–23.
24. Stagnaro-Green A, Rovet J. Maternal thyroid function in pregnancy – a tale of two tails. Nat Rev Endocrinol. 2016;12(2):110. https://doi.org/10.1038/nrendo.2015.228. Epub 2015 Dec 18. Erratum for: Nat Rev Endocrinol. 2016;12(1):10–1. https://doi.org/10.1038/nrendo.2015.212. PMID: 26678810.
25. Ji Y, Xu J, Su T, Lin L, Zhou S, Bao H, et al. Effect of levothyroxine treatment on fetal growth among women with mild subclinical hypothyroidism and thyroid peroxidase antibody negative: a cohort study. BMC Pregnancy Childbirth [Internet]. 2023;23(1):1–9. Available from: https://doi.org/10.1186/s12884-023-05676-5.
26. Korevaar TIM, Medici M, Visser TJ, Peeters RP. Thyroid disease in pregnancy: new insights in diagnosis and clinical management. Nat Rev Endocrinol [Internet]. 2017;13(10):610–22. Available from: https://doi.org/10.1038/nrendo.2017.93.
27. De Leo S, Lee SY, Braverman LE, Unit E, Sciences C. Hyperthyroidism: lancet review. Lancet. 2016;388(10047):906–18.
28. Khan I, Okosieme O, Lazarus J. Antithyroid drug therapy in pregnancy: a review of guideline recommendations. Expert Rev Endocrinol Metab [Internet]. 2017;12(4):269–78. Available from: https://doi.org/10.1080/17446651.2017.1338944.
29. Lee SY, Pearce EN. Testing, monitoring, and treatment of thyroid dysfunction in pregnancy. J Clin Endocrinol Metab. 2021;106(3):883–92. https://doi.org/10.1210/clinem/dgaa945. PMID: 33349844; PMCID: PMC7947825.
30. Elston MS, Tu'Akoi K, Meyer-Rochow GY, Tamatea JAU, Conaglen JV. Pregnancy after definitive treatment for Graves' disease – does treatment choice influence outcome? Aust N Z J Obstet Gynaecol. 2014;54(4):317–21.
31. Kahaly GJ, Bartalena L, Hegedüs L, Leenhardt L, Poppe K, Pearce SH. 2018 European thyroid association guideline for the management of graves' hyperthyroidism. Eur Thyroid J. 2018;7(4):167–86.
32. Stagnaro-Green A, Abalovich M, Alexander E, Azizi F, Mestman J, Negro R, et al. Guidelines of the American Thyroid Association for the diagnosis and management of thyroid disease during pregnancy and postpartum. Thyroid. 2011;21(10):1081–125.
33. Petca A, Dimcea DAM, Dumitrașcu MC, Șandru F, Mehedințu C, Petca RC. Management of hyperthyroidism during pregnancy: a systematic literature review. J Clin Med. 2023;12(5):1811.
34. Laurberg P, Bournaud C, Karmisholt J, Orgiazzi J. Management of Graves' hyperthyroidism in pregnancy: focus on both maternal and foetal thyroid function, and caution against surgical thyroidectomy in pregnancy. Eur J Endocrinol. 2009;160(1):1–8.
35. Karras S, Tzotzas T, Kaltsas T, Krassas GE. Pharmacological treatment of hyperthyroidism during lactation: review of the literature and novel data. Pediatr Endocrinol Rev. 2010;8(1):25–33.

36. Mioto VCB, de Castro Nassif Gomes Monteiro AC, De Camargo RYA, Borel AR, Catarino RM, Kobayashi S, et al. High prevalence of iodine deficiency in pregnant women living in adequate iodine area. Endocr Connect. 2018;7(5):762–7.
37. Scher J, Dabao C, Rukat C. Thyroid autoimmunity: the treatment of Hashimoto's disease, or the presence of antithyroid antibodies alone, in pregnancy. Am J Reprod Immunol. 2025;93(1):1–7.
38. Singh M, Wambua S, Lee SI, Okoth K, Wang Z, Fazla F, et al. Autoimmune diseases and adverse pregnancy outcomes: an umbrella review. Lancet (Lond, Engl) [Internet]. 2023;402:S84. Available from: https://doi.org/10.1016/S0140-6736(23)02128-1.
39. Zaccarelli-Marino MA, Dsouki NA, de Carvalho RP, Maciel RMB. Evaluation of anti-thyroperoxidase (A-TPO) and anti-thyroglobulin (A-Tg) antibodies in women with previous Hashimoto's thyroiditis during and after pregnancy. J Clin Med. 2024;13(15):4519.
40. Osinga JAJ, Derakhshan A, Karachaliou M, et al. Association of gestational thyroid function and thyroid autoimmunity with gestational diabetes: a systematic review and individual participant meta-analysis. Lancet Diabetes Endocrinol. 2025;13(8):651–61. https://doi.org/10.1016/S2213-8587(25)00068-3.
41. Wrońska K, Hałasa M, Szczuko M. The role of the immune system in the course of Hashimoto's thyroiditis: the current state of knowledge. Int J Mol Sci. 2024;25(13):6883.
42. Nguyen CT, Mestman JH. Postpartum thyroiditis. Clin Obstet Gynecol. 2019;62(2):359–64.
43. Erdő-Bonyár S, Simon D, Bajnok A, Nörenberg J, Serény-Litvai T, Várnagy Á, et al. Physiological changes in the levels of anti-cytokine autoantibodies in early pregnancy are missing in pregnant women with Hashimoto's thyroiditis. J Immunol Res. 2023;2023:5221658.
44. Minnetti M, Sada V, Feola T, Giannetta E, Pozza C, Gianfrilli D, et al. Selenium supplementation in pregnant women with autoimmune thyroiditis: a practical approach. Nutrients. 2022;14(11):1–14.
45. Bhakat B, Chakraborty SK, Das S, Mallick SI. A prospective study to evaluate the possible role of cholecalciferol supplementation on autoimmunity in Hashimoto's thyroiditis. J Indian Med Assoc. 2022;120(7):21–4.
46. Medenica S, Arjunan D, Mladenovic V, Zankovic N, Aksam S, Gluvic Z, et al. Thyroid nodules and thyroid cancer in pregnancy. Gynecol Endocrinol [Internet]. 2025;41(1). Available from: https://doi.org/10.1080/09513590.2025.2517878.
47. Yuk JS, Kim JM. Uterine fibroids increase the risk of thyroid goiter and thyroid nodules. Sci Rep [Internet]. 2022;12(1):1–10. Available from: https://doi.org/10.1038/s41598-022-10625-x.
48. Drui D, Briet C, Guerin C, Lugat A, Borson-Chazot F, Grunenwald S. SFE-AFCE-SFMN 2022 Consensus on the management of thyroid nodules: thyroid nodules and pregnancy. Ann Endocrinol (Paris) [Internet]. 2022;83(6):435–9. Available from: https://doi.org/10.1016/j.ando.2022.10.005.
49. Gao M, Chen Y, Zhang Y, Sun H, Zhang Q, Chen W, et al. Thyroglobulin can be a functional biomarker of iodine deficiency, thyroid nodules, and goiter in Chinese pregnant women. Asia Pac J Clin Nutr. 2020;29(1):27–34.
50. Ahn HY, Yi KH. Diagnosis and management of thyroid disease during pregnancy and postpartum: 2023 revised Korean Thyroid Association guidelines. J Bone Metab. 2023;38(3):289–94.
51. Papini E, Crescenzi A, D'Amore A, Deandrea M, De Benedictis A, Frasoldati A, et al. Italian guidelines for the management of non-functioning benign and locally symptomatic thyroid nodules. Endocr Metab Immune Disord Drug Targets. 2023;23(6):876–85.
52. Papini E, Negro R, Pinchera A, Guglielmi R, Baroli A, Beck-Peccoz P, et al. Thyroid nodule and differentiated thyroid cancer management in pregnancy. An Italian Association of Clinical Endocrinologists (AME) and Italian Thyroid Association (AIT) joint statement for clinical practice. J Endocrinol Investig. 2010;33(8):579–86.
53. Langdon J, Gupta A, Sharbidre K, Czeyda-Pommersheim F, Revzin M. Thyroid cancer in pregnancy: diagnosis, management, and treatment. Abdom Radiol [Internet]. 2023;48(5):1724–39. Available from: https://doi.org/10.1007/s00261-023-03808-1.

54. Perros P, Boelaert K, Colley S, Evans C, Evans RM, Gerrard Ba G, et al. Guidelines for the management of thyroid cancer. Clin Endocrinol (Oxf). 2014;81(SUPPL. 1):1–122.
55. Yu SS, Bischoff LA. Thyroid cancer in pregnancy. Semin Reprod Med. 2016;34(6):351–5.
56. Angell TE, Alexander EK. Thyroid nodules and thyroid cancer in the pregnant woman. Endocrinol Metab Clin North Am [Internet]. 2019;48(3):557–67. Available from: https://doi.org/10.1016/j.ecl.2019.05.003.
57. Sullivan SA. Thyroid nodules and thyroid cancer in pregnancy. Clin Obstet Gynecol. 2019;62(2):365–72. https://doi.org/10.1097/GRF.0000000000000431. PMID: 30925552.
58. Galofré JC, Riesco-Eizaguirre G, Álvarez-Escolá C. Clinical guidelines for management of thyroid nodule and cancer during pregnancy. Endocrinol Nutr (English Ed) [Internet]. 2014;61(3):130–8. Available from: https://doi.org/10.1016/j.endoen.2014.02.014.
59. Chinelatto LA, Hojaij FC, de Carlucci D, Cernea CR. Thyroid cancer surgical indication during pregnancy: systematic literature review and series of illustrative cases. Braz J Otorhinolaryngol. 2025;91(December 2024):2–6.
60. Lin JS, Aiello Bowles EJ, Williams SB, Morrison CC. Screening for thyroid cancer: updated evidence report and systematic review for the US preventive services task force. JAMA – J Am Med Assoc. 2017;317(18):1888–903.
61. Baruah MP, Kailey J, Ahmad I. Principles of ear nose and throat surgery for pregnant women. Br J Hosp Med. 2017;78(4):206–12.
62. Ruan D, Moalem J. Thyroid gland: pregnancy – a risk factor for thyroid surgery complications. Nat Rev Endocrinol. 2009;5(11):589–90.
63. Patel KN, Yip L, Lubitz CC, Grubbs EG, Miller BS, Shen W, et al. Executive summary of the American Association of Endocrine Surgeons guidelines for the definitive surgical management of thyroid disease in adults. Ann Surg. 2020;271(3):399–410.
64. Cleo Kenington J, Pellino G, Iqbal MR, Ahmed N, Chandima Halahakoon V, Zaborowski AM, et al. Guidelines on general surgical emergencies in pregnancy. Br J Surg [Internet]. 2024;111(3):1–17. Available from: https://doi.org/10.1093/bjs/znae051.
65. Wojtczak B, Kaliszewski K, Binko M, Sępek M, Mulek R, Rudnicki J, et al. Thyroid oncology in pregnancy. Ann Thyroid. 2020;5(5):0–2.
66. van der Spek AH, Bisschop PH. Universal screening for thyroid disease SHOULD NOT be recommended before and during pregnancy. Best Pract Res Clin Endocrinol Metab. 2020;34(4):101429. https://doi.org/10.1016/j.beem.2020.101429. Epub 2020 Jun 17. PMID: 32622828.
67. Hatting LC, Kristensen MØ, Lundgaard MH, Sørensen A, Andersen SL. Screening for thyroid disease in pregnancy: a study of Danish clinical practice. Thyroid Res [Internet]. 2023;16(1):1–9. Available from: https://doi.org/10.1186/s13044-023-00151-x.
68. Tužil J, Jiskra J, Koudelková M, Chloupková R, Hejcmanová K, Májek O, et al. Cost-effectiveness analysis of universal screening for subclinical hypothyroidism in pregnancy based on the Czech Nation-Wide Pilot Screening Program in light of current evidence. Value Health Reg Issues. 2025;49:101145.
69. Dosiou C, Barnes J, Schwartz A, Negro R, Crapo L, Stagnaro-Green A. Cost-effectiveness of universal and risk-based screening for autoimmune thyroid disease in pregnant women. J Clin Endocrinol Metab. 2012;97(5):1536–46.
70. Korevaar TIM, Dhillon-Smith R. Levothyroxine treatment in euthyroid women positive for thyroid peroxidase antibodies and recurrent pregnancy loss. Lancet Diabetes Endocrinol. 2022;10(5):299–301.
71. Díaz-Soto G, Largo E, Álvarez-Colomo C, Martínez-Pino I, de Luis D. Valores de referencia y cribado universal de la disfunción tiroidea en la mujer gestante. Endocrinol Nutr. 2014;61(6):336–8.
72. Khadilkar S. Thyroid-stimulating hormone values in pregnancy: cutoff controversy continues? J Obstet Gynaecol India. 2019;69(5):389–94. https://doi.org/10.1007/s13224-019-01272-w. Epub 2019 Sep 13. PMID: 31598039; PMCID: PMC6765031.

73. Korevaar TIM, Derakhshan A, Taylor PN, Meima M, Chen L, Bliddal S, et al. Association of thyroid function test abnormalities and thyroid autoimmunity with preterm birth: a systematic review and meta-analysis. JAMA – J Am Med Assoc. 2019;322(7):632–41.
74. Lazarus JH, Bestwick JP, Channon S, et al. Antenatal screening for hypothyroidism and childhood cognitive impairment. N Engl J Med. 2012;306(6):1–14.
75. Vaishnav S, Pandya D, Shrivastava R, Patel N, Phatak AG, Patel A. Early treatment will prevent feto-maternal complications in thyroid disorders during pregnancy: a prospective study. J Family Med Prim Care. 2023;12(12):3393–8. https://doi.org/10.4103/jfmpc.jfmpc_1185_23. Epub 2023 Nov 22. PMID: 38361867; PMCID: PMC10866218.
76. Tsourdi E, Anastasilakis AD. Parathyroid disease in pregnancy and lactation: a narrative review of the literature. Biomedicines. 2021;9(5):475. https://doi.org/10.3390/biomedicines9050475. PMID: 33925967; PMCID: PMC8145477.
77. Sullivan SA. Parathyroid diseases. Clin Obstet Gynecol. 2019;62(2):347–58.
78. Appelman-Dijkstra NM, Pilz S. Approach to the patient: management of parathyroid diseases across pregnancy. J Clin Endocrinol Metab. 2023;108(6):1505–13. https://doi.org/10.1210/clinem/dgac734. PMID: 36546344; PMCID: PMC10188304.
79. Wheeler BJ, Taylor BJ, de Lange M, Harper MJ, Jones S, Mekhail A, et al. A longitudinal study of 25-hydroxy vitamin D and parathyroid hormone status throughout pregnancy and exclusive lactation in New Zealand mothers and their infants at 45° S. Nutrients. 2018;10(1):1–12.
80. Avidime OM, Avidime S, Randawa AJ, Kawu MU, Mohammed A, Oweh OT. Physiological changes in serum calcium, phosphate, vitamin D, parathyroid hormone and calcitonin during pregnancy and lactation in randomised population of Zaria women. Niger J Physiol Sci. 2022;37(1):77–82.
81. Ma SS, Hu HL, Li JJ, Yin WJ, Tao RX, Zhu P. The role of parathyroid hormone during pregnancy on the relationship between maternal vitamin D deficiency and fetal growth restriction: a prospective birth cohort study. Br J Nutr. 2020;124(4):432–9.
82. Bollerslev J, Rejnmark L, Zahn A, Heck A, Appelman-Dijkstra NM, Cardoso L, et al. European expert consensus on practical management of specific aspects of parathyroid disorders in adults and in pregnancy: recommendations of the ESE Educational Program of Parathyroid Disorders (PARAT 2021). Eur J Endocrinol. 2022;186(2):R33–63.
83. Hysaj O, Marqués-Gallego P, Richard A, Elgizouli M, Nieters A, Quack Lötscher KC, Rohrmann S. Parathyroid hormone in pregnancy: vitamin D and other determinants. Nutrients. 2021;13(2):360. https://doi.org/10.3390/nu13020360. PMID: 33504033; PMCID: PMC7911996.
84. Salles JP. Bone metabolism during pregnancy. Ann Endocrinol (Paris). 2016;77(2):163–8. https://doi.org/10.1016/j.ando.2016.04.004. Epub 2016 May 2. PMID: 27157104.
85. Dochez V, Ducarme G. Primary hyperparathyroidism during pregnancy. Arch Gynecol Obstet. 2015;291(2):259–63.
86. Zhong H, Liao Q, Liu J, Chen X, Hu Y, Jian S, et al. Expert consensus on multidisciplinary approach to the diagnosis and treatment of primary hyperparathyroidism in pregnancy in China. Endocrine. 2023;82(2):282–95.
87. Bilezikian JP, Khan AA, Silverberg SJ, Fuleihan GEH, Marcocci C, Minisola S, et al. Evaluation and management of primary hyperparathyroidism: summary statement and guidelines from the fifth international workshop. J Bone Miner Res. 2022;37(11):2293–314.
88. Ali DS, Dandurand K, Khan AA. Hypoparathyroidism in pregnancy and lactation: current approach to diagnosis and management. J Clin Med. 2021;10(7):1378.
89. Miles B, Panchbhavi M, Mackey JD. Analysis of fracture incidence in 135 patients with pregnancy and lactation osteoporosis (PLO). Cureus. 2021;13(10):e19011. https://doi.org/10.7759/cureus.19011. PMID: 34824928; PMCID: PMC8610434.
90. Kaneshapillai A, Hettiaratchi U, Prathapan S, Liyanage G. Parathyroid hormone in Sri Lankan pregnant women: vitamin D and other determinants. PLoS One [Internet]. 2021;16(10 October):1–11. Available from: https://doi.org/10.1371/journal.pone.0258381.

91. Wang JJ, Yang Y, Wang YB, Song A, Jiang Y, Li M, et al. Pseudohypoparathyroidism during pregnancy and the postpartum period: a case series of five patients. Front Endocrinol (Lausanne). 2022;13(November):1–10.
92. Khan AA, Koch CA, Van Uum S, Baillargeon JP, Bollerslev J, Brandi ML, et al. Standards of care for hypoparathyroidism in adults: a Canadian and international consensus. Eur J Endocrinol. 2019;180(3):P1–22.
93. Hatswell BL, Allan CA, Teng J, Wong P, Ebeling PR, Wallace EM, et al. Management of hypoparathyroidism in pregnancy and lactation – a report of 10 cases. Bone Rep [Internet]. 2015;3:15–9. Available from: https://doi.org/10.1016/j.bonr.2015.05.005.
94. Gafni RI, Collins MT. Hypoparathyroidism. N Engl J Med. 2019;380(18):1738–47. https://doi.org/10.1056/NEJMcp1800213. PMID: 31042826.
95. Mantovani G, Bastepe M, Monk D, De Sanctis L, Thiele S, Ahmed SF, et al. Recommendations for diagnosis and treatment of pseudohypoparathyroidism and related disorders: an updated practical tool for physicians and patients. Horm Res Paediatr. 2021;93(3):182–96.
96. Bastepe M, Gensure RC. Hypoparathyroidism and pseudohypoparathyroidism. [Updated 2024 May 8]. In: Feingold KR, Ahmed SF, Anawalt B, et al., editors. Endotext [Internet]. South Dartmouth: MDText.com, Inc.; 2000. Available from: https://www.ncbi.nlm.nih.gov/books/NBK279165/.
97. Jüppner H. Molecular definition of pseudohypoparathyroidism variants. J Clin Endocrinol Metab. 2021;106(6):1541–52. https://doi.org/10.1210/clinem/dgab060. PMID: 33529330; PMCID: PMC8118362.
98. Sandler ML, Ho R, Xing MH, Gidumal S, Spitzer H, Levy JC, et al. Primary hyperparathyroidism during pregnancy treated with parathyroidectomy: a systematic review. Laryngoscope. 2021;131(8):1915–21.
99. Komarowska H, Bromińska B, Luftmann B, Ruchała M. Primary hyperparathyroidism in pregnancy – a review of literature. Ginekol Pol. 2017;88(5):270–5.
100. Pal R, Mukherjee S, Prasad TN, Bhadada SK. Pregnancy with primary hyperparathyroidism. Best Pract Res Clin Endocrinol Metab [Internet]. 2025;39(2):101983. Available from: https://doi.org/10.1016/j.beem.2025.101983.
101. Ali DS, Dandurand K, Khan AA. Primary hyperparathyroidism in pregnancy: literature review of the diagnosis and management. J Clin Med. 2021;10(13):2956.
102. Gallo S, McDermid JM, Al-Nimr RI, Hakeem R, Moreschi JM, Pari-Keener M, Stahnke B, Papoutsakis C, Handu D, Cheng FW. Vitamin D supplementation during pregnancy: an evidence analysis center systematic review and meta-analysis. J Acad Nutr Diet. 2020;120(5):898–924.e4. https://doi.org/10.1016/j.jand.2019.07.002. Epub 2019 Oct 25. PMID: 31669079.
103. Johansen-Bibby A, Girling J. Thyroid disorders and other endocrine disorders in pregnancy. Obstet Gynaecol Reprod Med. 2016;26(5):140–8.
104. Sperling MA, Angelousi A, Yau M. Autoimmune polyglandular syndromes. [Updated 2024 Jul 21]. In: Feingold KR, Ahmed SF, Anawalt B, et al., editors. Endotext [Internet]. South Dartmouth: MDText.com, Inc.; 2000. Available from: https://www.ncbi.nlm.nih.gov/books/NBK279152/.
105. Brown EM. Anti-parathyroid and anti-calcium sensing receptor antibodies in autoimmune hypoparathyroidism. Endocrinol Metab Clin North Am. 2009;38(2):437–45, x. https://doi.org/10.1016/j.ecl.2009.01.001. PMID: 19328421; PMCID: PMC2700354.
106. Kahaly GJ, Frommer L. Polyglandular autoimmune syndromes. J Endocrinol Investig. 2018;41(1):91–8. https://doi.org/10.1007/s40618-017-0740-9. Epub 2017 Aug 17. PMID: 28819917.
107. Laakso S, Holopainen E, Betterle C, Saari V, Vogt E, Schmitt MM, et al. Pregnancy outcome in women with APECED (APS-1): a multicenter study on 43 females with 83 pregnancies. J Clin Endocrinol Metab. 2022;107(2):E528–37.
108. Üsküdar Cansu D, Cansu GB, Yildirim R, Dinler M, Tekin E, Ak Sivrikoz İ, et al. Hypercalcemia in IgG4-related disease: coincidental or associated? Case based review. Rheumatol Int. 2022;42(7):1297–305.

109. Pliakos I, Chorti A, Moysidis M, Kotsovolis G, Kaltsas T, Pana A, et al. Parathyroid adenoma in pregnancy: a case report and systematic review of the literature. Front Endocrinol (Lausanne). 2022;13(October):1–12.
110. Hultin H, Hellman P, Lundgren E, Olovsson M, Ekbom A, Rastad J, et al. Association of parathyroid adenoma and pregnancy with preeclampsia. J Clin Endocrinol Metab. 2009;94(9):3394–9.
111. Sabbah N, Demar M, Sogbo F, Zappa M, Alsibai KD, Amroun H, et al. Recurrent vomiting and confusion in pregnancy: hypercalcaemia due to parathyroid adenoma. Lancet. 2023;402(10395):62–3.
112. Daglar HK, Kirbas A, Biberoglu E, Laleli B, Danisman N. Management of a multiple endocrine neoplasia type 1 during pregnancy: a case report and review of the literature. J Exp Ther Oncol. 2016;11(3):217–20. PMID: 28471129.
113. Kiernan CM, Grubbs EG. Surgical management of multiple endocrine neoplasia 1 and multiple endocrine neoplasia 2. Surg Clin North Am. 2019;99(4):693–709. https://doi.org/10.1016/j.suc.2019.04.015. Epub 2019 May 27. PMID: 31255200.
114. Tora R, Welch J, Sun J, Agarwal SK, Bell DA, Merino M, et al. Phenotypic profiling and molecular mechanisms in hyperparathyroidism-jaw tumor syndrome. J Clin Endocrinol Metab. 2023;108(12):3165–77.
115. Carpten JD, Robbins CM, Villablanca A, Forsberg L, Presciuttini S, Bailey-Wilsons J, et al. HRPT2, encoding parafibromin, is mutated in hyperparathyroidism-jaw tumor syndrome. Nat Genet. 2002;32(4):676–80.
116. Dematapitiya C, Perera C, Pathmanathan S, Subasinghe V, Anandagoda G, Dissanayaka V, et al. Parathyroid carcinoma during pregnancy: a novel pathogenic CDC73 mutation – a case report. BMC Endocr Disord [Internet]. 2022;22(1):2–7. Available from: https://doi.org/10.1186/s12902-022-01169-2.
117. Hirsch D, Kopel V, Nadler V, Levy S, Toledano Y, Tsvetov G. Pregnancy outcomes in women with primary hyperparathyroidism. J Clin Endocrinol Metab. 2015;100(5):2115–22.
118. Sharma SG, Levcine SN, Yatavelli RK, Shaha MA, Nathan CAO. Parathyroidectomy in first trimester of pregnancy. J Endocr Soc. 2020;4(3):bvaa015. https://doi.org/10.1210/jendso/bvaa015. PMID: 32133431; PMCID: PMC7049289.
119. Pothiwala P, Levine SN. Parathyroid surgery in pregnancy: review of the literature and localization by aspiration for parathyroid hormone levels. J Perinatol [Internet]. 2009;29(12):779–84. Available from: https://doi.org/10.1038/jp.2009.84.
120. Wilhelm SM, Wang TS, Ruan DT, Lee JA, Asa SL, Duh QY, et al. The American association of endocrine surgeons guidelines for definitive management of primary hyperparathyroidism. JAMA Surg. 2016;151(10):959–68.
121. Owen RP, Chou KJ, Silver CE, Beilin Y, Tang JJ, Yanagisawa RT, et al. Thyroid and parathyroid surgery in pregnancy. Eur Arch Oto-Rhino-Laryngol. 2010;267(12):1825–35.
122. Hemmingway A, Kenny LC, Malvisi L, Kiely ME. Exploring the concept of functional Vitamin D deficiency in pregnancy: impact of the interaction between 25-hydroxyVitamin D and parathyroid hormone on perinatal outcomes. Am J Clin Nutr [Internet]. 2018;108(4):821–9. Available from: https://doi.org/10.1093/ajcn/nqy150.
123. Kramer CK, Ye C, Hanley AJ, Connelly PW, Sermer M, Zinman B, et al. The relationship between parathyroid hormone and 25-hydroxyvitamin D during and after pregnancy. J Clin Endocrinol Metab. 2016;101(4):1729–36.
124. Vescini F, Borretta G, Chiodini I, Boniardi M, Carotti M, Castellano E, et al. Italian guidelines for the management of sporadic primary hyperparathyroidism. Endocrine Metab Immune Disord-Drug Targets. 2023;24(8):991–1006.
125. Calina D, Docea AO, Golokhvast KS, Sifakis S, Tsatsakis A, Makrigiannakis A. Management of endocrinopathies in pregnancy: a review of current evidence. Int J Environ Res Public Health. 2019;16(5):1–25.

Chapter 11
Neurological Diseases During Pregnancy

Yeliz Çiftçi

11.1 Introduction

Pregnancy is characterized by profound physiological, immunological, and hormonal changes that significantly influence the course and management of neurological diseases. During this period, conditions such as headache, epilepsy, demyelinating disorders, neuromuscular diseases, stroke, and movement disorders pose unique risks for both the mother and the fetus. Pregnancy-related hemodynamic alterations, increased coagulability, hormonal fluctuations, and changes in drug metabolism not only modify the clinical presentation of neurological disorders but also directly impact diagnostic and therapeutic decision-making.

Headaches are among the most common neurological complaints in pregnancy. While migraines often improve by the second trimester, secondary causes such as preeclampsia, cerebral venous thrombosis, or posterior reversible encephalopathy syndrome carry substantial risks for maternal morbidity and mortality. In women with epilepsy, the primary aim is to maintain seizure control while minimizing teratogenic risks. Drug selection, therapeutic drug monitoring, and dose adjustments throughout gestation remain central to management. In demyelinating diseases, such as multiple sclerosis and neuromyelitis optica spectrum disorders, preconception disease stabilization, continuity of therapy, and relapse prevention in the postpartum period are key considerations.

Although less common, neuromuscular disorders, such as myasthenia gravis or inherited neuropathies, can complicate pregnancy and delivery, sometimes with severe maternal or neonatal consequences. Likewise, maternal stroke, though relatively rare in young women, is three times more frequent during pregnancy and is associated with high mortality, particularly in the peripartum period. Movement

Y. Çiftçi (✉)
Izmir Bakircay University, Faculty of Medicine, Department of Neurology, Izmir, Turkey
e-mail: yeliz.ciftci@bakircay.edu.tr

© The Author(s), under exclusive license to Springer Nature Switzerland AG 2026

I. Karaca (ed.), *Managing Maternal Chronic Diseases for a Healthy Pregnancy*,
https://doi.org/10.1007/978-3-032-15221-3_11

disorders, including restless legs syndrome or chorea gravidarum, may also occur during pregnancy and significantly impair maternal quality of life. Therefore, the management of neurological diseases in pregnancy requires not only an understanding of the natural history of these conditions but also careful consideration of the physiological adaptations of pregnancy and the limitations they impose on diagnostic and therapeutic strategies. Diagnostic evaluation should be guided by clinical suspicion and supported with timely neuroimaging and laboratory investigations, while treatment planning must carefully balance maternal benefit against fetal safety. A multidisciplinary approach remains essential to achieve optimal maternal and neonatal outcomes.

11.2 Headaches

Migraine and other types of headaches are quite common clinical disorders during pregnancy. However, headaches are often not treated with adequate, safe, and effective methods in pregnancy, in which both physicians and patients have an instinct to avoid all kinds of medications. On the other hand, due to the increased risk of certain secondary headaches during pregnancy and after childbirth, obstetricians, family physicians, and neurologists should increase their awareness in this regard.

When a patient presents with headache complaints during pregnancy, a thorough inquiry should be conducted, and patients should be carefully evaluated for primary or secondary headaches.

11.2.1 Primary Headaches

In the first two trimesters of pregnancy, primary headaches usually become milder or improve. Most women (approximately 50%) experience improvement in headaches by the end of the first trimester, and more than 80% are headache-free by the end of the second trimester [1].

Tension-type headaches are the most common type of headache worldwide; however, due to their severity and the disability they cause, they are less likely to be the leading cause for hospital visits compared to migraines. The prevalence of migraines is three times higher in women of reproductive age than in men. Additionally, migraines have been associated with pregnancy-related hypertensive disorders, miscarriage, low birth weight, and preterm birth [2]. Cluster headache is a type of headache that is unilateral, does not switch sides, is short-lasting, comes in clusters, and is accompanied by autonomic symptoms. It is more common in men, and the frequency of its occurrence during pregnancy is low [3].

It is crucial to stress that whether a woman has a primary headache diagnosis before pregnancy or not, when a pregnant woman describes a headache, the clinician should be vigilant for secondary headaches due to the increased risks involved.

11.2.2 Secondary Headaches

When evaluating headache complaints during pregnancy and postpartum, a variety of secondary headache syndromes should be considered, including vascular and hypertensive disorders, cerebrospinal fluid (CSF) pressure issues (intracranial hypertension or hypotension), infections, and endocrine disorders (such as hypothyroidism and pituitary hemorrhage).

Cerebral venous thrombosis has been associated with hormonal changes in pregnancy, hypercoagulability, dehydration, and dural puncture during delivery [4, 5]. Headache is the most frequent complaint, and patients may present with focal neurological deficits, symptoms of eclampsia, papilledema, or epileptic seizures. The diagnosis is made with MR venography (contrast agents can be safely used in the postpartum period), and treatment is managed with LMWH.

Pregnancy-related hypertensive disorders require special attention. Preeclampsia is a serious clinical condition characterized by widespread endothelial damage, placental ischemia, and immune system changes during pregnancy. Since more extensive information on preeclampsia is provided in various sections of this book, details will not be discussed here. The key point to emphasize is that if sudden and severe headache occurs during pregnancy, especially accompanied by high blood pressure and proteinuria, preeclampsia should always be considered.

In a pregnant woman presenting with headache and encephalopathy (confusion, seizures, focal neurological deficits), cerebral imaging, especially showing edema in the posterior portions of the hemisphere, should strongly raise suspicion for posterior reversible encephalopathy syndrome (PRES). This is the radiological counterpart of endothelial dysfunction, and imaging findings (cerebral MRI) reflect secondary disruptions in cerebral autoregulation that arise in the setting of increased hydrostatic pressure and endothelial cell dysfunction [6].

Another pregnancy-related hypertensive disorder is reversible cerebral vasoconstriction syndrome (RCVS), which can present with a sudden, thunderclap-like headache and focal neurological deficits. Like PRES, RCVS is reversible unless permanent cerebral damage occurs or it becomes complicated [6].

Cerebrovascular events during pregnancy, whether hemorrhagic or ischemic strokes, may also present with headaches. When neck pain accompanies the headache, dissection of the neck vessels should be considered, and additional neurological signs should be sought. More detailed information on stroke during pregnancy will be discussed in later sections of this article.

Idiopathic intracranial hypertension can present with pulsatile tinnitus, refractory headache, and visual field narrowing. In cases where no other cause for the increase in CSF pressure is found, surgery (optic nerve fenestration) to protect the optic nerve and the placement of a ventriculoperitoneal shunt should not be delayed, if indicated. After dural puncture, a decrease in intracranial pressure may cause a headache that worsens upon standing, while lying down would worsen the headache in cases of increased intracranial CSF pressure.

Pituitary apoplexy, which involves hemorrhagic infarction of the pituitary gland, usually presents with a thunderclap-like headache.

11.2.3 Treatment

During the examination of all women of reproductive age, pregnancy plans should be inquired about when prescribing medication, and the teratogenic effects of medications should be discussed. In women receiving chronic headache treatment who are planning pregnancy, oral medications should be gradually reduced and discontinued before ovulation. In patients using monoclonal antibodies targeting calcitonin gene-related peptide (CGRP) activity, injections should be stopped approximately 5–6 months before pregnancy. The use of onabotulinumtoxin A injections during pregnancy is controversial, and the consensus is to avoid it.

When treating acute headaches during pregnancy, no medication should be considered completely safe for the fetus. The benefit-risk ratio should be considered, aiming to improve functionality and quality of life. The goal is to achieve reliable clinical benefit within 2 h.

Acetaminophen has long been considered safe during pregnancy and is frequently used for its analgesic effect. However, a 2020 review by the Agency for Healthcare Research and Quality, updated in 2021, suggested that metoclopramide, diphenhydramine, and triptans may be better first-line options than acetaminophen for the treatment of acute headache attacks during pregnancy [7]. It has been noted that the use of acetaminophen in the third trimester is associated with early closure of the ductus arteriosus, an increased incidence of respiratory tract infections during early childhood with frequent use, and a potential link to attention deficit hyperactivity disorder (ADHD) with prolonged use. In this context, it is recommended to avoid frequent use of acetaminophen during pregnancy. Metoclopramide, lidocaine, diphenhydramine, and ondansetron are recommended by some authorities [7, 8].

In the acute treatment of a migraine attack during pregnancy, second-line options include triptans, ibuprofen, corticosteroids, and prochlorperazine [7, 9, 10].

Ergot alkaloids should not be used during pregnancy. Similarly, direct CGRP receptor antagonists (ubrogepant and rimegepant) and serotonin 1F agonist lasmiditan are not recommended for use during pregnancy due to insufficient safety data.

In pain management, neuromodulation therapies such as transcranial magnetic stimulation, vagus nerve stimulation, trigeminal or occipital nerve stimulation, although having lower efficacy and challenges in accessibility due to their high costs, can be alternative options to medical treatments during pregnancy.

Chronic prophylactic pain treatments are used in the long-term management of primary headaches, which are frequent, severe, functionally impairing, and negatively affecting the quality of life. When considering the initiation of these treatments during pregnancy, safety and efficacy are important concerns. It should be kept in mind that many patients' headaches will decrease or improve during pregnancy, and therefore, decisions regarding chronic treatment should not be rushed.

The primary long-term preventive treatment options during pregnancy are propranolol and oral magnesium. Although fetal risks have been reported regarding the use of intravenous magnesium for more than 5 days in eclampsia and preeclampsia, no risks have yet been reported for oral magnesium [11].

In the Agency for Healthcare Research and Quality's review, calcium channel blockers and antihistamines have been recommended as first-line treatments for the prophylactic management of headaches during pregnancy [7]. There are some studies suggesting that when sufficient benefit cannot be achieved with these, onabotulinumtoxin A injections, CoQ10, antidepressants (SNRIs, tricyclics), and gabapentin may be considered, taking the benefit-risk ratio into account. However, it is important to highlight that there is insufficient safety data regarding onabotulinumtoxin A during pregnancy.

Similarly, due to a lack of sufficient data, new agents such as direct anti-CGRP monoclonal antibodies are not used during pregnancy. ACE inhibitors and angiotensin II receptor blockers are also avoided due to fetal risks. Valproic acid is contraindicated for migraine prophylaxis during pregnancy [11].

11.2.4 Breastfeeding

Generally, the treatment options during pregnancy show similar safety and efficacy data during breastfeeding as well. Additionally, since onabotulinumtoxin A has a large molecular weight, it would be appropriate to say that it is relatively safe during breastfeeding.

11.3 Epilepsy

Epileptic seizures are the most common major neurological complication during pregnancy, and epilepsy is one of the most common neurological diseases that requires continuous treatment throughout pregnancy [12]. Therefore, women of reproductive age with a diagnosis of epilepsy require specialized care during pregnancy.

The results of a cohort study in the United Kingdom, which included data from over one million pregnancies, have shown that the use of antiepileptic drugs (AEDs) in the first trimester does not increase the risk of miscarriage. The same study observed a dose-dependent increased risk of miscarriage in pregnancies of patients with epilepsy, with this risk being particularly prominent in those using valproate [13].

11.3.1 Fertility

The use of antiepileptic drugs (AEDs), especially polytherapy (the use of multiple AEDs) and certain medications like phenobarbital, can negatively affect fertility [14]. In addition, 2019 data from the U.S. Epilepsy Birth Control Registry showed that the live birth rate was higher in patients using lamotrigine (89.1%) compared to those using valproate (63.3%) [15].

11.3.2 Birth Control and Family Planning

Hormonal birth control pills are typically absorbed through the intestines and metabolized by the CYP3A4 enzyme. Some antiepileptic drugs (e.g., phenytoin, phenobarbital, carbamazepine) increase the production of the CYP3A4 enzyme, which rapidly metabolizes the estrogenic and progestogenic components of birth control pills. This reduces the effectiveness of the pills and increases the risk of contraceptive failure [16].

Some newer AEDs (e.g., felbamate, topiramate) have a weaker effect on the CYP3A4 enzyme and may have different effects on estrogen and progestin components. To reduce the risk of contraceptive failure, women with epilepsy who are taking enzyme-inducing AEDs are advised to use high-dose birth control pills. Additionally, using an additional method of contraception (e.g., condoms and spermicides or an intrauterine device (IUD)) is recommended [17]. Some AEDs, such as lamotrigine, levetiracetam, and zonisamide, which do not induce the CYP3A enzyme, are considered to have no significant impact on hormonal contraceptive methods. However, an important point should not be overlooked regarding lamotrigine. While progestin components do not alter lamotrigine serum levels, the estrogen component stimulates glucuronidation pathways, leading to a 40–60% decrease in lamotrigine levels. This reduction may increase the risk of seizures. Moreover, during the hormone-free week, lamotrigine levels may rise and reach toxic levels. To manage this interaction, the lamotrigine dose should be adjusted according to serum levels, or alternative methods such as an intrauterine device (IUD) should be considered [18].

Women with epilepsy are considered high-risk during pregnancy due to increased risks of certain obstetric and fetal complications, such as miscarriage, antepartum hemorrhage, gestational hypertension, preeclampsia, breech position, labor induction, cesarean delivery, and preterm birth. Moreover, seizures during pregnancy are dangerous not only due to the risk of seizure-related falls and trauma but also because of their potential to cause hypoxia and asphyxia in the fetus [19]. Most women with epilepsy do not experience a change in seizure frequency during pregnancy and childbirth, while only about 1–2% may see an increase in seizure frequency during labor [20].

During pregnancy, changes in plasma volume, a decrease in serum protein concentration, alterations in drug metabolism, and hormonal factors are expected to cause changes in blood levels of medications. To maximize seizure control during this period, it is recommended to monitor antiepileptic drug levels and adjust dosages frequently [19]. In 2019, the ILAE ranked antiepileptic drugs based on the extent of decrease in serum concentrations during pregnancy as follows: lamotrigine, levetiracetam, oxcarbazepine (40–70%), phenobarbital, phenytoin, topiramate, and zonisamide (30–60%), carbamazepine, and valproate (10–20%) [21]. It is known that women with epilepsy have an increased risk of hypertension and preeclampsia during pregnancy. In a meta-analysis of 17 studies, it was shown that the risk of gestational hypertension and preeclampsia in women with epilepsy is increased by 37% (odds ratio, 1.37; 95% confidence interval, 1.21–1.55) [19]. It has also been suggested that there is a relationship between the use of antiepileptic drugs and these hypertensive disorders; while lamotrigine and levetiracetam do not predispose to mild preeclampsia, valproate has been shown to increase the risk of mild preeclampsia [22].

Spontaneous miscarriage rates in pregnant women with epilepsy are associated with the level of development of countries. The lowest rate was reported in Norway, at 0.5% among women with epilepsy, compared to 0.3% in women without epilepsy; this data comes from a population-based study involving a total of 372,128 births [23]. Both epilepsy and the use of antiepileptic drugs are among the factors that increase the risk of preterm birth [24]. Uncontrolled seizure activity also increases the risk of preterm birth [25].

11.3.3 Congenital Malformation

The causes of congenital malformations are likely multifactorial, involving a combination of both endogenous and exogenous factors. The risk increases with antiepileptic drug use during early pregnancy, depending on the type and dose of the drugs used, whether the treatment is monotherapy or polytherapy, low maternal serum folate levels, and low maternal education level [26]. The most common malformations are cardiovascular system disorders, followed by musculoskeletal system disorders [27]. The most significant factor increasing this risk is the teratogenic effects of antiepileptic drugs. Valproate carries a particularly high risk of congenital malformations, as well as cognitive and behavioral disorders [28]. While some antiepileptic drugs (AEDs) have a lower risk profile (e.g., lamotrigine, levetiracetam), the risks of many newer AEDs (e.g., perampanel, brivaracetam) lack sufficient human pregnancy data [29].

A 2016 Cochrane Review meta-analysis evaluated the risk of congenital malformations associated with antiepileptic drugs (AEDs) used as monotherapy. The reported malformation risks, from lowest to highest, were as follows: gabapentin (1.47%), levetiracetam (1.77%), oxcarbazepine (2.39%), topiramate (4.28%), carbamazepine (4.93%), phenytoin (6.26%), phenobarbital (7.10%), primidone (8.49%), and valproate (10.93%) [30].

A case-control study by the European Surveillance of Congenital Anomalies (EUROCAT), covering 19 congenital anomaly registries and data from 3.8 million births, observed an increased risk of spina bifida with valproate (odds ratio, 12.7; 95% confidence interval, 7.7–20.7) and carbamazepine (odds ratio, 2.6; 95% confidence interval, 1.2–5.3). Carbamazepine and phenytoin have well-documented risks (neural tube defects, facial clefts), but their risks were lower than valproate [31, 32]. Topiramate carries a moderate risk, higher than newer AEDs but lower than older agents like phenytoin or carbamazepine. Its association with cleft palate and low birth weight warrants caution. Primidone and phenobarbital (barbiturates) are rarely used today due to high teratogenicity and neurodevelopmental risks [33].

In addition, children of mothers with epilepsy may experience various developmental deficits, such as impairments in language skills, cognitive capacity, and social-emotional functioning. While nearly all antiepileptic drugs (AEDs) have been implicated in cognitive deficits, valproate is most strongly associated with these outcomes. Children exposed to valproate in utero had IQ scores 8–11 points lower than those exposed to lamotrigine, carbamazepine, or phenytoin (NEAD Study) [34, 35]. It has also been reported that the risk of autism spectrum disorder (ASD) in children exposed to valproate in utero is 4.4%, compared to 1.5% in the general population [36]. Among the proposed mechanisms for neurodevelopmental risks of valproate could be histone deacetylase (HDAC) inhibition and GABAergic effects. Lamotrigine and levetiracetam are recommended as safer alternatives [37, 38].

Folic acid supplementation is critically important during pregnancy. During pregnancy, folate requirements increase by 5–10 times compared to nonpregnant women. Adequate periconceptional folate levels are essential for the structural and functional development of the fetal brain. Particularly in the early stages of pregnancy (the first 12 weeks), a daily intake of more than 400 mcg of folic acid is associated with better neurodevelopmental outcomes in children of mothers with epilepsy. Certain antiepileptic drugs (AEDs), especially those that induce cytochrome P450 enzymes, lower folate levels and can negatively impact the structural and functional development of the fetal brain. Early folic acid supplementation has been shown to help prevent not only major congenital malformations but also language delays and autistic traits linked to intrauterine exposure to antiepileptic drugs [39]. The American Academy of Neurology recommends that preconception folic acid supplementation be between 0.4 and 4 mg/day [12].

11.3.4 Breastfeeding

In a 2020 study examining the ratio of infant serum antiepileptic drug concentrations to maternal concentrations during breastfeeding, the reported ratios were 0.3% for oxcarbazepine, 5.3% for levetiracetam, 5.4% for carbamazepine-epoxide, 17.2%

for topiramate, 21.4% for valproic acid, 28.9% for lamotrigine, and 44.2% for zonisamide. The study emphasized that for all the drugs, the infant serum concentrations were significantly lower than the maternal serum concentrations [40]. Considering the physical and neurodevelopmental benefits of breast milk, it is widely accepted that breastfeeding is not harmful and should be strongly encouraged even in women with epilepsy who are using antiepileptic drugs.

11.4 Demyelinating CNS Diseases (Multiple Sclerosis and Neuromyelitis Optica Spectrum Disorders)

Multiple sclerosis (MS) is a chronic, demyelinating, inflammatory, and neurodegenerative autoimmune disease that disrupts the structural and functional integrity of myelin, axons, and neurons in the central nervous system. MS affects women of reproductive age three times more frequently than men and is often characterized clinically by relapses and remissions, along with progressive neurological functional loss. Up to 33% of women diagnosed with MS become pregnant after the onset of the disease [41].

Thanks to advancements in the pharmaceutical industry, treatment options for MS have significantly improved in recent years. The availability of numerous effective immunomodulatory and immunosuppressive therapies approved by the FDA and EMA has provided reassurance to clinicians. However, for most of these treatments, dosage and frequency adjustments—or even complete discontinuation—are required during pregnancy. This necessitates careful planning and close monitoring of medication regimens in women of reproductive age diagnosed with MS.

Recent studies indicate that, with well-managed care, women with MS can experience a healthy pregnancy and successfully breastfeed. In women with MS, the frequency of relapses decreases during pregnancy; however, in about one-third of patients, an increase in relapse rates has been reported within the first 3–6 months after delivery [42]. On the other hand, it been reported that mothers with MS have a slightly higher likelihood of giving birth to babies with lower birth weight compared to mothers without MS (3.4% vs. 2.8%) [43].

The second most common demyelinating disease affecting young adults, primarily involving the spinal cord and optic nerves, is neuromyelitis optica spectrum disorders (NMOSD). This condition affects women nine times more frequently than men, and in most patients, antibodies against the aquaporin-4 protein found in astrocytes are detected. Unlike MS, disease activity in NMOSD has been reported to increase even during pregnancy, and obstetric complications are also observed more frequently [44].

Intrapartum and postpartum outcomes are closely related to disease stability during the year prior to pregnancy in patients with MS or NMOSD [45]. Therefore, planned pregnancy and achieving disease stabilization before conception are strongly recommended. Highly active disease should be well-controlled before, during, and after pregnancy using effective disease-modifying therapies (DMTs).

11.4.1 Disease-Modifying Therapies

Among the DMTs that can be used in MS treatment, first-line injectable agents such as glatiramer acetate and interferon-betas do not require a washout period and can be used until conception, and even during pregnancy depending on the clinician's judgment.

Among oral medications are S1P receptor modulators, fumarates, teriflunomide, and cladribine. All of these should be discontinued during pregnancy. S1P receptor modulators are recommended to be stopped 2 months before conception; however, due to the risk of rebound inflammatory activity, bridging therapy with anti-CD20 treatments or natalizumab is advised. Fumarates are also agents that do not require a washout period and can be used until pregnancy occurs. Teriflunomide must be cleared from the body with a rapid elimination protocol before conception, due to its teratogenic and fetotoxic effects.

Patients receiving cladribine can plan pregnancy 6 months after completing the treatment course (i.e., in the 18th month). Anti-CD20 monoclonal antibodies (ocrelizumab, rituximab) should be discontinued 2–3 months before planning a pregnancy.

Due to the high risk of rebound and the absence of demonstrated obstetric or fetal risks, natalizumab may be used—with extended dosing intervals of 6–8 weeks—up to the 32nd week of pregnancy.

Azathioprine, used in the treatment of NMOSD, can be continued throughout pregnancy. Methotrexate is recommended to be discontinued 1 month before conception, and mycophenolate mofetil 6 weeks before. Monoclonal antibodies, such as inebilizumab, rituximab, and eculizumab, should be stopped 2 months before conception; however, in cases where maternal risks outweigh fetal risks, it has been reported that these treatments may be continued during pregnancy with informed risk acceptance. Tocilizumab and satralizumab should be discontinued 2–3 months prior to conception [46].

11.4.2 Relapse Treatment

During pregnancy, if an MS relapse suspicion arises and new neurological symptoms develop, MRI can be performed outside of the first trimester, if possible. When deciding on relapse treatment, if possible, methylprednisolone, prednisone, and prednisolone should be preferred, as they are inactivated by placental 11-β-hydroxysteroid dehydrogenase and do not pass into the fetal circulation outside the first trimester. The use of high-dose steroids in the second and third trimesters has been associated with pregnancy-related hypertension, preeclampsia, intrauterine growth restriction (IUGR), and low birth weight. Therefore, treatment decisions should be made carefully and considered in cases where new neurological and/or functional disabilities develop [47, 48].

When a woman with NMOSD develops a suspected relapse during pregnancy, intravenous methylprednisolone treatment is primarily recommended. In cases of steroid-resistant relapses, IVIG (0.4 g/kg/day) or plasmapheresis are suggested as options [49].

After delivery, close follow-up should be conducted to monitor both visible and nonvisible clinical symptoms neurologically, as well as to track both clinical and silent inflammation.

11.4.3 Breastfeeding

Breastfeeding should be encouraged due to its benefits for both the mother and the child. If gadolinium-enhanced MRI is performed, milk should be pumped and discarded 6–8 h after the injection. The transfer of large molecules such as glatiramer acetate and interferon-beta to breast milk is minimal and considered negligible. The transfer of monoclonal antibodies to breast milk has also been reported at low levels. There is insufficient safety data regarding the use of oral disease-modifying therapies (DMTs) during breastfeeding [46, 50].

Due to the very limited data on pregnancy in relation to central nervous system involvement in Behçet's disease, ADEM, Susac syndrome, and various rheumatologic diseases, these topics will not be discussed in detail here.

11.5 Neuromuscular Diseases

Neuromuscular diseases constitute a broad group of disorders that include lower motor neuron disorders, peripheral neuropathies, neuromuscular junction disorders, and muscle diseases, encompassing various genetic or acquired conditions. Preconception counseling should be provided for genetic disorders, and medication adjustments should be made prior to pregnancy for acquired conditions under treatment. Close monitoring is essential during pregnancy and in the postpartum period for potential disease exacerbations.

11.5.1 Peripheral Neuropathies

One of the most common hereditary neuropathies is Charcot-Marie-Tooth (CMT) disease. Distal motor and sensory involvement in all extremities typically begins in the first to third decade, with gait disturbances gradually accompanied by hand and foot deformities. Although conflicting reports have been published in the literature, an increased fetal risk is not expected in pregnant women with CMT [51]. During pregnancy, one-third of women with CMT may experience a worsening of disease symptoms [52]. There is no specific feature related to the type of anesthesia during delivery; the mode of delivery should be decided by the clinician based on the patient's clinical condition, muscle strength, and fatigue level.

Autoimmune neuropathies may have occurred before pregnancy, but they can also present during pregnancy or after delivery. Women who are still undergoing treatment due to previous peripheral neuropathy should have their treatment regimen adjusted before pregnancy, and disease stabilization should be achieved prior to pregnancy.

Guillain-Barré syndrome (GBS) is a clinical condition, most commonly presenting as acute inflammatory demyelinating polyneuropathy (AIDP), typically triggered by an infection (such as C. jejuni, CMV, and EBV) several weeks prior. It is characterized by rapidly progressing bilateral weakness in the extremities and sometimes facial muscles, paresthesias, and loss of reflexes. The highest level of disability is reached approximately 2–8 weeks after the onset of symptoms, and progression ceases after 8 weeks [53]. Diagnosis is established based on clinical findings, albuminocytologic dissociation in the CSF, and electrophysiological studies. While no difference has been reported in the incidence of GBS during pregnancy, interestingly, an increased frequency has been noted within the first month postpartum [54]. IVIG or plasmapheresis may be preferred for treatment.

Chronic inflammatory demyelinating polyneuropathy (CIDP) is an inflammatory autoimmune neuropathy typically characterized by painless proximal and distal muscle weakness, sensory disturbances, and hypo/areflexia lasting more than 8 weeks. The diagnosis is made based on clinical findings, electrophysiological tests, and increased protein levels in the CSF [55]. Corticosteroids, IVIg, and plasmapheresis can be used in the treatment of CIDP relapses during pregnancy. In women who are on long-term immunosuppressive therapy, medications such as rituximab, cyclosporine, cyclophosphamide, and mycophenolate mofetil should be discontinued before pregnancy. Azathioprine can be continued during pregnancy [56].

Focal neuropathies are clinical conditions that can frequently occur during pregnancy. Hormonal changes, musculoskeletal system changes, weight gain, and fluid retention are considered responsible. Carpal tunnel syndrome and cubital tunnel syndrome are typically treated with conservative approaches, such as avoiding repetitive movements and using night splints. Rarely, especially during prolonged labor, positional compression can lead to secondary fibular neuropathy, obturator neuropathy, femoral neuropathy, and lumbar radiculopathy. Treatment is also conservative. Interestingly, Bell's palsy is reported to occur three times more frequently during pregnancy. It is most common in the third trimester and in the first month following delivery. Oral steroids and antiviral agents are used in treatment [57].

11.5.2 Neuromuscular Junction Disorders

Myasthenia gravis is an autoimmune disease that disrupts neuromuscular junction communication, leading to fluctuating weakness in the skeletal muscles. It can be classified into ocular, bulbar, or generalized MG depending on the affected area. In 85% of patients, antibodies against the acetylcholine receptor (AChR) are detected. Diagnosis is made using clinical findings, serology, and electrophysiological tests. When diagnosed during pregnancy, a chest CT for thymoma can be postponed until after delivery unless there is serious suspicion. If necessary, a chest MRI can be performed. Thymectomy should be deferred to elective conditions [58].

In symptomatic treatment, pyridostigmine is considered safe during pregnancy. If symptom control is insufficient, steroids can be used, and steroid-sparing agents such as azathioprine and cyclosporine can be administered for long-term treatment. Agents like mycophenolate mofetil, cyclophosphamide, and methotrexate, which are used in long-term immunosuppressive therapy for MG, should not be used during pregnancy, and treatment adjustment prior to pregnancy is necessary. Although real-world data has not reported major anomalies in infants exposed to rituximab and eculizumab in utero, caution is advised [59, 60].

If symptoms can be controlled with pyridostigmine and/or corticosteroids, this represents the optimal scenario for management during pregnancy. Due to the risk of myasthenic exacerbation or crisis, discontinuation of steroid-sparing agents during pregnancy is not recommended unless necessary. Likewise, initiation of such agents in pregnancy is not urgent, since they require prolonged time to achieve full effect [61]. In the case of preeclampsia/eclampsia, beta-blockers, calcium channel blockers, and magnesium should be used with caution, as they may cause myasthenic exacerbation. Safer agents, such as hydralazine, should be preferred. When infection treatment is required, antibiotics that do not lead to neuromuscular transmission disturbances should be selected.

During delivery, non-depolarizing agents, neuromuscular blockers, narcotics, and general anesthesia should be avoided. Regional anesthesia is considered safe. The mode of delivery should be decided by the clinician based on the patient's muscle strength and level of fatigue.

After delivery, neonates should be closely monitored for neonatal myasthenia (a temporary myasthenic condition caused by maternal antibodies transferred to the baby) during the first 48 h [58].

During breastfeeding, pyridoxine, corticosteroid doses of 20 mg/g or lower, IVIG, plasmapheresis, azathioprine, cyclosporine, and eculizumab are considered relatively safe.

11.5.3 Myopathies

Acquired autoimmune inflammatory myopathies (such as polymyositis, dermatomyositis, and inclusion body myositis) are rare during the reproductive age. However, it has been reported that there is no disease worsening during pregnancy, and in fact, clinical improvement is observed in half of the patients, with remission occurring after pregnancy [62].

In women diagnosed with myotonic dystrophy, a type of adult-onset muscular dystrophy, the infertility rate is high, and it has been reported that complications such as spontaneous abortions, ectopic pregnancies, preterm labor, peripartum hemorrhage, and placenta previa are more common during pregnancy. Both striated and smooth muscles (including the uterus) are affected. When maternal transmission leads to anticipation, congenital myotonic dystrophy may occur in the baby, presenting with a more severe clinical picture and potentially manifesting as polyhydramnios during pregnancy [63]. General anesthesia should be avoided during delivery; regional anesthesia should be preferred. The mode of delivery should be selected by the clinician based on the patient's muscle strength and fatigue level [64].

In women diagnosed with limb-girdle muscular dystrophy or mitochondrial myopathy, assisted delivery may be required due to a decrease in proximal muscle strength. Generally, regional anesthesia should be preferred.

11.6 Stroke

The incidence of maternal stroke is reported to be three times higher than in non-pregnant women of the same age group, at 30 per 100,000. Half of these pregnancy-related stroke cases are hemorrhagic strokes. The highest risk period for maternal stroke is reported to be the peripartum period and the first 1–2 weeks following delivery [65]. Due to factors such as advancing maternal age, increasing obesity, smoking, pregnancy-related hypertension, and hypercoagulable states, the number of pregnancy-related stroke cases has increased over the years.

Stroke increases maternal mortality by 100 times [66]. Unfortunately, maternal hemorrhagic stroke outcomes are fatal in up to 50% of cases [67]. On the other hand, outcomes of maternal ischemic stroke are somewhat more favorable. Women who experience acute ischemic stroke during pregnancy or the postpartum period and receive acute reperfusion therapy have good outcome rates like those of non-pregnant women of the same age group [68].

The pathophysiology of maternal stroke requires careful consideration of the physiological changes that occur during pregnancy. The increase in cardiac output, augmented venous capacitance because of pregnancy hormones, systemic vasodilation, and increased vascular compliance raise the risk of venous stasis. Meanwhile, increased sympathetic vasomotor activation raises the risk of reversible cerebral vasoconstriction syndrome. With intravascular volume expansion, the serum levels of certain clotting factors decrease, and along with a shift toward a procoagulant state in the body, there is a tendency toward thrombosis [69]. Additionally, changes in the immune system that begin after conception, as well as maternal infections, have been identified as separate risk factors for maternal stroke [70, 71].

Preeclampsia can lead to both hemorrhagic and ischemic cerebrovascular complications through various mechanisms, including RCVS, PRES, spontaneous cervical artery dissection, cerebral venous thrombosis, arterial ischemic stroke, SAH, and ICH [72].

The etiology of acute ischemic infarcts that develop during pregnancy and the postpartum period is often due to cardioembolism and paradoxical embolism resulting from a patent foramen ovale or peripartum events. Cervical artery dissection should also be considered as a cause of stroke in young women.

The most common cause of intracerebral hemorrhage during pregnancy is hypertensive disease of pregnancy. Less frequently, hemorrhage from an existing aneurysm or AV malformation may occur. Hemorrhagic cerebral infarcts secondary to cerebral venous thrombosis can also be seen. Factors that predispose to cerebral venous thrombosis during pregnancy include dehydration, obesity, preeclampsia, infections, underlying factor deficiencies, and dural puncture [4, 69]. In pregnancy, subarachnoid hemorrhage most commonly develops secondary to reversible cerebral vasoconstriction syndrome (RCVS). This condition, RCVS, is characterized by temporary, multifocal, segmental, non-vasculitic vasospasm of large and medium-sized cerebral arteries. Although the condition is reversible, it may leave permanent neurological deficits due to prolonged cerebral ischemia [73]. Patients with frequent migraine attacks, hypertension, thrombophilia, or a history of previous stroke should be considered high-risk for maternal stroke and should be monitored with blood pressure checks during pregnancy and the postpartum period.

A history of previous stroke does not constitute an indication for cesarean delivery, but in patients who have experienced an acute stroke, cesarean delivery is recommended due to the risk of hemorrhagic conversion [70].

11.6.1 Treatment

In cases of suspected acute stroke during pregnancy, if rapid access to MRI is not available, a brain CT should be performed urgently for differential diagnosis of ischemic or hemorrhagic stroke. When there is suspicion of large artery occlusion or rupture, CT angiography is recommended [74].

Early treatment of acute ischemic stroke during pregnancy does not contraindicate intravenous thrombolytic therapy. Alteplase and tenecteplase do not cross the placenta [75]. When indicated, mechanical thrombectomy should not be withheld [76].

In the treatment of acute hemorrhagic stroke, controlling bleeding (if appropriate, through endovascular or surgical methods), effective blood pressure control (labetalol, methyldopa, long-acting nifedipine), correction of coagulopathy, and prevention and treatment of complications such as vasospasm, hydrocephalus, raised intracranial pressure (ICP), and seizures should be considered.

In cases of increased intracranial pressure, the goal should be to avoid hypotension, ensure adequate cerebral perfusion pressure, and provide analgesia and sedation. Low-dose hyperosmolar therapy (0.25–0.5 g/kg) with mannitol can be administered [77].

The diagnosis, treatment, and follow-up of maternal stroke require a high level of awareness, a multidisciplinary approach involving obstetricians, neurologists, neurosurgeons, anesthesiologists, radiologists, and pediatricians, along with close monitoring. While minimizing fetal risks, the goal should be to protect maternal health and reduce morbidity and mortality.

11.7 Movement Disorders

Movement disorders and pregnancy co-occurrence, although not common, require awareness and knowledge regarding the dual effects of medical treatments and potential issues during pregnancy and childbirth. Hyperkinetic (chorea, dystonia, essential tremor, tics, myoclonus, restless legs syndrome, etc.) and hypokinetic (e.g., Parkinson's disease) movement disorders may be observed.

Essential tremor, the most common movement disorder in the population, can also occur in pregnant women, though not frequently. This clinical condition, often with a family history, does not pose maternal or fetal risks. Propranolol and primidone, the recommended treatments, are considered contraindicated during pregnancy due to their teratogenic effects. Other treatment options, such as gabapentin and topiramate, are not recommended for the treatment of essential tremor during pregnancy, considering the benefit-risk balance [78].

The most common movement disorder during pregnancy is restless legs syndrome (RLS). It typically manifests later in the day during rest, with restlessness in the legs and a strong urge to move them, which is relieved by standing up and walking. Primary RLS is often associated with a family history, while secondary RLS has been linked to various conditions such as iron deficiency anemia, diabetic peripheral neuropathy, chronic kidney disease, and pregnancy [79]. The incidence of restless legs syndrome (RLS) during pregnancy has been reported to be around 25%, and it typically occurs in the third trimester. In most cases, it disappears after childbirth. The efficacy of dopaminergic medications in the treatment of RLS has been demonstrated, and reports on a limited number of pregnant women and a few cases suggest that these medications do not pose a fetal risk [80].

Chorea can be described as random, sudden, short-lived muscle contractions that can occur in any part of the body. It may involve the facial, trunk, or distal limb muscles. One of the secondary causes is pregnancy (chorea gravidarum). Basal ganglia strokes, diabetes mellitus, drug use, Wilson's disease, and Huntington's disease should be ruled out in differential diagnosis [81]. Risk factors include a history of rheumatic fever, systemic lupus erythematosus (SLE), antiphospholipid antibody

(APA) syndrome, and encephalitis. It often begins after the first trimester and can rarely have a severe course, in which case treatment is recommended. Dopamine receptor blockers are used in treatment. Since the teratogenic effects in human pregnancies have not been clearly demonstrated, patients should be informed about the potential side effects [82].

Dystonia is a movement disorder characterized by involuntary, repetitive, and sustained muscle contractions that result in twisting or turning movements in a specific direction and pattern. Simultaneous contraction of agonist and antagonist muscles occurs. Early onset increases the likelihood of generalized dystonia. Most cases of primary hereditary dystonia exhibit autosomal dominant (AD) inheritance. During pregnancy, dystonia often presents acutely as a secondary condition due to commonly used antiemetics. However, rare cases of pregnancy-induced dystonia not related to medication (dystonia gravidarum) have also been reported. It is generally accepted that pregnancy does not have negative effects on dystonia [83]. Dystonia treatment includes the use of levodopa, as well as baclofen and trihexyphenidyl. It is thought that the use of levodopa during pregnancy does not pose major fetal risks. Although data on its use during pregnancy is limited, it has been reported that when high doses of baclofen are used during pregnancy, withdrawal symptoms may occur in the newborn after birth [84]. Caution should also be exercised when using benzodiazepines. They can cause withdrawal symptoms in the newborn after delivery and may also lead to difficulties such as weakness in sucking during breastfeeding, as they pass into breast milk. Although small case series and case reports regarding the use of onabotulinumtoxin A during pregnancy have not reported serious fetal risks, its use during pregnancy is not recommended. Deep brain stimulation (DBS) for dystonia is considered not to pose fetal or maternal risks [85]. In pregnant women who have undergone DBS, if delivery is to be by cesarean section, it is recommended to use a bipolar electrocautery, and to keep electronic devices at least 15 cm away from the DBS stimulator and cables. The use of short-wave (27 MHz) and microwave (2.54 GHz) diathermy for wound healing, as well as therapeutic ultrasound (1–5 MHz), is contraindicated in cases with DBS [86, 87].

Idiopathic Parkinson's disease is a neurodegenerative, progressive disorder characterized by bradykinesia, rigidity, resting tremor, and postural instability. Considering the characteristic distribution of age and gender, the coexistence of pregnancy and Parkinson's disease is rare, and the literature data on this topic is based solely on case reports or small case series. There are case reports indicating that levodopa, carbidopa, benserazide, pramipexole, and ropinirole, which are used in the treatment of Parkinson's disease, do not pose fetal risks. Amantadine should not be used during pregnancy [88].

Acknowledgments I would like to express my profound gratitude to Professor Bedile Irem Tiftikcioglu, M.D., HOD of Neurology, for her scientifically insightful, critical, and constructive contributions during the preparation of this review.

References

1. van Casteren DS, van den Brink AM, Terwindt GM. Migraine and other headache disorders in pregnancy. Handb Clin Neurol. 2020;172:187–99.
2. Skajaa N, Szepligeti SK, Xue F, Sorensen HT, Ehrenstein V, Eisele O, et al. Pregnancy, birth, neonatal, and postnatal neurological outcomes after pregnancy with migraine. Headache. 2019;59(6):869–79.
3. Fischera M, Marziniak M, Gralow I, Evers S. The incidence and prevalence of cluster headache: a meta-analysis of population-based studies. Cephalalgia. 2008;28(6):614–8.
4. Guner D, Tiftikcioglu BI, Uludag IF, Oncel D, Zorlu Y. Dural puncture: an overlooked cause of cerebral venous thrombosis. Acta Neurol Belg. 2015;115(1):53–7.
5. Liang ZW, Gao WL, Feng LM. Clinical characteristics and prognosis of cerebral venous thrombosis in Chinese women during pregnancy and puerperium. Sci Rep. 2017;7:43866.
6. Lucia M, Viviana M, Alba C, Giulia D, Carlo DR, Porpora MG, et al. Neurological complications in pregnancy and the puerperium: methodology for a clinical diagnosis. J Clin Med. 2023;12(8):2994.
7. Saldanha IJ, Roth JL, Chen KK, Zullo AR, Adam GP, Konnyu KJ, et al. Management of primary headaches in pregnancy. AHRQ comparative effectiveness reviews. Rockville: Agency for Healthcare Research and Quality; 2020.
8. Parker SE, Van Bennekom C, Anderka M, Mitchell AA, National Birth Defects Prevention Study. Ondansetron for treatment of nausea and vomiting of pregnancy and the risk of specific birth defects. Obstet Gynecol. 2018;132(2):385–94.
9. Burch R. Epidemiology and treatment of menstrual migraine and migraine during pregnancy and lactation: a narrative review. Headache. 2020;60(1):200–16.
10. Ephross SA, Sinclair SM. Final results from the 16-year sumatriptan, naratriptan, and treximet pregnancy registry. Headache. 2014;54(7):1158–72.
11. Rayhill M. Headache in pregnancy and lactation. Continuum (Minneap Minn). 2022;28(1):72–92.
12. Harden CL, Pennell PB, Koppel BS, Hovinga CA, Gidal B, Meador KJ, et al. Practice parameter update: management issues for women with epilepsy--focus on pregnancy (an evidence-based review): vitamin K, folic acid, blood levels, and breastfeeding: report of the Quality Standards Subcommittee and Therapeutics and Technology Assessment Subcommittee of the American Academy of Neurology and American Epilepsy Society. Neurology. 2009;73(2):142–9.
13. Forbes H, Madley-Dowd P, Ahlqvist V, Campbell J, Davies NM, Liebling R, et al. First-trimester use of antiseizure medications and the risk of miscarriage: a population-based cohort study. J Neurol Neurosurg Psychiatry. 2024;95(8):693–703.
14. Sukumaran SC, Sarma PS, Thomas SV. Polytherapy increases the risk of infertility in women with epilepsy. Neurology. 2010;75(15):1351–5.
15. MacEachern DB, Mandle HB, Herzog AG. Infertility, impaired fecundity, and live birth/pregnancy ratio in women with epilepsy in the USA: findings of the Epilepsy Birth Control Registry. Epilepsia. 2019;60(9):1993–8.
16. Harden CL, Leppik I. Optimizing therapy of seizures in women who use oral contraceptives. Neurology. 2006;67(12 Suppl 4):S56–8.
17. Stephen LJ, Harden C, Tomson T, Brodie MJ. Management of epilepsy in women. Lancet Neurol. 2019;18(5):481–91.
18. Li Y, Meador KJ. Epilepsy and pregnancy. Continuum (Minneap Minn). 2022;28(1):34–54.
19. Viale L, Allotey J, Cheong-See F, Arroyo-Manzano D, McCorry D, Bagary M, et al. Epilepsy in pregnancy and reproductive outcomes: a systematic review and meta-analysis. Lancet. 2015;386(10006):1845–52.
20. Battino D, Tomson T, Bonizzoni E, Craig J, Lindhout D, Sabers A, et al. Seizure control and treatment changes in pregnancy: observations from the EURAP epilepsy pregnancy registry. Epilepsia. 2013;54(9):1621–7.

21. Tomson T, Battino D, Bromley R, Kochen S, Meador K, Pennell P, et al. Management of epilepsy in pregnancy: a report from the International League Against Epilepsy Task Force on Women and Pregnancy. Epileptic Disord. 2019;21(6):497–517.
22. Danielsson KC, Borthen I, Morken NH, Gilhus NE. Hypertensive pregnancy complications in women with epilepsy and antiepileptic drugs: a population-based cohort study of first pregnancies in Norway. BMJ Open. 2018;8(4):e020998.
23. Borthen I, Eide MG, Veiby G, Daltveit AK, Gilhus NE. Complications during pregnancy in women with epilepsy: population-based cohort study. BJOG. 2009;116(13):1736–42.
24. Soontornpun A, Choovanichvong T, Tongsong T. Pregnancy outcomes among women with epilepsy: a retrospective cohort study. Epilepsy Behav. 2018;82:52–6.
25. Artama M, Gissler M, Malm H, Ritvanen A, Drug and Pregnancy Group. Effects of maternal epilepsy and antiepileptic drug use during pregnancy on perinatal health in offspring: nationwide, retrospective cohort study in Finland. Drug Saf. 2013;36(5):359–69.
26. Tomson T, Battino D, Bonizzoni E, Craig J, Lindhout D, Perucca E, et al. Comparative risk of major congenital malformations with eight different antiepileptic drugs: a prospective cohort study of the EURAP registry. Lancet Neurol. 2018;17(6):530–8.
27. Meador K, Reynolds MW, Crean S, Fahrbach K, Probst C. Pregnancy outcomes in women with epilepsy: a systematic review and meta-analysis of published pregnancy registries and cohorts. Epilepsy Res. 2008;81(1):1–13.
28. Pettie MA, Wilkin-Krug LCM, Ellenbroek B. Pre- and postnatal valproate exposure affects brain development. Curr Top Behav Neurosci. 2025;75:43–68.
29. Practice Guideline from the AAN, AES, SMFM, Pack AM, Oskoui M, Roberson SW, Donley DK, et al. Teratogenesis, perinatal, and neurodevelopmental outcomes after in utero exposure to antiseizure medication. Epilepsy Curr. 2025:15357597241258514.
30. Weston J, Bromley R, Jackson CF, Adab N, Clayton-Smith J, Greenhalgh J, et al. Monotherapy treatment of epilepsy in pregnancy: congenital malformation outcomes in the child. Cochrane Database Syst Rev. 2016;11(11):CD010224.
31. Jentink J, Loane MA, Dolk H, Barisic I, Garne E, Morris JK, et al. Valproic acid monotherapy in pregnancy and major congenital malformations. N Engl J Med. 2010;362(23):2185–93.
32. Jentink J, Dolk H, Loane MA, Morris JK, Wellesley D, Garne E, et al. Intrauterine exposure to carbamazepine and specific congenital malformations: systematic review and case-control study. BMJ. 2010;341:c6581.
33. Vajda FJE, O'Brien TJ, Graham JE, Hitchcock AA, Perucca P, Lander CM, et al. The teratogenesis risk associated with antiseizure medication duotherapy in women with epilepsy. Epilepsy Res. 2024;200:107316.
34. Oyen N, Vollset SE, Eide MG, Bjerkedal T, Skjaerven R. Maternal epilepsy and offsprings' adult intelligence: a population-based study from Norway. Epilepsia. 2007;48(9):1731–8.
35. Baker GA, Bromley RL, Briggs M, Cheyne CP, Cohen MJ, Garcia-Finana M, et al. IQ at 6 years after in utero exposure to antiepileptic drugs: a controlled cohort study. Neurology. 2015;84(4):382–90.
36. Christensen J, Gronborg TK, Sorensen MJ, Schendel D, Parner ET, Pedersen LH, et al. Prenatal valproate exposure and risk of autism spectrum disorders and childhood autism. JAMA. 2013;309(16):1696–703.
37. Meador KJ, Pennell PB, May RC, Van Marter L, McElrath TF, Brown C, et al. Fetal loss and malformations in the MONEAD study of pregnant women with epilepsy. Neurology. 2020;94(14):e1502–11.
38. Meador KJ, Cohen MJ, Loring DW, Matthews AG, Brown C, Robalino CP, et al. Cognitive outcomes at age 3 years in children with fetal exposure to antiseizure medications (MONEAD study) in the USA: a prospective, observational cohort study. Lancet Neurol. 2023;22(8):712–22.
39. Bjork M, Riedel B, Spigset O, Veiby G, Kolstad E, Daltveit AK, et al. Association of folic acid supplementation during pregnancy with the risk of autistic traits in children exposed to antiepileptic drugs in utero. JAMA Neurol. 2018;75(2):160–8.

40. Birnbaum AK, Meador KJ, Karanam A, Brown C, May RC, Gerard EE, et al. Antiepileptic drug exposure in infants of breastfeeding mothers with epilepsy. JAMA Neurol. 2020;77(4):441–50.
41. Hsu S, Balan A, Bove R. Topical review: lactation and use of DMTs in women with MS. Mult Scler. 2024;30(13):1578–91.
42. Vukusic S, Hutchinson M, Hours M, Moreau T, Cortinovis-Tourniaire P, Adeleine P, et al. Pregnancy and multiple sclerosis (the PRIMS study): clinical predictors of post-partum relapse. Brain. 2004;127(Pt 6):1353–60.
43. Chen YH, Lin HL, Lin HC. Does multiple sclerosis increase risk of adverse pregnancy outcomes? A population-based study. Mult Scler. 2009;15(5):606–12.
44. D'Souza R, Wuebbolt D, Andrejevic K, Ashraf R, Nguyen V, Zaffar N, et al. Pregnancy and neuromyelitis optica spectrum disorder – reciprocal effects and practical recommendations: a systematic review. Front Neurol. 2020;11:544434.
45. Das G, Damotte V, Gelfand JM, Bevan C, Cree BAC, Do L, et al. Rituximab before and during pregnancy: a systematic review, and a case series in MS and NMOSD. Neurol Neuroimmunol Neuroinflamm. 2018;5(3):e453.
46. Bove RM, Houtchens MK. Pregnancy management in multiple sclerosis and other demyelinating diseases. Continuum (Minneap Minn). 2022;28(1):12–33.
47. Galati A, Brown ES, Bove R, Vaidya A, Gelfand J. Glucocorticoids for therapeutic immunosuppression: clinical pearls for the practicing neurologist. J Neurol Sci. 2021;430:120004.
48. Battin M, Bevan C, Harding J. Growth in the neonatal period after repeat courses of antenatal corticosteroids: data from the ACTORDS randomised trial. Arch Dis Child Fetal Neonatal Ed. 2012;97(2):F99–105.
49. Wind M, Gaasbeek AGA, Oosten LEM, Rabelink TJ, van Lith JMM, Sueters M, et al. Therapeutic plasma exchange in pregnancy: a literature review. Eur J Obstet Gynecol Reprod Biol. 2021;260:29–36.
50. Langer-Gould AM. Pregnancy and family planning in multiple sclerosis. Continuum (Minneap Minn). 2019;25(3):773–92.
51. Pisciotta C, Calabrese D, Santoro L, Tramacere I, Manganelli F, Fabrizi GM, et al. Pregnancy in Charcot-Marie-Tooth disease: data from the Italian CMT national registry. Neurology. 2020;95(24):e3180–9.
52. Rudnik-Schoneborn S, Thiele S, Walter MC, Reinecke L, Sereda M, Schoneborn R, et al. Pregnancy outcome in Charcot-Marie-Tooth disease: results of the CMT-NET cohort study in Germany. Eur J Neurol. 2020;27(8):1390–6.
53. Leonhard SE, Mandarakas MR, Gondim FAA, Bateman K, Ferreira MLB, Cornblath DR, et al. Diagnosis and management of Guillain-Barre syndrome in ten steps. Nat Rev Neurol. 2019;15(11):671–83.
54. Meenakshi-Sundaram S, Swaminathan K, Karthik SN, Bharathi S. Relapsing Guillain-Barre syndrome in pregnancy and postpartum. Ann Indian Acad Neurol. 2014;17(3):352–4.
55. Van den Bergh PYK, van Doorn PA, Hadden RDM, Avau B, Vankrunkelsven P, Allen JA, et al. European Academy of Neurology/Peripheral Nerve Society guideline on diagnosis and treatment of chronic inflammatory demyelinating polyradiculoneuropathy: report of a joint task force-second revision. J Peripher Nerv Syst. 2021;26(3):242–68.
56. Birru Talabi M, Clowse MEB. Antirheumatic medications in pregnancy and breastfeeding. Curr Opin Rheumatol. 2020;32(3):238–46.
57. Evangelista V, Gooding MS, Pereira L. Bell's palsy in pregnancy. Obstet Gynecol Surv. 2019;74(11):674–8.
58. Hamel J, Ciafaloni E. An update: myasthenia gravis and pregnancy. Neurol Clin. 2018;36(2):355–65.
59. Perrotta K, Kiernan E, Bandoli G, Manaster R, Chambers C. Pregnancy outcomes following maternal treatment with rituximab prior to or during pregnancy: a case series. Rheumatol Adv Pract. 2021;5(1):rkaa074.
60. Vu T, Harvey B, Suresh N, Farias J, Gooch C. Eculizumab during pregnancy in a patient with treatment-refractory myasthenia gravis: a case report. Case Rep Neurol. 2021;13(1):65–72.

61. Massey JM, Gable KL. Neuromuscular disorders and pregnancy. Continuum (Minneap Minn). 2022;28(1):55–71.
62. Pinal-Fernandez I, Selva-O'Callaghan A, Fernandez-Codina A, Martinez-Gomez X, Rodrigo-Pendas J, Perez-Lopez J, et al. "Pregnancy in adult-onset idiopathic inflammatory myopathy": report from a cohort of myositis patients from a single center. Semin Arthritis Rheum. 2014;44(2):234–40.
63. Edmundson C, Guidon AC. Neuromuscular disorders in pregnancy. Semin Neurol. 2017;37(6):643–52.
64. Johnson NE, Hung M, Nasser E, Hagerman KA, Chen W, Ciafaloni E, et al. The impact of pregnancy on myotonic dystrophy: a registry-based study. J Neuromuscul Dis. 2015;2(4):447–52.
65. Swartz RH, Cayley ML, Foley N, Ladhani NNN, Leffert L, Bushnell C, et al. The incidence of pregnancy-related stroke: a systematic review and meta-analysis. Int J Stroke. 2017;12(7):687–97.
66. Elgendy IY, Gad MM, Mahmoud AN, Keeley EC, Pepine CJ. Acute stroke during pregnancy and puerperium. J Am Coll Cardiol. 2020;75(2):180–90.
67. Scott CA, Bewley S, Rudd A, Spark P, Kurinczuk JJ, Brocklehurst P, et al. Incidence, risk factors, management, and outcomes of stroke in pregnancy. Obstet Gynecol. 2012;120(2 Pt 1):318–24.
68. Leffert LR, Clancy CR, Bateman BT, Cox M, Schulte PJ, Smith EE, et al. Treatment patterns and short-term outcomes in ischemic stroke in pregnancy or postpartum period. Am J Obstet Gynecol. 2016;214(6):723 e1–11.
69. Zhang X, Fang K, Zhang Y, Song J, Wang R, Ji X, et al. Cerebral venous thrombosis during pregnancy and postpartum: a systematic review and meta-analysis. Int J Stroke. 2025;20:17474930251355751.
70. Miller EC. Maternal stroke associated with pregnancy. Continuum (Minneap Minn). 2022;28(1):93–121.
71. Esenwa CC, Elkind MS. Inflammatory risk factors, biomarkers and associated therapy in ischaemic stroke. Nat Rev Neurol. 2016;12(10):594–604.
72. Miller EC, Vollbracht S. Neurology of preeclampsia and related disorders: an update in neuro-obstetrics. Curr Pain Headache Rep. 2021;25(6):40.
73. McDermott M, Miller EC, Rundek T, Hurn PD, Bushnell CD. Preeclampsia: association with posterior reversible encephalopathy syndrome and stroke. Stroke. 2018;49(3):524–30.
74. Puac P, Rodriguez A, Vallejo C, Zamora CA, Castillo M. Safety of contrast material use during pregnancy and lactation. Magn Reson Imaging Clin N Am. 2017;25(4):787–97.
75. Powers WJ, Rabinstein AA, Ackerson T, Adeoye OM, Bambakidis NC, Becker K, et al. Guidelines for the early management of patients with acute ischemic stroke: 2019 update to the 2018 guidelines for the early Management of acute ischemic stroke: a guideline for healthcare professionals from the American Heart Association/American Stroke Association. Stroke. 2019;50(12):e344–418.
76. Ladhani NNN, Swartz RH, Foley N, Nerenberg K, Smith EE, Gubitz G, et al. Canadian stroke best practice consensus statement: acute stroke management during pregnancy. Int J Stroke. 2018;13(7):743–58.
77. Godoy DA, Robba C, Paiva WS, Rabinstein AA. Acute intracranial hypertension during pregnancy: special considerations and management adjustments. Neurocrit Care. 2022;36(1):302–16.
78. Ba F, Miyasaki JM. Movement disorders in pregnancy. Handb Clin Neurol. 2020;172:219–39.
79. Anguizola D, Garcia Aragon A, Moncada B, Garcia-Borreguero D. Restless legs syndrome: neurochemistry and therapy. Semin Neurol. 2025;45:368.
80. Dostal M, Weber-Schoendorfer C, Sobesky J, Schaefer C. Pregnancy outcome following use of levodopa, pramipexole, ropinirole, and rotigotine for restless legs syndrome during pregnancy: a case series. Eur J Neurol. 2013;20(9):1241–6.
81. Maia DP, Fonseca PG, Camargos ST, Pfannes C, Cunningham MC, Cardoso F. Pregnancy in patients with Sydenham's Chorea. Parkinsonism Relat Disord. 2012;18(5):458–61.

82. Gentile S. Antipsychotic therapy during early and late pregnancy. A systematic review. Schizophr Bull. 2010;36(3):518–44.
83. Trender-Gerhard I, Sweeney MG, Schwingenschuh P, Mir P, Edwards MJ, Gerhard A, et al. Autosomal-dominant GTPCH1-deficient DRD: clinical characteristics and long-term outcome of 34 patients. J Neurol Neurosurg Psychiatry. 2009;80(8):839–45.
84. Ratnayaka BD, Dhaliwal H, Watkin S. Drug points: neonatal convulsions after withdrawal of baclofen. BMJ. 2001;323(7304):85.
85. Mehanna R, Tarakad A, Taneff LY, Furr Stimming E. Pregnancy in dystonia or Tourette's patients with DBS. Fourteen news cases and a review of the literature. Mov Disord Clin Pract. 2025;12(1):82–8.
86. Paluzzi A, Bain PG, Liu X, Yianni J, Kumarendran K, Aziz TZ. Pregnancy in dystonic women with in situ deep brain stimulators. Mov Disord. 2006;21(5):695–8.
87. Balaz M, Buril J, Kunst J, Hrabovsky D, Hajda S, Chrastina J. Deep brain stimulation during pregnancy and delivery: review of current literature. J Neurol Surg A Cent Eur Neurosurg. 2023;84(3):275–80.
88. Lehn AC, Lee JY, Sciacca G, Patterson S, Morton A, Pun P, et al. The management of Parkinson's disease before, during and after pregnancy-an MDS Scientific Issues Committee review. Mov Disord Clin Pract. 2025. https://doi.org/10.1002/mdc3.70289.

Chapter 12
Understanding and Addressing Musculoskeletal Challenges in Pregnancy

Filiz Meryem Sertpoyraz

12.1 Introduction

Pregnancy is one of the periods during which the female body undergoes the most comprehensive physiological changes. In this process, not only the reproductive system but also all organ systems—especially the cardiovascular, respiratory, endocrine, and musculoskeletal systems—are affected to varying degrees. Changes in the musculoskeletal system, in particular, may lead to painful syndromes that directly impact maternal quality of life as pregnancy advances. Postural adaptations, hormonal fluctuations, weight gain, and fluid retention collectively increase susceptibility to a range of musculoskeletal problems.

The most common musculoskeletal conditions encountered during pregnancy include low back pain, carpal tunnel syndrome, chondromalacia patella, transient osteoporosis of the hip, osteonecrosis of the femoral head, and muscle cramps. Beyond limiting daily activities, these conditions can disrupt sleep quality and precipitate psychosocial challenges. Thus, the pain experienced in pregnancy has physical, emotional, and social dimensions.

Accurately understanding pregnancy-related musculoskeletal changes and the clinical entities they provoke is essential for designing preventive strategies and appropriate treatment plans. Patient education, postural modifications, structured exercise programs, and physiotherapeutic interventions suffice in most cases, whereas medical or surgical treatments may be required in selected situations. Consequently, a holistic, multidisciplinary approach to musculoskeletal problems in pregnancy is a cornerstone of safeguarding both maternal and fetal health.

F. M. Sertpoyraz (✉)
Izmir Bakircay University, Faculty of Medicine, Department of Physical Medicine and Rehabilitation, Izmir, Turkey
e-mail: filiz.sertpoyraz@bakircay.edu.tr

© The Author(s), under exclusive license to Springer Nature Switzerland AG 2026

I. Karaca (ed.), *Managing Maternal Chronic Diseases for a Healthy Pregnancy*,
https://doi.org/10.1007/978-3-032-15221-3_12

12.2 Musculoskeletal Changes During Pregnancy

Pregnancy induces widespread physiological alterations across all maternal systems, with the musculoskeletal system being particularly affected due to its association with painful syndromes that can significantly impair maternal quality of life. Approaches to managing these pain syndromes must consider both maternal well-being and fetal safety, often requiring a multidisciplinary strategy.

The anatomical and physiological adaptations observed in pregnancy are essential for meeting the developmental needs of both the mother and the fetus, ensuring maternal homeostasis and optimal fetal growth. Changes in estrogen and relaxin levels play a key role in musculoskeletal adaptations, leading to ligamentous laxity, soft tissue edema, weight gain, and secondary postural alterations of the spine.

In addition, cardiovascular and respiratory adjustments are also of clinical importance. To meet fetal demands, maternal heart rate increases, while peripheral vascular resistance decreases, promoting cardiopulmonary adaptation. Respiratory changes include increased tidal volume, oxygen consumption, and ventilatory capacity [1]. The musculoskeletal changes in pregnancy are multifactorial. The progressive enlargement of the uterus shifts the maternal center of gravity anteriorly, leading to postural adaptations such as increased lumbar lordosis and thoracic cage expansion. Concurrently, gestational weight gain imposes additional mechanical load on the spine, pelvis, and lower extremities, further contributing to discomfort and pain. Increased fluid retention, particularly during the third trimester, results in soft tissue edema and may predispose to entrapment neuropathies and reduced joint mobility. In addition, hormonal influences—most notably elevated estrogen and relaxin levels—induce connective tissue laxity, which enhances pelvic joint mobility but also increases susceptibility to musculoskeletal strain and instability.

12.2.1 Alterations in Center of Gravity and Postural Changes

With the progressive enlargement and increased weight of the uterus, the maternal center of gravity—normally located at the level of the second sacral vertebra—shifts anteriorly. This anterior displacement, combined with the increased abdominal load, necessitates compensatory postural adaptations, most notably an increase in lumbar lordosis to maintain balance. The accentuation of lumbar lordosis induces biomechanical changes both proximally and distally: abdominal muscles become elongated with a loss of tone, while lumbar extensor muscles shorten and demonstrate increased tension.

As a consequence, anterior pelvic tilt develops, accompanied by knee hyperextension and excessive load on the medial aspect of the foot, which promotes pronation. To compensate for exaggerated lumbar lordosis, thoracic kyphosis increases, resulting in rounded shoulders and a forward head posture. These alterations are further associated with shortening of the pectoral muscles, elongation of the rhomboids, and cervical spine dysfunction. Additionally, reliance on an upper thoracic breathing pattern contributes to hyperactivity of the scalene muscles, which may predispose to thoracic outlet syndrome. Collectively, these postural modifications create muscular imbalances and joint dysfunctions, some of which may persist until approximately the 12th postpartum week [2, 3].

12.2.2 *Weight Gain*

Gestational weight gain contributes to increased mechanical loading on the lumbar spine, pelvic joints, and lower extremities. These regions, already influenced by hormonal and postural changes, are subjected to additional strain, which may exacerbate discomfort and predispose to musculoskeletal pain.

12.2.3 *Increased Fluid Retention*

Enhanced fluid retention during pregnancy can lead to a variety of musculoskeletal problems. Most commonly observed in the third trimester, edema in the lower extremities reduces joint range of motion and contributes to discomfort. Moreover, fluid accumulation, in combination with postural changes, is an important factor in the development of entrapment neuropathies.

12.2.4 *Hormonal Changes*

Hormonal alterations in pregnancy, particularly elevated levels of estrogen, progesterone, endogenous cortisol, and especially relaxin, produce distinct changes in connective tissue. Relaxin softens cartilage, increases ligamentous laxity, and induces synovial proliferation. These effects result in relaxation and hypermobility of the pelvic girdle joints, while simultaneously imposing greater mechanical stress on the sacroiliac joints as well as the pelvic and lumbar vertebral articulations.

12.3 Preexisting Musculoskeletal Pain Conditions Before Pregnancy

Low back pain is reported to be more common in women with preexisting musculoskeletal disorders such as spondylolisthesis, vertebral degeneration, or lumbar disc disease prior to pregnancy. Lumbar discopathy present before conception may worsen during gestation, existing scoliosis may progress, and coccydynia that had previously resolved can reappear during pregnancy [4, 5].

The musculoskeletal pain conditions most frequently observed in pregnancy are listed below [6]:

1. Low back pain
2. Nerve compression syndromes
3. De Quervain's tenosynovitis
4. Soft tissue pain syndromes
5. Chondromalacia patella
6. Rectus diastasis
7. Progression of scoliosis
8. Avascular necrosis of the femoral head
9. Transient osteoporosis of the hip in pregnancy
10. Leg cramps

12.3.1 Low Back Pain

Low back pain is the most common musculoskeletal problem encountered during pregnancy. Recent studies report a prevalence of 40.5%, with rates of 28.3% in the first trimester, 36.8% in the second trimester, and 47.8% in the third trimester. The primary etiological factors include ligamentous laxity, postural changes, and increased biomechanical loading. Pregnancy-related low back pain typically begins around the 6th month of gestation and may persist until 6 months postpartum [7]. It is often associated with sleep disturbances and can negatively affect daily activities and overall quality of life [8].

12.3.1.1 Causes of Low Back Pain

Sacroiliac Joint Dysfunction

The sacroiliac joint is responsible for 10–25% of low back pain cases. Studies indicate that sacroiliac joint dysfunction accounts for posterior pelvic and low back pain in 20–80% of pregnant women [5]. The pain may radiate to the hip, groin, and lower extremities. Diagnosis relies on clinical evaluation and provocation tests. Sacral sulcus tenderness is a frequent finding, and the Gillet test is commonly used. In this test, the examiner places a finger on the posterior superior iliac spine while the patient lifts the affected leg; lack of expected movement indicates dysfunction.

Pelvic Relaxation

Pelvic relaxation refers to pain originating from the symphysis pubis and/or sacroiliac joints associated with pregnancy or delivery. Risk factors include multiparity, abnormal fetal presentation, congenital anomalies, and ligamentous laxity during pregnancy. Pelvic relaxation often coexists with sacroiliac joint dysfunction.

Magnetic resonance imaging can aid diagnosis, although clinical findings remain key. Symptoms include pain in the sacroiliac joint, pubic symphysis, and medial thigh. Tenderness on palpation of the pubic bone and/or sacroiliac joint and a positive Trendelenburg test are common findings.

Lumbar Discopathy
Pregnancy has been reported as an independent risk factor for postpartum lumbar disc herniation. Preexisting disc disease may become symptomatic during pregnancy, leading to pain syndromes [4, 5, 8].

Spondylolisthesis
Spondylolisthesis, characterized by anterior displacement of one vertebra over the one below, can be exacerbated during pregnancy due to hormonal changes—particularly relaxin-induced connective tissue laxity—combined with weight gain and postural adaptations. It is most commonly observed at the lumbosacral junction, particularly at L5–S1. In pregnant women, spondylolisthesis may aggravate low back pain, cause radicular symptoms extending to the lower extremities, and significantly impair daily activities. Preexisting spondylolisthesis may become symptomatic or progress during pregnancy. Diagnosis is based on clinical assessment and imaging, while management is primarily conservative. Patient education, postural correction, and exercise programs are the mainstay of treatment. Surgical intervention is rarely required but may be considered in cases of severe neurological deficits within a multidisciplinary framework.

Coccydynia
Coccydynia refers to pain localized to the coccyx, the terminal portion of the sacrum. In pregnancy, the enlarging uterus exerts pressure on the pelvic floor and coccyx, while excessive strain or trauma during labor can trigger symptoms. Prolonged labor, difficult delivery, and instrumental interventions such as forceps are recognized risk factors. Women with preexisting coccygeal pathology may also experience recurrence or worsening of symptoms during gestation. Clinically, pain is aggravated by sitting and accentuated when rising to a standing position. Conservative management is preferred, including posture modification, specialized cushions, analgesics, and physiotherapy. In rare refractory cases, interventional procedures may be required.

Postural Low Back Pain
Postural back pain results from mechanical stress secondary to accentuated thoracic and lumbar lordosis during pregnancy. The pain is typically mechanical in nature, worsens with movement, and improves with rest [9].

12.3.1.2 Management of Low Back Pain

The primary goals in the management of pregnancy-related low back pain are effective pain control, reduction of functional limitations in daily activities, and improvement of overall quality of life. Therapeutic strategies include patient education, rest and activity modification, structured exercise programs, lumbar–abdominal or pelvic supports, physiotherapeutic modalities, relaxation techniques, massage, acupuncture, kinesiotherapy, chiropractic care, yoga, and pharmacological interventions.

Patient Education
Weight control should be encouraged, and pregnant women should be informed about musculoskeletal adaptations and proper body mechanics. Educational programs aim to prevent and reduce painful conditions by providing reassurance and guidance. Patients should be advised to remain active, continue daily routines as tolerated, and engage in individualized exercise programs when appropriate. Emphasis on posture correction and regular physical activity is also critical for preventing both antenatal and postpartum pain [5, 8, 9].

Rest
Rest is frequently employed during acute pain episodes to alleviate symptoms. However, prolonged bed rest is discouraged, as it may lead to muscle weakness, joint stiffness, and circulatory problems. Rest should therefore be brief and performed in positions that minimize discomfort. Lateral decubitus positioning—particularly on the left side—has been shown to enhance uteroplacental perfusion and relieve pressure on the lumbar and pelvic regions. Adequate mattress support and the use of pillows under the lumbar spine and hips to maintain a neutral posture may facilitate pain relief. Clinical practice guidelines recommend avoiding complete immobilization; instead, controlled mobilization combined with short periods of rest and exercise is more effective. Hence, rest should be viewed as part of a comprehensive treatment approach rather than as a stand-alone therapy.

Exercise
Both individual and group-based exercise programs are recommended for the prevention and treatment of low back pain in pregnancy. These may include aerobic, strengthening, and stretching routines, performed on land or in water. Evidence from meta-analyses suggests that exercise interventions reduce pain, improve functional capacity, and decrease sick leave associated with pregnancy-related back pain. Recent studies have also highlighted the beneficial effect of music-accompanied exercise sessions [5]. Exercises are particularly useful for postural low back pain and sacroiliac joint dysfunction. Stretching is emphasized for shortened muscles, while strengthening is recommended for elongated or weakened muscle groups. Specific examples include supine bridge exercises and isometric abdominal contractions for sacroiliac dysfunction, gluteus medius and maximus strengthening to stabilize pelvic joints, and pelvic tilt exercises to preserve lumbar and hip muscle strength. Correct body mechanics during lifting, carrying, and posture adjustment are equally important for long-term pain control.

Yoga
Yoga incorporates breathing techniques, stretching, and relaxation practices that improve joint mobility, flexibility, muscle strength and endurance, balance, concentration, and self-confidence, while simultaneously promoting psychological

well-being. Prenatal yoga has demonstrated benefits in reducing anxiety, depression, stress, low back pain, and sleep disturbances among pregnant women. Although data in high-risk pregnancies remain limited, existing studies suggest improvements in maternal outcomes. Initiating yoga during pregnancy is considered safe, with high maternal and fetal tolerance [10, 11].

Progressive Muscle Relaxation

Progressive muscle relaxation is a technique designed to reduce stress responses and perceived pain by systematically relaxing major muscle groups, often combined with deep breathing exercises. It has been shown to provide both physical and psychological benefits in pregnant populations [12].

Mechanical Supports

Mechanical supports such as lumbar and pelvic braces are commonly used in pregnant women with painful conditions. These devices restrict spinal motion, stabilize the lumbar spine and pelvis, reduce mechanical loading, and provide additional warmth and massage effects. Examples include the Ozzlo pillow—a wedge-shaped support that relieves nocturnal pain when placed under the abdomen in lateral decubitus—and trochanteric belts, which have been found effective in alleviating symptoms of pelvic insufficiency [10]. Specially designed pelvic support belts for pregnant women are frequently used in cases of pubic symphysis separation and sacroiliac dysfunction, providing both structural support and symptom relief [11, 12].

Physiotherapeutic Modalities and Medical Treatment

Superficial Heat and Cold Therapy

Localized application of superficial heat or cold can provide symptomatic relief. According to the gate control theory, cold application inhibits sensory nerve conduction, reduces catecholamine levels, and increases endorphin release, thereby elevating the pain threshold and decreasing pain intensity. Heat therapy exerts similar effects; however, direct application to the uterus and abdominal region should be avoided [13].

Transcutaneous Electrical Nerve Stimulation (TENS)

TENS is a noninvasive therapeutic modality primarily used to alleviate pain by delivering electrical impulses to peripheral nerves via surface electrodes placed over the painful region. It is believed to inhibit nociceptive transmission by activating inhibitory interneurons in the substantia gelatinosa of the spinal cord and/or by engaging descending pain modulation pathways. Clinical studies have shown that TENS improves pain and functional outcomes in pregnant women with low back pain and reduces work absenteeism, with no reported adverse effects on either the mother or fetus [14–16]. Its use is generally recommended after the second trimester. Additionally, intrapartum use of TENS has been associated with shorter labor duration and reduced need for postpartum analgesics [17].

Acupuncture

Acupuncture involves the insertion of fine needles at specific meridian points to promote energy flow ("Qi") and stimulate endogenous opioid release. Although its safety and efficacy during pregnancy remain debated, existing studies report that acupuncture may be effective and safe for low back and pelvic pain, with no significant adverse fetal effects [18, 19]. Nevertheless, serious organic pathology must be excluded before initiating treatment, and a careful risk–benefit analysis along with informed patient consent is essential.

Massage, Mobilization, and Manipulation

Myofascial release and deep connective tissue massage may be beneficial for soft tissue imbalances. In cases of sacroiliac subluxation, gentle manipulative techniques have been shown to relieve low back pain, while forceful or aggressive manipulations are discouraged. Osteopathic manipulative therapy—encompassing stretching, gentle pressure, and resistance techniques—has been reported in a meta-analysis to significantly reduce pain and improve functional disability in pregnant women, although the evidence is of moderate quality [14, 19].

Kinesio Taping

Kinesio tape is an elastic therapeutic tape widely used in sports injuries and musculoskeletal disorders. By lifting the skin, it is thought to improve blood and lymphatic flow, reduce pain, and support muscles and joints. A meta-analysis demonstrated that kinesio taping reduced pregnancy-related low back pain within the first week of use, promoted functional recovery, and could be safely applied during the second and third trimesters. Except for rare allergic reactions, it is considered free of major side effects, which makes it an attractive adjunctive therapy [20, 21].

Pharmacological Therapy

Acetaminophen remains the first-line analgesic for pregnancy-related low back pain. Depending on the trimester, other medications such as ibuprofen, diclofenac, metamizole, and opioids may be considered with caution, though special care must be taken when prescribing NSAIDs in the third trimester [22]. Analgesics that can be used during different trimesters of pregnancy are shown in Table 12.1. COX-2 inhibitors are not recommended. For neuropathic pain, tricyclic antidepressants (e.g., amitriptyline) and serotonin-norepinephrine reuptake inhibitors, such as duloxetine and venlafaxine, are considered safe options.

Surgical Treatment

Surgical intervention plays a very limited role in the management of low back pain during pregnancy, as the vast majority of cases are attributable to mechanical, hormonal, and postural changes that can be effectively controlled with conservative measures. However, in rare instances, surgery may become necessary in the presence of severe neurological deficits, progressive motor weakness, or impairment of bladder and bowel function. In the literature, acute cauda equina syndrome secondary to lumbar disc herniation is considered one of the few absolute indications for surgical management during pregnancy.

When surgical treatment is indicated, both maternal and fetal safety must be prioritized, with careful attention to anesthesia selection, surgical positioning, and intraoperative monitoring. Decisions regarding surgical intervention should ideally be made within a multidisciplinary framework involving obstetrics, orthopedics or neurosurgery, anesthesiology, and neonatology teams. Outside of such urgent indications, surgery may only be considered in rare cases where conservative treatment fails and severe, disabling pain significantly impairs maternal quality of life.

12.3.2 Nerve Compression Syndromes

12.3.2.1 Carpal Tunnel Syndrome

Carpal tunnel syndrome (CTS) is the most common peripheral nerve entrapment disorder affecting the upper extremity, particularly in women. During pregnancy, it represents the second most frequent musculoskeletal pain condition after low back pain. CTS occurs most commonly in the third trimester (63%), followed by the second (26%) and first trimesters (11%). The underlying pathophysiology is attributed to elevated levels of estrogen, aldosterone, cortisol, prolactin, and glucose, in combination with gestational weight gain and fluid retention. In particular, impaired venous return and edema at the level of the carpal ligament play a central role in median nerve compression [23].

Symptoms may be unilateral or bilateral and typically worsen with activity, presenting as pain in the hand, wrist, and radiocarpal joint. Paresthesia and tingling due to compression and ischemia of the median nerve are common, often accompanied by nocturnal pain and numbness that disturb sleep and impair quality of life, especially during the third trimester. These symptoms may also impose additional physical and psychological burden on the pregnant patient. On physical examination, pain and sensory deficits are observed along the distribution of the median nerve, with possible thenar muscle atrophy and reduced grip strength.

Diagnosis is based on clinical history, physical examination, ultrasound, and electrophysiological studies. High-frequency ultrasonography, in particular, is considered safe and reliable during pregnancy. Its noninvasive nature, wide availability, low cost, short examination time, and absence of patient discomfort make it an attractive diagnostic tool. Sonographic findings supportive of CTS include increased cross-sectional area of the median nerve, a hypoechoic pattern due to neural edema,

Table 12.1 Analgesics that can be used during different trimesters of pregnancy

	First trimester	Second trimester	Third trimester
First-line option	Paracetamol Ibuprofen	Paracetamol Ibuprofen	Paracetamol
Second choice	Diclofenac	Diclofenac	—
Third choice	Metamizole	Metamizole	—

and a characteristic "hourglass" appearance of the nerve beneath the transverse carpal ligament [24].

12.3.2.2 Brachial Plexus Pain

Brachial plexus pain in pregnancy is a neuropathic condition that may develop as a result of postural changes and biomechanical adaptations in the shoulder girdle and cervical spine. Increased lumbar lordosis and thoracic kyphosis, accompanied by forward displacement of the head, can cause muscular imbalance in the shoulder girdle and hypertonicity of the scalene muscles, leading to mechanical compression of the brachial plexus. Clinically, this condition manifests particularly in the third trimester with symptoms of upper extremity pain radiating from the neck and shoulder, paresthesia, and muscle weakness.

12.3.2.3 Meralgia Paresthetica

Meralgia paresthetica is an entrapment neuropathy caused by compression of the lateral femoral cutaneous nerve (n. cutaneus femoralis lateralis) beneath the inguinal ligament. In pregnancy, the enlarging uterus, increased abdominal pressure, weight gain, and postural alterations predispose this nerve to compression. Clinically, patients present with numbness, burning, tingling, and sometimes superficial pain localized to the anterolateral aspect of the thigh. The condition is reported more frequently in the second half of pregnancy, with symptoms closely related to increased intra-abdominal pressure.

12.3.2.4 Tibial Posterior Nerve Compression

Tibial posterior nerve compression is a peripheral entrapment neuropathy that may occur in the advanced stages of pregnancy, predominantly due to lower extremity edema. The nerve becomes compressed as it passes behind the medial malleolus at the ankle. Patients typically report numbness, burning, tingling, and pain on the plantar surface of the foot and toes. Symptoms are aggravated by prolonged standing or walking. Fluid retention and circulatory changes during pregnancy are considered the primary etiological factors. On physical examination, a positive Tinel's sign at the medial malleolus supports the diagnosis. Management is generally conservative, including edema reduction strategies, rest, proper footwear, cold application, and light exercises. Orthotic support may be beneficial in refractory cases. Pharmacological options are limited during pregnancy; therefore, treatment relies primarily on non-pharmacological methods.

12.3.2.5 Intercostal Neuralgia

Intercostal neuralgia is occasionally observed in the third trimester, presenting as intermittent pain along the anterior margin of the lower ribs, typically unilateral. The condition arises from mechanical stretching of the costal joint soft tissues due to upward displacement of the uterus within the abdominal cavity. Management is conservative and includes local heat and cold application, combined with breathing exercises, which enhance therapeutic efficacy.

12.3.2.6 Thoracic Outlet Syndrome

Thoracic outlet syndrome (TOS) occurs as a result of compression of the brachial plexus, subclavian vein, and/or subclavian artery between the clavicle and the first rib. Contributing factors include extension of the upper cervical vertebrae, kyphotic alignment of the lower cervical and upper thoracic vertebrae, elevation of the first rib, internal rotation of the glenohumeral joint, forward head posture, and spasm of the scalene muscles. Clinically, patients present with pain and paresthesia in the upper extremity, often accompanied by circulatory disturbances such as edema and skin color changes.

Management of entrapment neuropathies, including TOS, is generally conservative. Standard approaches consist of patient education, rest and splinting, nerve and tendon gliding exercises, vitamin supplementation, nonsteroidal anti-inflammatory drugs (NSAIDs), and oral or injectable corticosteroids. In severe cases, decompression surgery may be considered. Patient education is an important component, focusing on pathophysiology, symptom recognition, and precautions during pregnancy and the postpartum period. In carpal tunnel syndrome, for example, patients should be advised to avoid wrist flexion activities, rest the affected hand, and use splints to maintain the wrist in a neutral position. Nerve and tendon gliding techniques may enhance venous return, reduce local edema, and improve neural conduction, and these exercises can be safely performed at home once proper instruction is given. Kinesio taping is another adjunctive option, with reported benefits including improved mobility and stability, reduced edema and muscle tension, and modulation of pain pathways [25].

For refractory or acutely exacerbated cases, pharmacological treatment may be required. Acetaminophen is generally considered the first-line option, while ibuprofen may be cautiously used after the 30th week of pregnancy [26]. Corticosteroid therapy, most often with dexamethasone acetate, has been reported as safe and effective in controlling symptoms, particularly in acute third-trimester carpal tunnel syndrome, where it may provide temporary relief until delivery [27]. Among physical therapy modalities, laser therapy has been shown to reduce local inflammation and alleviate pain, while phonophoresis can enhance the transdermal absorption of topical agents such as corticosteroids. Both techniques have demonstrated efficacy in decreasing pain and clinical symptoms of carpal tunnel syndrome [28].

12.3.3 De Quervain's Tenosynovitis

De Quervain's tenosynovitis is a common soft tissue disorder during pregnancy and, in particular, the postpartum period. Clinically, affected women present with pain and tenderness localized to the radial side of the wrist, typically aggravated by activities such as prolonged infant carrying, repetitive hand movements during breastfeeding, or grasping maneuvers while holding the baby. Additional findings may include reduced grip strength, discomfort when pinching or grasping with the thumb, and occasional swelling along the radial aspect of the wrist.

The Finkelstein test is widely used in diagnosis; the maneuver reproduces characteristic pain when the thumb is placed inside the fist and the wrist is forced into ulnar deviation. Most cases can be managed conservatively with rest, wrist splinting, stretching exercises, and application of cold compresses. In persistent or severe cases, corticosteroid injections may be considered, though pharmacological interventions during pregnancy and lactation require cautious evaluation and careful risk–benefit assessment.

12.3.4 Soft Tissue Pain

Soft tissue–related pain is relatively common in pregnancy, with both hormonal and mechanical changes playing key roles in its pathogenesis. Elevated levels of estrogen and relaxin contribute to connective tissue laxity and reduced joint stability, while increased fluid retention promotes edema within the soft tissues. These physiological changes predispose pregnant women to muscular strain, tension, and the development of trigger points.

As pregnancy progresses, the growing uterus and maternal weight gain alter the center of gravity, necessitating postural adaptations. Stretching of the abdominal muscles, increased load on the paraspinal and lumbar musculature, and muscular imbalance around the cervical and shoulder girdle regions contribute to soft tissue pain, most commonly localized to the lower back, pelvic girdle, and cervical spine. Clinically, such pain presents with muscle tenderness, tension, trigger points, pain exacerbated by movement, and functional limitation. Literature indicates that myofascial pain syndromes are particularly prominent during the second and third trimesters, predominantly in the lumbar and pelvic regions. These symptoms may impair sleep quality, restrict daily activities, and negatively affect overall quality of life. Additionally, trapezius and cervical muscle tension associated with postural imbalance may precipitate headaches and neck pain.

Management focuses primarily on conservative measures. Postural education, ergonomic modifications, regular stretching and relaxation exercises, and light aerobic activity are generally beneficial. Adjunctive interventions may include physiotherapeutic modalities such as heat and cold application, transcutaneous electrical nerve stimulation (TENS), ultrasound, manual therapy, and massage.

Pharmacological therapy is limited and should be reserved for cases requiring additional symptom control, with careful consideration of safe agents during pregnancy. Thus, management of soft tissue pain in pregnancy should be individualized, multimodal, and symptom-directed.

12.3.5 Chondromalacia Patella

Chondromalacia patella is characterized by softening, fibrillation, or ulceration of the cartilage on the posterior surface of the patella, presenting clinically with anterior knee pain. Symptoms are typically exacerbated by prolonged sitting, knee flexion, and extension. Conservative treatment is the first-line approach and includes activity modification, rest, cold application, use of patellar-stabilizing braces, patellofemoral joint mobilization, and quadriceps-strengthening exercises. Surgical intervention is considered only in cases where conservative measures fail to achieve adequate symptom relief [29].

12.3.6 Rectus Diastasis

Rectus diastasis refers to an abnormal widening of the linea alba, resulting in excessive separation between the two rectus abdominis muscles. Parity is the most frequently reported etiological factor. During pregnancy, elevated levels of estrogen, progesterone, and relaxin contribute to tissue laxity and reduced supportive function of the connective tissue. The condition is often observed when the rectus abdominis contracts against gravity, such as during the transition from a supine to a sitting position [30].

Rectus diastasis has two major clinical consequences. The first is aesthetic impairment of the abdominal contour, and the second is functional issues such as poor posture and low back pain. In severe cases, rectus diastasis may predispose to back pain, compromise abdominal wall integrity, and even increase the risk of fetal injury. Malpresentation and inefficient abdominal contractions during labor and delivery have also been associated with this condition. Noninvasive prenatal management aims to preserve abdominal muscle strength and prevent progression of diastasis.

Conservative therapy is considered the first-line approach. Although limited studies have investigated the role of exercise therapy in rectus diastasis, its principal advantage is being a noninvasive intervention. Regular exercise before pregnancy appears to reduce the risk of diastasis and narrow the inter-rectus distance [31]. After delivery, abdominal exercises are routinely recommended for women with rectus diastasis. Other nonsurgical interventions include aerobic exercise, postural and back-care education, and the use of external supports such as corsets or Tubigrip bandages [32].

12.3.7 Progression of Scoliosis

The course of preexisting scoliosis during pregnancy remains variable, although most studies suggest that mild to moderate curvatures do not exert a significant adverse impact on pregnancy or delivery. Nevertheless, hormonal changes leading to connective tissue laxity, weight gain, and postural adaptations may predispose some patients to curve progression. The risk is particularly higher in women with severe or structural scoliosis, where increased lumbar lordosis and mechanical loading during pregnancy can exacerbate deformity. Clinically, this may manifest as worsening back pain, accentuated postural imbalance, and, in rare cases, respiratory restriction. Regular follow-up with clinical examinations and imaging, when necessary, is important for monitoring deformity. Management is primarily conservative, focusing on patient education, postural correction strategies, and exercise programs. Surgical intervention is rarely indicated during pregnancy but may be considered in cases of rapid progression or the presence of severe neurological symptoms, requiring a multidisciplinary approach.

12.3.8 Avascular Necrosis of the Femoral Head

Avascular necrosis (AVN) of the femoral head is a syndrome resulting from impaired blood supply, leading to osteocyte and bone marrow cell death, subchondral bone collapse, and progressive necrosis of the femoral head. In pregnancy, venous congestion, hypercoagulability, and elevated cortisol levels have been implicated as contributing risk factors. AVN represents an important cause of hip, pelvic, and groin pain in pregnant women, most commonly presenting in the late third trimester or postpartum with sudden and severe hip pain. Clinically, the affected hip demonstrates restricted and painful movements. Magnetic resonance imaging (MRI) is considered the gold standard for early diagnosis, typically revealing focal defects in the femoral head and neck, subchondral changes, and diffuse bone marrow edema. MRI is also essential for differentiating AVN from transient osteoporosis of the hip [33].

Management depends on the stage of the disease. In the early phase, conservative strategies such as joint rest, partial weight-bearing with crutches, cold application, and analgesics are recommended. Isometric exercises are prescribed to preserve muscle strength, while passive and assisted range-of-motion exercises aim to maintain joint mobility. In cases unresponsive to conservative management or in advanced disease stages, surgical interventions may be necessary. Options include bone grafting, core decompression, intertrochanteric osteotomy, and, in severe cases, total hip arthroplasty [33].

12.3.9 Transient Osteoporosis of the Hip in Pregnancy

Transient osteoporosis of the hip (TOH) is a rare condition that typically emerges in the last trimester of pregnancy or the early postpartum period. The etiology and pathophysiology of pregnancy-associated osteoporosis remain unclear. While osteoporosis is classically linked to estrogen deficiency, pregnancy is a state of excessive estrogen production. The condition, which is usually unilateral, is thought to result from impaired venous return and bone marrow edema [34]. Reported risk factors include genetic predisposition, physical inactivity, poor nutrition, low body weight, family history of fractures, and vitamin D deficiency. Clinically, affected women present in the third trimester with unilateral or bilateral hip pain, gait disturbance, and limping in the absence of trauma. Although hip range of motion is often preserved, rotation movements are painful, and in advanced cases, fractures may occur. Differential diagnosis is essential, particularly to distinguish TOH from avascular necrosis of the femoral head and pubic symphysis dysfunction.

MRI is considered the most reliable diagnostic modality, capable of detecting bone marrow edema and signal abnormalities within 48 hours of symptom onset. Imaging features include intermediate signal intensity on T1-weighted sequences, low signal intensity in affected regions, and high signal intensity on T2-weighted sequences. Unlike AVN, TOH is characterized by the absence of subchondral collapse [34].

The primary goals of treatment are pain control and fracture prevention. First-line preventive strategies include balanced nutrition, regular physical activity, and prophylactic calcium (600–1500 mg/day) and vitamin D (800–880 IU/day) supplementation. Once diagnosed, discontinuation of breastfeeding and supplementation with calcium and vitamin D have been shown to improve bone mineral density, with reported increases of 6% per month and up to 9.5% within 2–4 years [35]. Conservative management includes joint rest, non-weight-bearing or partial weight-bearing with crutches, wheelchair use if necessary, exercises to prevent contractures, and the use of mild analgesics such as acetaminophen or NSAIDs [35, 36]. These approaches aim to reduce pain and prevent microfractures but do not alter the natural course of the disease.

Oral and intravenous bisphosphonates and other antiresorptive agents are contraindicated during pregnancy and lactation due to their potential effects on fetal skeletal development, including growth restriction, premature delivery, transient neonatal hypocalcemia, and spontaneous abortion [37]. Calcitonin, however, does not cross the placenta and has been reported to reduce symptom duration, making it a relatively safe therapeutic option in pregnancy [37]. Calcium and vitamin D supplementation are generally recommended, particularly in early stages, as no pregnancy-related contraindications have been reported.

Surgical management may be considered in cases of femoral neck fractures. While surgical intervention may be lifesaving in displaced fractures, conservative therapy is usually preferred for subcapital fractures. In most cases, symptoms resolve within the first 2 months postpartum, and MRI findings typically return to normal within 3–6 months after delivery [38]. Despite causing significant pain and functional limitation, the overall prognosis of pregnancy-associated TOH is favorable.

12.3.10 Leg Cramps

Leg cramps are painful, involuntary muscle contractions that most commonly occur in the calves and thighs during the second half of pregnancy. Their prevalence has been reported to range between 15% and 30%. These cramps typically present at night, disrupting sleep and contributing to discomfort in pregnant women. Although the exact etiology remains unclear, several mechanisms have been proposed, including calcium or magnesium deficiency, ischemia, nerve root compression, and reduced physical activity.

Management focuses on conservative strategies. Walking, warm baths, and stretching exercises such as knee extension and ankle dorsiflexion can effectively alleviate cramps. Magnesium supplementation has also been recommended for pregnant women experiencing frequent cramps, with evidence suggesting beneficial effects in symptom reduction [39].

References

1. Brook G, Coldron Y, Evans G, Gulliford G, Haslam J, Hawkes R. Physiotherapy in women's health. Tidy's Physiother. 2008:113–44.
2. To WW, Wong MW. Factors associated with back pain symptoms in pregnancy and the persistence of pain 2 years after pregnancy. Acta Obstet Gynecol Scand. 2003;82(12):1086–91. https://doi.org/10.1046/j.1600-0412.2003.00235.x.
3. Beyaz EA, Özcan E. Painful conditions arising from musculoskeletal system during pregnancy and therapeutic management. Turk J Phys Med Rehabil. 2005;51(2):65–8.
4. McCarthy TA, Simonds AH, Velez S, Spaeth AM. Meeting exercise guidelines during pregnancy associates with less lumbopelvic disability and fear avoidance. Womens Health (Lond). 2025;21:17455057251321019. https://doi.org/10.1177/17455057251321019.
5. Liddle SD, Pennick V. Interventions for preventing and treating low-back and pelvic pain during pregnancy. Cochrane Database Syst Rev. 2015;2015(9):CD001139. https://doi.org/10.1002/14651858.
6. Lan Q, Fu ACL, McKay MJ, et al. The association between musculoskeletal pain during pregnancy and pregnancy outcomes: a systematic review and meta-analyses. Eur J Obstet Gynecol Reprod Biol. 2024;294:180–90. https://doi.org/10.1016/j.ejogrb.2024.01.027.
7. Salari N, Mohammadi A, Hemmati M, Hasheminezhad R, Kani S, Shohaimi S, Mohammadi M. The global prevalence of low back pain in pregnancy: a comprehensive systematic review and meta-analysis. BMC Pregnancy Childbirth. 2023;23(1):830. https://doi.org/10.1186/s12884-023-06151-x.
8. Koukoulithras I Sr, Stamouli A, Kolokotsios S, et al. The effectiveness of non-pharmaceutical interventions upon pregnancy-related low back pain: a systematic review and meta-analysis. Cureus. 2021;13(1):e13011. https://doi.org/10.7759/cureus.13011.

9. Conder R, Zamani R, Akrami M. The biomechanics of pregnancy: a systematic review. J Funct Morphol Kinesiol. 2019;4(4):72. https://doi.org/10.3390/jfmk4040072.
10. Babbar S, Shyken J. Yoga in pregnancy. Clin Obstet Gynecol. 2016;59(3):600–12. https://doi.org/10.1097/GRF.0000000000000210.
11. Martins RF, Pinto e Silva J. An exercise method for the treatment of lumbar and posterior pelvic pain in pregnancy. Rev Bras Ginecol Obstet. 2005;27:275–82.
12. Abera M, Hanlon C, Daniel B, et al. Effects of relaxation interventions during pregnancy on maternal mental health, and pregnancy and newborn outcomes: a systematic review and meta-analysis. PLoS One. 2024;19(1):e0278432. https://doi.org/10.1371/journal.pone.0278432.
13. French SD, Cameron M, Walker BF, Reggars JW, Esterman AJ. A Cochrane review of superficial heat or cold for low back pain. Spine (Phila Pa 1976). 2006;31(9):998–1006. https://doi.org/10.1097/01.brs.0000214881.10814.64.
14. Zhu F, Zhang M, Wang D, et al. Yoga compared to non-exercise or physical therapy exercise on pain, disability, and quality of life for patients with chronic low back pain: a systematic review and meta-analysis of randomized controlled trials. PLoS One. 2020;15(9):e0238544. https://doi.org/10.1371/journal.pone.0238544.
15. Quittan M, Bily W, Crevenna R, et al. Transcutaneous Electrical Nerve Stimulation (TENS) in patients with pregnancy-induced low back pain and/or pelvic girdle pain. Phys Med Rehabil Kurortmed. 2016;26(02):91–5. https://doi.org/10.1055/s-0035-1565058.
16. Keskin EA, Onur O, Keskin HL, et al. Transcutaneous electrical nerve stimulation improves low back pain during pregnancy. Gynecol Obstet Investig. 2012;74(1):76–83. https://doi.org/10.1159/000337720.
17. Bulguroglu M, Bulguroglu HI, Degirmenci B, et al. Effectiveness of a prenatal pilates program on ligamentous laxity and joint hypermobility in pregnant women: a dual-center randomized controlled trial. BMC Pregnancy Childbirth. 2025;25(1):897. https://doi.org/10.1186/s12884-025-08082-1.
18. Pai MYB, Hohl A, Souza LRC, Mendes MV, Sampaio LCS, Tsai AWW. Acupuncture for pregnancy-related pain in the lower back and posterior pelvic girdle. Rev Assoc Med Bras (1992). 2023;69(suppl 1):e2023S101. https://doi.org/10.1590/1806-9282.2023S101.
19. Koukoulithras I Sr, Stamouli A, Kolokotsios S, Plexousakis M Sr, Mavrogiannopoulou C, Koukoulithras I, Plexousakis M. The effectiveness of non-pharmaceutical interventions upon pregnancy-related low back pain: a systematic review and meta-analysis. Cureus. 2021;13(1):e13011.
20. Xue X, Chen Y, Mao X, et al. Effect of kinesio taping on low back pain during pregnancy: a systematic review and meta-analysis. BMC Pregnancy Childbirth. 2021;21(1):712. https://doi.org/10.1186/s12884-021-04197-3.
21. Güner A, Altan L, Kasapoğlu AM. The effectiveness of the low-power laser and kinesiotaping in the treatment of carpal tunnel syndrome, a pilot study. Rheumatol Int. 2018;38(5):895–904. https://doi.org/10.1007/s00296-018-4020-6.
22. Marhofer D, Jaksch W, Aigmüller T, et al. Schmerztherapie in der Schwangerschaft : Eine expertInnenbasierte interdisziplinäre Konsensus-Empfehlung [Pain management during pregnancy: an expert-based interdisciplinary consensus recommendation]. Schmerz. 2021;35(6):382–90. German. https://doi.org/10.1007/s00482-021-00571-4.
23. Cîmpeanu MC, Roman N, Grigorescu S, et al. Management of "De novo" carpal tunnel syndrome in pregnancy: a narrative review. J Pers Med. 2024;14(3):240. https://doi.org/10.3390/jpm14030240.
24. Hamoda R, Osman D, Hamada A, et al. Effect of myofascial release on electrophysiological and clinical measures of pregnant women with carpal tunnel syndrome. Physiother Q. 2019;27(1):18–24. https://doi.org/10.5114/pq.2019.83057.
25. Carlson H, Colbert A, Frydl J, Arnall E, Elliot M, Carlson N. Current options for nonsurgical management of carpal tunnel syndrome. Int J Clin Rheumtol. 2010;5(1):129–42. https://doi.org/10.2217/IJR.09.63.

26. Burke FD, Ellis J, McKenna H, Bradley MJ. Primary care management of carpal tunnel syndrome. Postgrad Med J. 2003;79(934):433–7. https://doi.org/10.1136/pmj.79.934.433.
27. Gooding MS, Evangelista V, Pereira L. Carpal tunnel syndrome and meralgia paresthetica in pregnancy. Obstet Gynecol Surv. 2020;75(2):121–6. https://doi.org/10.1097/OGX.0000000000000745.
28. Burke FD, Bradley MJ, Sinha S, et al. Primary care management of patients with carpal tunnel syndrome referred to surgeons: are non-operative interventions effectively utilised? Postgrad Med J. 2007;83(981):498–501. https://doi.org/10.1136/pgmj.2007.058206.
29. Habusta SF, Coffey R, Ponnarasu S, Mabrouk A, Griffin EE. Chondromalacia patella. In: StatPearls [Internet]. Treasure Island: StatPearls Publishing; 2023. PMID: 29083563.
30. Chen B, Zhao X, Hu Y. Rehabilitations for maternal diastasis recti abdominis: an update on therapeutic directions. Heliyon. 2023;9(10):e20956. https://doi.org/10.1016/j.heliyon.2023.e20956.
31. Keshwani N, McLean L. Ultrasound imaging in postpartum women with diastasis recti: intrarater between-session reliability. J Orthop Sports Phys Ther. 2015;45(9):713–8. https://doi.org/10.2519/jospt.2015.5879.
32. Sheppard S. The role of transversus abdominus in post partum correction of gross divarication recti. Man Ther. 1996;1(4):214–6. https://doi.org/10.1054/math.1996.0272.
33. Montella BJ, Nunley JA, Urbaniak JR. Osteonecrosis of the femoral head associated with pregnancy. A preliminary report. J Bone Joint Surg Am. 1999;81(6):790–8. https://doi.org/10.2106/00004623-199906000-00006.
34. Galanis A, Dimopoulou S, Karampinas P, et al. The correlation between transient osteoporosis of the hip and pregnancy: a review. Medicine (Baltimore). 2023;102(41):e35475. https://doi.org/10.1097/MD.0000000000035475.
35. Korompilias AV, Karantanas AH, Lykissas MG, Beris AE. Bone marrow edema syndrome. Skeletal Radiol. 2009;38(5):425–36. https://doi.org/10.1007/s00256-008-0529-1.
36. Kibbi L, Touma Z, Khoury N, Arayssi T. Oral bisphosphonates in treatment of transient osteoporosis. Clin Rheumatol. 2008;27(4):529–32. https://doi.org/10.1007/s10067-007-0766-z.
37. Truszczyńska A, Walczak P, Rapała K. Transient peripartum osteoporosis of the femoral head in first and third pregnancy. J Clin Densitom. 2012;15(4):467–71. https://doi.org/10.1016/j.jocd.2012.02.010.
38. Morton A, Savard-Heppel J. Transient osteoporosis of the hip in pregnancy. Obstet Med. 2024;17(4):188–93. https://doi.org/10.1177/1753495X241236222.
39. Garrison SR, Korownyk CS, Kolber MR, Allan GM, Musini VM, Sekhon RK, Dugré N. Magnesium for skeletal muscle cramps. Cochrane Database Syst Rev. 2020;9(9):CD009402. https://doi.org/10.1002/14651858.

Chapter 13
Dermal Wellness: Managing Skin Conditions Throughout Motherhood

Meltem Türkmen

13.1 Introduction

Pregnancy is one of the most special periods in human life. While a healthy baby is brought into the world, the mother undergoes numerous changes. All body systems experience a series of physiological alterations in order to adapt to this new state, and among the few organs where these changes can be directly observed are the skin, hair, and nails. Recognizing these physiological changes accurately is essential for anticipating the alterations a pregnant woman may encounter, distinguishing them from pathological conditions, and implementing appropriate management while ensuring maternal and fetal well-being. Additionally, it is important to understand how preexisting chronic dermatological diseases behave during pregnancy, to adapt to necessary treatment modifications, and to manage potential exacerbations. Familiarity with these specific changes during pregnancy is crucial for providing effective care throughout this unique period.

13.2 Physiological Changes in Pregnancy

Physiological changes affecting the skin and its appendages during pregnancy are frequently mistaken for pathological conditions. Therefore, recognizing skin changes specific to pregnancy is crucial for preventing unnecessary investigations and maternal anxiety. Most of these physiological changes resolve spontaneously after delivery, and a conservative approach is generally sufficient [1].

M. Türkmen (✉)
University of Health Sciences, Faculty of Medicine, Department of Dermatology, Izmir, Turkey

© The Author(s), under exclusive license to Springer Nature Switzerland AG 2026

I. Karaca (ed.), *Managing Maternal Chronic Diseases for a Healthy Pregnancy*,
https://doi.org/10.1007/978-3-032-15221-3_13

Temporary modifications in the immune system, metabolism, and hormonal profile during pregnancy result in various alterations such as pigmentary changes, changes in hair and nails, vascular changes, and modifications in eccrine and apocrine gland activity [2].

13.2.1 Pigmentary Changes

13.2.1.1 Hyperpigmentation

Hyperpigmentation of the skin and mucous membranes is the most common physiological change, observed in approximately 85–90% of pregnant women. It typically appears as diffuse and mild pigmentation, most notably in areas that are physiologically darker, such as the periumbilical area, genital region, perineum, axillae, inner thighs, neck, and areola. In many women, darkening of the midline of the abdomen from the suprapubic region to the umbilicus, known as linea nigra, is observed. This pigmentation commonly extends from the umbilicus to the pubic symphysis [1, 3, 4].

Pigmentation during pregnancy is due to elevated levels of α- and β-melanocyte-stimulating hormones, progesterone, estrogen, and β-endorphins, which stimulate melanocytes and promote melanin synthesis. Additionally, placental lipids may activate tyrosinase enzyme, further enhancing melanin production [2, 3].

In individuals with darker skin tones, pigmentation lines following the peripheral cutaneous nerves (Voigt or Futcher's lines) may become more pronounced, particularly on the posterolateral aspects of the legs and upper arms [2, 3].

13.2.1.2 Melasma

Also referred to as chloasma or the "mask of pregnancy," melasma presents as symmetric, well-demarcated patches varying from light to dark brown, typically affecting the face. It often appears during the second half of pregnancy and is seen in approximately one-third of women using oral contraceptives. It can manifest in malar, mandibular, or central facial patterns [3].

Melasma is associated with genetic predisposition, sun exposure, cosmetic use, and increased levels of melanocyte-stimulating hormones, progesterone and estrogen. Histologically, it is classified based on whether melanin accumulation occurs in the epidermis or dermis. Approximately 90% of cases regress within 1 year postpartum. In persistent cases, treatment with topical hydroquinone or tretinoin is recommended. During pregnancy, sun protection and avoidance of irritating cosmetics are essential [2].

13.2.2 Nevi

Although it was previously believed that melanocytic nevi darken during pregnancy, studies have shown this occurs infrequently and requires further investigation [5]. While color changes are rare, slight enlargement in the diameter of nevi, particularly in areas subject to skin stretching such as the breasts and abdomen, may be observed [6]. Dermoscopic changes in nevi, such as thickening of the pigment network, an increase in the number of vessels, are considered normal, provided there are no clinical signs suggestive of melanoma [5, 6]. However, any nevus with suspicious features should undergo biopsy and histopathologic examination, regardless of gestational age [7].

13.2.3 Vascular Structures

Increased venous pressure can lead to edema, most commonly affecting the lower extremities but occasionally involving the face and hands. This benign edema typically resolves with leg elevation and bed rest or compression stockings. Persistent edema, particularly involving the face and hands, may indicate preeclampsia and warrants further investigation [1].

Elevated estrogen levels during pregnancy increase the number and visibility of telangiectasias, including spider angiomas and nevoid telangiectasias, particularly in light-skinned patients [8].

Pyogenic granuloma of pregnancy, also called granuloma gravidarum or pregnancy tumor, is a benign capillary hemangioma presenting as a rapidly growing, lobulated, pedunculated lesion ranging from pink to red to purple. This painless lesion occurs in 0.5–5% of pregnant women and may bleed but generally resolves spontaneously postpartum [2].

13.2.4 Mucosa

Increased blood flow, vascularity, and edema during pregnancy lead to softening and a bluish discoloration of the vagina and cervix, known, respectively, as Goodell's and Chadwick's signs. The presence of varicosities in the vulva and vagina, referred to as Jacquemier's sign, is also frequently observed. Additionally, hemangiomas have been commonly reported to develop in the vulvovaginal mucosa during pregnancy. The tendency toward constipation and prolonged straining during labor predisposes pregnant women to hemorrhoids [9].

From the second month of pregnancy onward, hyperemia and edema of the gingival tissues can occur, leading to pregnancy gingivitis. Mucosal pyogenic granulomas of pregnancy may also develop on the lips and gingiva. Decreased salivary flow may result in xerostomia, while nasal and sinus hyperemia can cause congestion [1, 2].

13.2.5 Glands

During pregnancy, eccrine and sebaceous gland activity generally increases, whereas apocrine gland activity decreases. The increase in eccrine gland activity is observed throughout the body, except on the palms, and may clinically manifest as hyperhidrosis and miliaria.

Increased sebaceous gland activity promotes the enlargement of Montgomery's tubercles, which are small papules located around the areolae that provide lubrication for breastfeeding [1, 2].

13.2.6 Connective Tissue

Hormonal changes, increased mechanical tension, and genetic predisposition lead to the degradation of dermal connective tissue during pregnancy, resulting in the formation of striae distensae (stretch marks). These affect more than 63% of pregnant women and represent one of the most frequently reported dermatologic changes of gestation. They typically appear during the third trimester as pink or purple atrophic bands following skin tension lines on the breasts, abdomen, hips, buttocks, and thighs. Over time, these striae become lighter and less noticeable but rarely disappear completely. Preexisting lesions such as neurofibromas, keloid scars, leiomyomas, dermatofibromas, and lipodystrophies may worsen during pregnancy [2].

13.2.7 Hair

During pregnancy, hirsutism and/or hypertrichosis may occur. Women with darker hair are more likely to develop noticeable hair growth on the upper lip, chin, cheeks, suprapubic area, and along the midline. While soft and fine hairs generally regress postpartum, terminal, coarse, and dark hairs tend to persist [1, 10].

Studies using trichoscan analysis have demonstrated increased hair shaft diameter and a prolonged anagen phase during pregnancy, resulting in a higher proportion of anagen-phase hairs by the end of gestation [1].

Following delivery, hormonal changes lead to a synchronized transition of hair follicles into the telogen phase, causing diffuse hair shedding several months after birth—a condition known as telogen effluvium. This typically resolves within 6–15 months postpartum, as hair growth cycles gradually return to an asynchronous pattern [11].

13.2.8 Nails

The most common nail changes observed during pregnancy include leukonychia, onycholysis, onychoshizia (lamellar splitting), and ingrown toenails. Additionally, increased nail growth, melanonychia, and subungual keratosis have also been reported [2].

Symmetrical, smooth, longitudinal hyperpigmentation of the nails may occur during pregnancy and typically regresses postpartum. However, cases of irregular pigmentation involving the cuticle should be carefully evaluated for possible melanoma [1, 2].

13.2.9 Breasts

Throughout pregnancy, breast development leads to tenderness, the appearance of prominent veins, striae formation, areolar enlargement and darkening, and increased nipple sensitivity and erection. Hyperpigmentation of the nipple and areola, as well as the enlargement of Montgomery's tubercles, is commonly observed. Another notable change is pregnancy-associated hyperkeratosis of the nipple and areola, which presents as bilateral, yellow-to-brown hyperkeratotic and/or papular lesions affecting the superior portion of the nipple. This condition may persist into the postpartum period and can be difficult to manage [12].

13.3 Pregnancy-Specific Dermatoses

In 2006, Ambros-Rudolph and colleagues classified pregnancy-specific dermatoses into four main groups. These are polymorphic eruption of pregnancy (PEP), pemphigoid gestationis (PG), atopic eruption of pregnancy (AEP), intrahepatic cholestasis of pregnancy (IHCP) (Table 13.1) [13].

13.3.1 Polymorphic Eruption of Pregnancy

Also referred to as pruritic urticarial papules and plaques of pregnancy (PUPPP), polymorphic eruption of pregnancy typically develops late in gestation (between the 36th and 39th weeks) and, more rarely, immediately postpartum [14]. With an estimated incidence of 1 in 200 pregnancies, it is the most common pregnancy-specific dermatosis.

Its exact etiology remains unclear; however, it is thought to be associated with factors that increase abdominal distension, such as excessive weight gain, multiple

Table 13.1 Pregnancy-specific dermatoses

Condition	Typical onset	Key clinical features	Diagnosis	Fetal risk	Recurrence	Management
Polymorphic eruption of pregnancy (PEP)	Late third trimester; rarely postpartum	Urticarial papules/plaques starting in striae; periumbilical sparing	Clinical; IF negative	No	Uncommon	Emollients; low–mid potency topical corticosteroids; antipruritics; short oral steroids if refractory
Pemphigoid gestationis (PG)	Second–third trimester; may flare postpartum	Intensely pruritic plaques → tense vesicles/bullae; often periumbilical	DIF linear C3/IgG at BMZ; ELISA to BP180	Yes (preterm, low birth weight; transient neonatal lesions)	Yes; may relate to OCPs	Topical or systemic corticosteroids; monitor postpartum flares
Atopic eruption of pregnancy (AEP)	First–second trimester (often earlier than others)	E-type: Eczematous flexural/face; P-type: Pruritic papules on extensor surfaces	Clinical	No	Variable	Skin care, emollients, topical steroids/photoprotection; manage itch
Intrahepatic cholestasis of pregnancy (ICP)	Second–third trimester	No primary lesions; nocturnal pruritus (palms/soles), secondary excoriations	Serum bile acids >10 μmol/L; LFTs; resolution postpartum	Yes (risk rises with bile acids; fetal distress/preterm)	Yes (including with OCPs)	UDCA 10–15 mg/kg/day; topical antipruritics; obstetric co-management

gestation, and macrosomia. Increased occurrence has also been reported in primiparous women, in cesarean deliveries, and in pregnancies with male fetuses. Recently, authors have suggested that it may represent a Th2-mediated hypersensitivity reaction to skin-resident bacteria and fungi, mediated by IL-9 and IL-33 [15].

The typical clinical feature is urticarial plaques beginning along abdominal striae, with relative sparing of the periumbilical area. Papules may coalesce to form plaques, which can extend to the trunk, buttocks, and extremities. The face, palms, soles, and periumbilical region remain unaffected. Target-like lesions, small vesicles, and polycyclic papules may also occur, and the eruption may persist for 4–6 weeks [14, 15].

Diagnosis is made clinically. It is essential to differentiate the condition from pemphigoid gestationis, as the urticarial phase of pemphigoid can be mistaken for polymorphic eruption of pregnancy. If the diagnosis is uncertain and/or pemphigoid gestationis is suspected, a skin biopsy with immunofluorescence studies should be performed. Histopathological findings are nonspecific, and both direct immunofluorescence (DIF) and indirect immunofluorescence (IF) are negative [14, 15].

The goal of treatment is symptom relief. Topical antipruritics, emollients, low- to mid-potency corticosteroid creams, and loose-fitting, nonallergenic cotton clothing are recommended. In refractory cases, low-dose oral corticosteroids may be used. Significant improvement is usually observed after delivery. There is no effect on fetal or maternal prognosis, and recurrence in subsequent pregnancies is uncommon [15].

13.3.2 *Pemphigoid Gestationis*

Pemphigoid gestationis (PG) is a rare autoimmune subepidermal blistering disorder that shares clinical and histopathological features with bullous pemphigoid. It most commonly presents in the second or third trimester of pregnancy (between the 21st and 28th weeks) but may, rarely, occur postpartum. In subsequent pregnancies, onset tends to occur earlier and follow a more severe course. Recurrences have also been reported during the menstrual cycle and with oral contraceptive use. PG is associated with fetal risks such as preterm delivery, low birth weight, and transient neonatal skin lesions [15, 16].

The disease is caused by maternal IgG autoantibodies targeting the NC16a domain of the BP180 (also known as BPAG2 or type XVII collagen) transmembrane antigen located in the basement membrane zone of the skin and in the chorionic and amniotic epithelium.

Clinically, PG typically begins with intensely pruritic erythematous urticarial papules and plaques, followed by the development of tense vesicles and bullae. Lesions may appear polymorphic and resemble erythema multiforme. Most cases begin in the periumbilical region and extend to the abdomen, lower extremities, palms, and soles. Oral mucosa is typically spared. The pre-bullous phase can resemble polymorphic eruption of pregnancy; immunofluorescence is used for differentiation [15].

Because clinical findings alone may be nonspecific, diagnosis relies on histopathology, immunofluorescence, and ELISA testing. Direct immunofluorescence (DIF) is considered the most sensitive and specific test for confirming PG, revealing linear deposition of C3 and IgG along the basement membrane zone.

Histopathology of early lesions shows papillary dermal edema with a lymphocytic infiltrate and variable numbers of eosinophils. Examination of an intact blister reveals a subepidermal split without acantholysis.

Mild, localized disease can be managed with topical corticosteroids and supportive skin care. Systemic corticosteroids are the mainstay of treatment for severe disease. The only criterion in the literature distinguishing mild from severe PG is the extent of body surface area involvement (<10% vs. >10%). Postpartum flares may occur; therefore, treatment should be continued until stable remission is achieved after delivery [15, 16].

13.3.3 Atopic Eruption of Pregnancy

Atopic eruption of pregnancy (AEP) is a clinical condition in which there is either the exacerbation of preexisting atopic dermatitis or its new onset during pregnancy. What makes this condition a pregnancy-specific dermatosis is the fact that approximately 80% of patients have no prior history of atopy [17]. Symptoms generally develop earlier than in other pregnancy dermatoses (first and second trimesters), although in patients without a prior atopic history, onset may occur later [18].

Ambros-Rudolph et al. classified AEP into two phenotypes: E-type (eczema type): Classical distribution of eczematous lesions involving the face, neck, presternal area, and flexural surfaces. P-type (prurigo type): Clusters of small, pruritic, erythematous papules primarily affecting the extensor surfaces of the extremities and the trunk [18].

AEP poses no maternal or fetal risk, and clinical improvement is typically observed postpartum. Treatment focuses on symptom relief and includes gentle cleansing products, nonallergenic cotton clothing, and the use of emollients.

13.3.4 Intrahepatic Cholestasis of Pregnancy

Intrahepatic cholestasis of pregnancy (ICP) typically occurs in the second or third trimester and initially presents with pruritus in the absence of primary skin lesions. Its etiology remains incompletely understood, with genetic, hormonal, environmental, and immunologic factors all implicated [19, 20].

Clinically, the pruritus—often more intense at night—may initially be limited to the palms and soles. Secondary skin changes due to scratching, such as excoriations, papules, and erosions, may subsequently appear. Jaundice occurs in approximately 20% of cases, typically developing 2–4 weeks after the onset of pruritus.

Although diagnostic criteria are not universally standardized, ICP is generally defined by pruritus that resolves after delivery and a serum bile acid concentration > 10 μmol/L. Liver function tests may also be elevated [18].

Treatment aims to control pruritus and reduce elevated bile acid levels. Ursodeoxycholic acid (UDCA) at a dosage of 10–15 mg/kg/day is the mainstay of therapy. Emollients, topical antipruritics, and antihistamines may be used for symptomatic relief. Pruritus typically improves within 48 h postpartum, although normalization of bile acid levels may take 2–4 weeks. Serum bile acid concentrations ≥100 μmol/L are associated with increased risks of preterm birth, perinatal mortality, and fetal distress [18].

13.4 Management of Psoriasis in Pregnancy

Psoriasis is an inflammatory dermatosis that can affect the skin, joints, and internal organs. The highest incidence occurs between the ages of 30 and 40, which includes the reproductive years. Given its association with comorbidities such as metabolic syndrome, cardiovascular involvement, and depressive disorder, effective disease management is crucial [20].

The course of psoriasis during pregnancy is unpredictable—cases of both improvement and exacerbation have been reported—necessitating an individualized treatment approach [21]. The most common phenotype in pregnancy is plaque psoriasis, characterized by well-demarcated erythematous lesions covered with silvery scales.

In the third trimester, impetigo herpetiformis (pustular psoriasis of pregnancy) may occur, presenting with erythematous patches and plaques involving intertriginous areas such as the axillae and breasts, with centrifugal spread and pustules at the plaque margins. One-third of patients have no prior history of psoriasis. Unlike classical psoriasis, mutations in the IL36RN gene have been reported. Hypocalcemia, hypoalbuminemia, and secondary hypoparathyroidism have been described as possible contributing factors.

Diagnosis is based on clinical findings, as no specific diagnostic test exists. Histopathological features may include parakeratosis, subcorneal neutrophilic pustules in the upper epidermis, and the presence of neutrophil nuclei. Both direct and indirect immunofluorescence tests are negative.

In pustular psoriasis of pregnancy, calcium and albumin levels should be closely monitored. Treatment options include topical corticosteroids and short courses of systemic corticosteroids (0.5–1 mg/kg/day). In resistant cases, systemic cyclosporine (2.5–3.5 mg/kg/day) and narrowband UVB therapy may be used.

For psoriasis not specific to pregnancy, first-line treatment consists of topical corticosteroids, provided lesions remain controlled and optimal dosages are

Table 13.2 Conventional treatments of psoriasis during pregnancy

Therapy	Modality	Key considerations in pregnancy
Emollients	Topical	Foundation of care; safe throughout pregnancy
Topical corticosteroids	Topical	Use lowest effective potency/amount; avoid very high cumulative doses
Calcipotriol	Topical	Consider in limited areas if alternatives fail; data limited
Narrowband UVB	Phototherapy	Useful for widespread disease; monitor folate; advise photoprotection
Cyclosporine	Systemic	Consider for severe/refractory disease; needs close monitoring
Methotrexate	Systemic	Contraindicated (teratogenic)
Acitretin	Systemic	Contraindicated (retinoid embryopathy)

Table 13.3 Biological treatments of psoriasis during pregnancy

Biological agent	
Certolizumab pegol	First choice during pregnancy and breastfeeding. Does not cross the placenta
Etanercept	It can cross the placenta. It is generally well-tolerated. There have been cases reported of it causing VACTERL syndrome
Adalimumab	Can cross the placenta. No malformation/negative pregnancy results were found
Infliximab	Can cross the placenta
Ustekinumab/ secukinumab	Avoid electively in pregnancy when alternatives exist; limited data

maintained. In more extensive disease, narrowband UVB phototherapy—either alone or combined with topical corticosteroids—can be considered a safe option. Cumulative UVB dose should be monitored, as exceeding threshold levels has been associated with decreased folic acid levels. To prevent neural tube defects, daily supplementation with 5–6 mg folic acid is recommended during UVB therapy [22] (Table 13.2) .

Third-line therapies are indicated for severe psoriasis. Systemic agents such as methotrexate and acitretin are teratogenic and contraindicated during pregnancy.

Much of the safety data on biologic agents in pregnancy comes from their use in rheumatoid arthritis and inflammatory bowel disease. In the management of psoriasis in pregnant patients, adalimumab, etanercept, and infliximab may be used [23] (Table 13.3).

The Organisation of Teratology and Information Specialists project found no correlation between these agents and an increased risk of congenital malformations. However, monoclonal antibody levels in umbilical cord blood were found to be similar to those in maternal blood. This high fetal serum concentration has been associated in case reports with potential fetal and neonatal immunosuppression. For this reason, discontinuation of TNF-α inhibitors by the 30th week of gestation is recommended [24].

Certolizumab pegol—a PEGylated, Fc-free anti-TNF agent—does not cross the placenta and can be used safely during pregnancy. It is the only biologic with clinical trial data specifically supporting its potential use in pregnant patients [23].

13.5 Management of Atopic Dermatitis During Pregnancy

During pregnancy, the maternal immune system shifts toward a Th2-dominant response to promote tolerance toward the fetus. Atopic dermatitis (AD) itself is a Th2-mediated disease and is the most common skin condition observed during pregnancy, frequently experiencing exacerbations during the second and third trimesters [17].

AD has a significant negative impact on quality of life. Pruritus, sleep disturbances, and social isolation are common and are associated with higher rates of depression. Therapies that reduce AD symptoms have been shown to produce parallel improvements in depressive symptoms.

For first-line therapy, non-fluorinated topical corticosteroids (prednisolone and methylprednisolone) are preferred, as they are metabolized by placental 11-β-hydroxysteroid dehydrogenase and are thus considered safer. Total cumulative use should not exceed 300 g during pregnancy. Overuse can cause cutaneous atrophy and increased transepidermal absorption, potentially leading to systemic adverse effects [17, 25]. Although there is limited research on topical calcineurin inhibitors, topical use has not been associated with systemic accumulation. In pregnant transplant recipients, systemic doses far exceeding those used for AD have not been linked to malformations [26].

Narrowband UVB phototherapy exerts local immunosuppressive, immunomodulatory, and anti-inflammatory effects on the skin barrier. Previous studies have not shown an increased risk of adverse birth outcomes in women exposed to high cumulative UVB doses. However, treatment may increase the risk of melasma in pregnancy; facial photoprotection is therefore recommended [27].

Systemic corticosteroids are not considered teratogenic, but the European Task Force on Atopic Dermatitis (ETFAD) recommends limiting their use to short courses, with daily doses not exceeding 0.5 mg/kg body weight [28]. Prednisolone and methylprednisolone are preferred due to placental metabolism. Treatment should be as brief as possible, and vitamin D supplementation is advised to prevent osteopenia. Breastfeeding is not contraindicated; the infant's exposure is estimated at approximately 0.1% of the maternal therapeutic dose [29].

Cyclosporine and azathioprine are generally not recommended due to insufficient safety data. Methotrexate is contraindicated during pregnancy and lactation. For teratogenic drugs such as methotrexate and mycophenolate, a preconception washout period of 3 months is advised for both mothers and fathers [17].

Dupilumab, a recombinant IgG4 monoclonal antibody that inhibits IL-4Rα—a component of both IL-4 and IL-13 receptors—blocks signaling from both cytokines [17]. Because IgG4 is actively transported across the placenta, dupilumab should be avoided during pregnancy [30].

Table 13.4 Topical treatments of acne during pregnancy

Topical agent	Rationale/notes in pregnancy
Azelaic acid	Anti-inflammatory; safe across trimesters; useful for PIH
Benzoyl peroxide	Low systemic absorption; acceptable throughout gestation.
Sodium sulfacetamide	Limited data but likely safe; alternative when intolerance exists
Clindamycin (topical)	Acceptable in pregnancy/lactation; avoid application to areolae when breastfeeding
Erythromycin (topical)	Acceptable; consider resistance patterns
Metronidazole (topical)	Acceptable; no adverse fetal signals in topical use
Dapsone (topical)	Avoid near-term and during lactation due to theoretical risks
Salicylic/glycolic acids	Spot or limited-area use; avoid prolonged occlusion
Topical retinoids	Avoid (teratogenic potential with vitamin A analogs)

13.6 Managing Acne During Pregnancy

Pregnancy is a period in which severe acne can also be observed, and its management can be challenging due to restrictions on many of the medications commonly used for treating severe disease [31]. Treatment of acne during pregnancy is summarized in Table 13.4.

13.7 Conclusion and Clinical Recommendations

During pregnancy, childbirth, and breastfeeding, skin changes in the female body are shaped by the interaction of hormonal, immune-related, and psychological factors. Dermatological monitoring during this period is important not only for clinical diagnosis and treatment but also for supporting the mother's quality of life.

Comprehensive monitoring of skin health during the reproductive period should span from preconception to the postpartum phase. This approach enables the early recognition and appropriate management of physiological changes (hyperpigmentation, striae, vascular changes), inflammatory conditions (acne, eczema flares), and autoimmune processes (lupus, pemphigoid gestationis, etc.).

Postpartum dermatological changes should also be carefully addressed. Common findings during this period include postpartum hair loss (telogen effluvium), persistent pigmentation, striae retaining their red-purple appearance, and newly developed acneiform eruptions. In addition, contact dermatitis, periareolar irritation, and eczema related to breastfeeding are important considerations in postpartum skin health follow-up. Given that these complaints often overlap with motherhood-related anxieties, providing dermatological care in conjunction with psychological support is highly valuable.

A multidisciplinary follow-up approach is ideal, particularly in complex or treatment-resistant cases. Collaboration among dermatologists, obstetricians, family physicians, and—when necessary—psychologists/psychiatrists enhances both treatment outcomes and patient satisfaction. This teamwork maintains a delicate balance that prioritizes both fetal safety and maternal health.

An empathetic and supportive approach helps mothers make sense of and accept the changes in their bodies. The impact of skin changes on self-esteem, body image, and social life should not be underestimated. Physicians adopting not only diagnostic and therapeutic but also morale-boosting and educational roles can make this natural yet challenging period more manageable for mothers.

References

1. Motosko CC, Bieber AK, Pomeranz MK, et al. Physiologic changes of pregnancy: a review of the literature. Int J Womens Dermatol. 2017;3(4):219–24.
2. Tyler KH. Physiological skin changes during pregnancy. Clin Obstet Gynecol. 2015;58(1):119–24.
3. Bieber AK, Martires KJ, Stein JA, et al. Pigmentation and pregnancy. Obstet Gynecol. 2017;129(1):168–73.
4. Cohen PR. Linea Nigra: case report of a woman with a pregnancy-associated linear streak of cutaneous hyperpigmentation on her abdomen from the umbilicus to the pubic symphysis. Cureus. 2023;6(15):48408.
5. Bieber AK, Martires KJ, Driscoll MS, et al. Nevi and pregnancy. J Am Acad Dermatol. 2016;75(4):661–6.
6. Aktürk AS, Bilen N, Bayrämgürler D, et al. Dermoscopy is a suitable method for the observation of the pregnancy-related changes in melanocytic nevi. J Eur Acad Dermatol Venereol. 2007;21:1086–90.
7. Goldberg D, Maloney M. Dermatologic surgery and cosmetic procedures during pregnancy and the postpartum period. Dermatol Ther. 2013;26:321–30.
8. Fernandes LB, do Amaral WN. Clinical study of skin changes in low and high risk pregnant women. An Bras Dermatol. 2015;90:822–6.
9. Soutou B, Aractingi S. Skin disease in pregnancy. Best Pract Res Clin Obstet Gynaecol. 2015;29:732–40.
10. Geraghty LN, Pomeranz MK. Physiologic changes and dermatoses of pregnancy. Int J Dermatol. 2011;50:771–82.
11. Gizlenti S, Ekmekci TR. The changes in the hair cycle during gestation and the post-partum period. J Eur Acad Dermatol Venereol. 2014;28:878–81.
12. William Higgins H, Jenkins J, Horn TD, Kroumpouzos G. Pregnancy-associated hyperkeratosis of the nipple: a report of 25 cases. JAMA Dermatol. 2013;149:722–6.
13. Ambros-Rudolph CM, Müllegger RR, Vaughan-Jones SA, et al. The specific dermatoses of pregnancy revisited and reclassified: results of a retrospective two-center study on 505 pregnant patients. J Am Acad Dermatol. 2006;54:395–404.
14. Zejnullahu VA, Zejnullahu VA. Polymorphic eruption of pregnancy. Dermatol Rep. 2023;15:9546.
15. Carvalho MLR, Magalhães GM, Leite HV. Update on specific dermatoses of pregnancy. Rev Assoc Med Bras (1992). 2023;69(suppl 1):e2023S109. https://doi.org/10.1590/1806-9282.2023S109.
16. Chapsa M, Heyne S, Schneiderat S, Beissert S, Günther C. Pemphigoid gestationis. Aktuelle Derm. 2018;44:256–9. https://doi.org/10.1055/a-0596-3447.

17. Heilskov S, Deleuran MS, Vestergaard C. Immunosuppressive and Immunomodulating therapy for atopic dermatitis in pregnancy: an appraisal of the literature. Dermatol Ther (Heidelb). 2020;10(6):1215–28. https://doi.org/10.1007/s13555-020-00457-w.
18. Teixeira V, Coutinho I, Gameiro R, Vieira R, Gonçalo M. Dermatoses específicas da gravidez [Specific dermatoses of pregnancy]. Acta Med Port. 2013;26(5):593–600.
19. Beard MP, Millington GW. Recent developments in the specific dermatoses of pregnancy. Clin Exp Dermatol. 2012;37(1):1–4; quiz 5. https://doi.org/10.1111/j.1365-2230.2011.04173.x.
20. Rademaker M, Agnew K, Andrews M, et al. Psoriasis in those planning a family, pregnant or breast-feeding. The Australasian Psoriasis Collaboration. Australas J Dermatol. 2018;59(2):86–100. https://doi.org/10.1111/ajd.12641.
21. Murase JE, Chan KK, Garite TJ, et al. Hormonal effect on psoriasis in pregnancy and post partum. Arch Dermatol. 2005 May;141(5):601–6. https://doi.org/10.1001/archderm.141.5.601.
22. Bae YS, Van Voorhees AS, Hsu S, National Psoriasis Foundation, et al. Review of treatment options for psoriasis in pregnant or lactating women: from the Medical Board of the National Psoriasis Foundation. J Am Acad Dermatol. 2012;67(3):459–77. https://doi.org/10.1016/j.jaad.2011.07.039.
23. Simionescu AA, Danciu BM, Stanescu AMA. State-of-the-art review of pregnancy-related psoriasis. Medicina (Kaunas). 2021;57(8):804. https://doi.org/10.3390/medicina57080804.
24. Puig L, Barco D, Alomar A. Treatment of psoriasis with anti-TNF drugs during pregnancy: case report and review of the literature. Dermatology. 2010;220(1):71–6. https://doi.org/10.1159/000262284.
25. Murase JE, Heller MM, Butler DC. Safety of dermatologic medications in pregnancy and lactation: part I. Pregnancy. J Am Acad Dermatol. 2014;70(3):401.
26. Jain AB, Reyes J, Marcos A, et al. Pregnancy after liver transplantation with tacrolimus immunosuppression: a single center's experience update at 13 years. Transplantation. 2003;76(5):827–32. https://doi.org/10.1097/01.TP.0000084823.89528.89.
27. El-Saie LT, Rabie AR, Kamel MI, et al. Effect of narrowband ultraviolet B phototherapy on serum folic acid levels in patients with psoriasis. Lasers Med Sci. 2011;26(4):481–5. https://doi.org/10.1007/s10103-011-0895-0.
28. Vestergaard C, Wollenberg A, Barbarot S, et al. European task force on atopic dermatitis position paper: treatment of parental atopic dermatitis during preconception, pregnancy and lactation period. J Eur Acad Dermatol Venereol. 2019;33(9):1644–59. https://doi.org/10.1111/jdv.15709.
29. Ost L, Wettrell G, Björkhem I, Rane A. Prednisolone excretion in human milk. J Pediatr. 1985;106(6):1008–11. https://doi.org/10.1016/s0022-3476(85)80259-6.
30. Koren G, Ornoy A. The role of the placenta in drug transport and fetal drug exposure. Expert Rev Clin Pharmacol. 2018;11(4):373–85. https://doi.org/10.1080/17512433.2018.1425615.
31. Ly S, Kamal K, Manjaly P, Barbieri JS, Mostaghimi A. Treatment of acne vulgaris during pregnancy and lactation: a narrative review. Dermatol Ther (Heidelb). 2023;13(1):115–30. https://doi.org/10.1007/s13555-022-00854-3.

Chapter 14
Pregnancy and Perinatal Infections

Aslı Akdöner

14.1 Introduction

During pregnancy, every infection affects two patients simultaneously: the mother and, via the placenta, the fetus. The type of pathogen (viral, bacterial, fungal, protozoal), the timing of exposure (trimester), and the degree of maternal viremia/bacteremia determine outcomes that range from miscarriage to neurodevelopmental sequelae, preterm birth, or intrauterine death [1, 2]. Rubella, CMV, parvovirus B19, and Zika carry teratogenic risks in early pregnancy, whereas perinatal transmission of HBV/HCV is most pronounced around the time of delivery. Intrapartum exposure is critical for HSV, maternal colonization drives the risk in GBS, and infections such as toxoplasmosis and malaria demonstrate gestational age–dependent risk profiles that require tailored rather than uniform management.

Modern practice prioritizes prevention as the first step: Completion of immunization in reproductive-aged women, preconceptional counseling, safe food and water, vector control, and adherence to infection-control measures among healthcare providers are fundamental components. Timely and targeted antenatal screening strategies (e.g., HBsAg/HBV DNA, anti-HCV/HCV RNA, syphilis serology, GBS colonization), coupled with early diagnosis; appropriate isolation and prophylaxis (e.g., HBIG plus birth-dose HBV vaccination, immunoprophylaxis after varicella exposure); and trimester- and pathogen-specific safe therapeutic protocols can markedly improve maternal–fetal outcomes.

Diagnostic evaluation relies on ultrasonographic and Doppler assessment of fetal well-being, molecular confirmation from fetal blood or amniotic fluid in selected

A. Akdöner (✉)
Dokuz Eylul University, Faculty of Medicine, Department of Obstetrics and Gynecology, Izmir, Turkey
e-mail: asli.akdoner@deu.edu.tr

© The Author(s), under exclusive license to Springer Nature Switzerland AG 2026

I. Karaca (ed.), *Managing Maternal Chronic Diseases for a Healthy Pregnancy*,
https://doi.org/10.1007/978-3-032-15221-3_14

patients, and careful monitoring of maternal condition through laboratory and imaging studies. Multidisciplinary collaboration among obstetrics, neonatology, infectious diseases, microbiology, radiology, and public health is indispensable.

Ultimately, the goal in managing pregnancy and perinatal infections is not only to cure the mother but also to prevent transmission, reduce vertical spread, minimize long-term sequelae, and ensure the sustainable health of the mother–infant dyad. This chapter aims to provide clinicians with a practical roadmap by systematically reviewing the epidemiology, pathogenesis, and clinical features of relevant pathogens, together with current evidence on screening, diagnostic strategies, preventive measures, and therapeutic principles.

14.2 Viral Infections

14.2.1 Viral Hepatitis Infections

14.2.1.1 Hepatitis A

Hepatitis A virus (HAV) is an RNA virus primarily spread through the fecal-oral pathway, either by direct interpersonal contact or by ingestion of contaminated food resulting from poor sanitation. HAV is endemic worldwide and hyperendemic in some regions with poor sanitation. The World Health Organization reported 12,500 hepatitis A cases in 2018 [3]. Acute hepatitis A infection generally does not progress to a chronic disease due to its self-limiting nature. Lifelong immunity is acquired following recovery through the production of hepatitis A-specific immunoglobulin G. The likelihood of hepatitis A being transmitted perinatally to the fetus is considered minimal. Therefore, during pregnancy, the primary concern is providing supportive care for the mother [4–6]. Treatment of acute hepatitis A infection includes supportive measures such as hydration, antiemetics, antipyretics, and proper nutrition. However, due to the risk of preterm birth, close monitoring is important. As of now, an effective antiviral treatment specifically directed against HAV has not been identified [7]. Nevertheless, in the case of exposure during pregnancy, a single dose of immunoglobulin prophylaxis is recommended [3]. Although data in pregnant cases is limited, immunoglobulin prophylaxis administered within 14 days after exposure has been shown to provide passive and temporary immunity, with an efficacy rate of 80–90%. Highly effective and safe vaccines for active immunity have been available for about 25 years. Available inactivated vaccines include both monovalent preparations and combined formulations with hepatitis B. Vaccine administration is the same for pregnant women as for nonpregnant individuals. It is recommended for women who live in or plan to travel to endemic areas and who have low immunity. In cases where immunoglobulin is not accessible, vaccination can also be used for post-exposure prophylaxis. Newborns can acquire passive immunity for several months through the transplacental transfer of antibodies [3, 8].

14.2.1.2 Hepatitis B

Hepatitis B virus (HBV) infection continues to represent a major global public health issue, with an estimated 240 million individuals affected worldwide. Each year, approximately 786,000 deaths are attributed to HBV-related liver disorders. Chronic HBV infection constitutes a principal etiological factor for the development of liver cirrhosis, hepatic failure, and hepatocellular carcinoma. Among pregnant women, hepatitis B antigen positivity varies based on maternal race and ethnicity, ranging between 0.6% and 5.8% [9–12]. The incubation period of HBV infection may last up to 120 days on average. Although acute HBV infection carries an approximately 10% risk of perinatal transmission, it is not associated with teratogenic effects or an increased incidence of spontaneous abortion. Vertical transmission most frequently occurs during the perinatal phase as a result of neonatal exposure to maternal blood and body fluids at birth. Pregnant women with HBV DNA concentrations exceeding 200,000 IU/mL are at substantially greater risk of transmitting the virus vertically, whereas this risk is significantly reduced in infants who receive adequate prophylaxis when maternal viral loads remain below this threshold. Without vaccination, the risk of chronic disease in exposed newborns is about 90%, compared to 5–10% in adults [13–16].

The World Health Organization (WHO) advises that pregnant women who test positive for hepatitis B virus (HBV) and exhibit viral loads exceeding 5.3 $\log_{10}$ IU/mL (or > 200,000 IU/mL) should receive tenofovir prophylaxis beginning at the 28th week of gestation and continuing until delivery. In addition, three postpartum vaccine doses are recommended to further minimize the risk of vertical transmission [17]. Moreover, for women who commence antiviral therapy during pregnancy due to elevated viral load, it is recommended that treatment be maintained for 6 to 12 weeks postpartum to prevent hepatitis B flares and to decrease the likelihood of disease progression and cirrhosis [18].

Newborns, especially those born to mothers who are positive for hepatitis B surface antigen (HBsAg), remain at risk of acquiring hepatitis B infection until the vaccination series is completed. Consequently, the most crucial measure in preventing vertical transmission is the prompt immunization of the neonate. The efficacy of prophylaxis largely depends on the timely administration of both immunoglobulin and the initial vaccine dose at birth [19, 20]. The WHO recommends administering the birth dose of the vaccine within the first 24 h after delivery [21]. To identify potential cases of vertical transmission or vaccine failure, serologic testing for HBsAg and anti-HBs is advised between 9 and 12 months of age—approximately 2 to 3 months after completion of the primary vaccination schedule [22].

14.2.1.3 Hepatitis C

Worldwide, the prevalence of hepatitis C virus (HCV) infection is estimated to range from 0.73% to 1.46%. Based on 2019 data, the prevalence among women of reproductive age differs across countries, with an overall mean of approximately

0.78% [23, 24]. Universal antenatal screening programs enable the identification of nearly all cases of HCV infection. The screening process begins with testing for hepatitis C immunoglobulin G antibodies (anti-HCV), and if the result is positive, confirmatory testing with HCV RNA is performed. A negative anti-HCV result generally excludes active or prior HCV infection [25–27].

There is literature suggesting that hepatitis C infection may be associated with adverse obstetric outcomes such as gestational diabetes, gestational hypertension, preterm birth, low birth weight, and certain congenital malformations. Vertical transmission can occur in pregnant carriers of hepatitis C. While the risk is negligible in women who are HCV RNA-negative, it has been shown that temporary maternal viremia can still result in vertical transmission [28, 29]. The primary determinant of perinatal hepatitis C virus transmission is believed to be the infection of maternal peripheral blood mononuclear cells, a risk that is particularly elevated among women who use intravenous drugs [30].

At present, no effective vaccine exists for HCV infection, and the initiation of antiviral therapy during pregnancy remains a subject of debate [31]. Concerning the mode of delivery, available evidence indicates that cesarean section does not decrease the risk of vertical transmission; therefore, HCV infection alone is not considered an indication for operative delivery. Similarly, breastfeeding has not been associated with a higher risk of maternal-to-infant transmission, and discontinuation of breastfeeding is not advised for women with HCV infection [31–33].

14.2.1.4 Hepatitis D

Hepatitis D virus (HDV) infection manifests either as a coinfection or as a superinfection in individuals already affected by chronic HBV infection. Its global prevalence remains low, approximately 0.2%, and therefore routine antenatal screening is not currently recommended. The risk of vertical transmission is minimal, and the management approach during pregnancy parallels that of hepatitis B infection [8, 34].

14.2.1.5 Hepatitis E

Hepatitis E is one of the most common causes of acute hepatitis and there are regions where it is endemic [35]. Hepatitis E infection can manifest itself in a wide range of conditions during pregnancy, from mild subclinical disease to fulminant hepatic failure [4]. Although hepatitis E virus (HEV) infection, similar to hepatitis A, commonly presents as an acute hepatitis, it differs in that it may follow a more severe clinical course during pregnancy and is associated with significant maternal and fetal morbidity and mortality [36, 37]. Hepatitis E infection can cause anicteric hepatitis, acute hepatic failure, premature birth and related complications in newborns. For this reason, close neonatal follow-up is required in the case of maternal hepatitis E infection. Mother-to-child transmission of HEV may occur either in utero or during the peripartum period, with reported transmission rates ranging from 33% to 100%. Maternal viral load has been identified as a key determinant influencing the likelihood of vertical transmission [38–40]. Although ribavirin is an antiviral agent with potential efficacy against HEV, its administration during pregnancy is contraindicated due to well-documented teratogenic effects. Therefore, the treatment of hepatitis E infection during pregnancy is primarily supportive care. It is thought that preventing hepatitis E infection in endemic areas will make the main difference. For this purpose, vaccination can be administered. However, there are no sufficient studies on the safety of hepatitis E vaccine in this age group and in pregnant women [41–43].

14.2.2 Parvovirus

Human parvovirus B19 is recognized as the etiologic agent of erythema infectiosum, commonly known as fifth disease, a prevalent viral illness of childhood. Parvovirus B19 can affect approximately 1–5% of pregnant women [44, 45]. Although symptoms such as polyarthralgia and rash may be seen in pregnant women, the infection is asymptomatic in 30–50% of cases. Vertical transmission occurs in approximately 33–51% of cases [46]. In most instances, affected fetuses remain asymptomatic and achieve spontaneous recovery. Nevertheless, in certain cases, severe complications such as fetal hydrops, miscarriage, or intrauterine fetal demise may develop [47, 48].

Parvovirus B19 infection is recognized as one of the primary etiologic factors of nonimmune hydrops fetalis. Its pathogenesis is linked to the virus's tropism for erythroid progenitor cells and its capacity to traverse the placental barrier. Within infected fetal cells, parvovirus B19 triggers apoptosis, thereby reducing the lifespan of erythrocytes and resulting in reticulocytopenic fetal anemia. Additionally, viral myocarditis has been proposed as another pathogenic mechanism, potentially causing hydrops fetalis through decreased myocardial contractility and subsequent fetal cardiac failure [49, 50].

Accurate diagnosis and management of congenital parvovirus B19 infection are critically important for improving perinatal outcomes. Most affected fetuses are identified through ultrasonographic or Doppler findings indicative of fetal anemia, including ascites, cardiomegaly, hydrops, and increased peak systolic velocity in the middle cerebral artery. Therefore, identifying women suspected of parvovirus B19 infection is essential to improve fetal survival. Management typically involves either delivery of the fetus or intrauterine blood transfusion, which forms the cornerstone of prenatal treatment for parvovirus B19 infection [51, 52].

14.2.3 Cytomegalovirus

Cytomegalovirus (CMV) is among the most prevalent causes of congenital infection globally and represents the leading nongenetic cause of intellectual disability and sensorineural hearing loss in children. The prevalence of CMV infection during pregnancy varies between 0.05% and 1%, depending on maternal CMV seroprevalence. According to current literature, there is no proven treatment for CMV infection in pregnant women [53–55]. Due to the lack of an effective treatment for CMV, routine antenatal screening is not recommended. However, screening may be considered in pregnant women presenting with influenza-like symptoms or with ultrasound findings suggestive of CMV infection [56–58]. Maternal viremia can lead to transplacental transmission, infecting both the placenta and the fetus. CMV replicates within placental cytotrophoblasts and continues to multiply in various fetal and embryonic tissues [59]. Congenital cytomegalovirus (CMV) infection is a major contributor to nonhereditary sensorineural hearing loss, neurodevelopmental impairment, growth restriction, and visual deficits. In severe cases, it may also result in fetal or neonatal death [53, 60]. The timing of intrauterine transmission—particularly when it occurs during the early weeks of gestation—is the strongest predictor of symptomatic congenital CMV, influencing both neonatal presentation and long-term neurodevelopmental outcomes [61].

Confirmation of maternal infection and detection of suspicious fetal ultrasound findings are crucial for identifying potentially infected fetuses. Ultrasound is a noninvasive tool capable of detecting major structural anomalies, though its sensitivity is limited. Suspicious but nonspecific ultrasound findings associated with fetal CMV infection include: periventricular calcifications, cerebral ventriculomegaly, echogenic fetal bowel, microcephaly, cerebellar hypoplasia, hepatosplenomegaly, polymicrogyria, periventricular (pseudo) cysts, mega cisterna magna, periventricular echogenicity, abnormal amniotic fluid volume, fetal growth restriction, ascites or pleural effusion, hydrops, and placental enlargement [62–65].

According to the literature, the definitive method for diagnosis is the detection of CMV DNA by PCR. The most commonly used method for this is amniocentesis. Cordocentesis is another option, though both methods have similar sensitivity and specificity. However, cordocentesis carries a higher risk of complications [66–68].

Antiviral treatment for congenital CMV infection during pregnancy is not recommended [69, 70]. Regarding delivery, congenital CMV infection is not a contraindication for vaginal birth. However, if the fetal condition is unstable or non-reassuring, a cesarean delivery may be planned. As long as the newborn is stable, breastfeeding is not contraindicated. It may only be withheld in very low-birth-weight infants who may be at higher risk of developing severe sepsis due to CMV [69, 71].

14.2.4 Measles, Rubella, and Mumps

Measles, rubella, and mumps viruses are vaccine-preventable viral infections that can cause significant harm to nonimmune pregnant women, as well as to their fetuses and/or newborns upon exposure [72–80]. Among these, rubella infection is considered the most dangerous, with the most severe complications [74, 75, 77, 78].

Rubella, a member of the *Togaviridae* family, is transmitted via contact with infected respiratory droplets and spreads through the nasopharyngeal route. After transmission, the virus replicates in the nasopharynx and regional lymph nodes. In adult patients, rubella infection can be asymptomatic in about 50% of cases or present with nonspecific symptoms during the prodromal phase [81–83]. Compared to measles and mumps, rubella poses a greater risk during pregnancy [82].

Diagnosis of maternal rubella infection is primarily laboratory-based, involving the detection of immunglobulin (Ig) M and IgG antibodies, IgG avidity testing, and reverse transcriptase (RT)-PCR of nasopharyngeal secretions to identify the virus [84, 85]. If rubella infection occurs during the first 12 weeks of pregnancy, congenital rubella syndrome (CRS) develops in about 90% of infected fetuses. The risk decreases to around 20% between weeks 16 and 20, and beyond this point, while intrauterine transmission can still occur, the risk of CRS significantly drops [86, 87]. Rubella infection during embryogenesis may lead to the classic CRS triad of cataracts, cardiac anomalies, and sensorineural deafness, along with other defects. These anomalies can be classified as transient, permanent, or late-onset.

- Transient findings: thrombocytopenic purpura, low birth weight, hemolytic anemia, meningoencephalitis, and hepatosplenomegaly.
- Permanent findings: microphthalmia, cataracts, hearing loss, retinopathy, cardiac defects, central nerve system (CNS) abnormalities, and craniofacial malformations.
- Late-onset findings: endocrine, neurological, and cardiovascular disorders [88–90].

Prenatal diagnosis of congenital rubella is confirmed by detecting IgM antibodies in fetal blood or chorionic villi [84, 91]. Management depends on the gestational age at the time of infection [92].

Measles, a highly contagious RNA virus from the *Paramyxoviridae* family [72, 76], is not teratogenic like rubella. However, it can cause serious maternal and pregnancy complications, including pneumonia, miscarriage, stillbirth, low birth weight, and preterm birth. If exposure occurs within 10 days postpartum, neonatal measles may develop through vertical transmission [93, 94]. Management of measles in pregnancy is similar to that in nonpregnant women and involves supportive care. Intravenous immunoglobulin (IVIG) is recommended post-exposure. Since the MMR vaccine is contraindicated during pregnancy, it is not administered at that time. However, nonimmune women are advised to receive the vaccine postpartum, and breastfeeding is not a contraindication to vaccination [95].

Mumps, like measles, is an RNA virus from the *Paramyxoviridae* family [73, 76, 79]. Some studies have shown that mumps infection may increase the risk of miscarriage [96, 97]. However, mumps has not been associated with an increased risk of fetal anomalies [98]. A few studies have suggested a potential association between maternal mumps infection and endocardial fibroelastosis in fetuses [99, 100].

14.2.5 Varicella

The varicella-zoster virus (VZV), a member of the *Herpesviridae* family, can cause significant maternal and fetal complications when acute infection occurs during pregnancy. Vertical transmission may lead to serious adverse pregnancy and neonatal outcomes. The greatest risk to the newborn is observed when maternal infection develops within the period spanning 5 days before to 2 days after delivery. In rare cases, in utero transmission can occur during primary maternal infection. If transmission happens within the first 20 weeks of pregnancy, it may result in fetal loss, intrauterine growth restriction, hydrops, limb abnormalities, microcephaly, and other neurological defects—a condition known as congenital varicella syndrome (CVS) [101].

The diagnosis of CVS is established by identifying VZV DNA in fetal blood or amniotic fluid using PCR, in conjunction with supportive ultrasonographic findings [102]. Neonatal varicella typically presents within the first 5–10 days after birth with fever and generalized vesicular rash. In mild cases, the rash resolves within 7–10 days; however, in rare cases, the infant may develop disseminated disease, including varicella pneumonia, hepatitis, and meningoencephalitis [103].

To prevent CVS, nonimmune pregnant women exposed to the virus should receive post-exposure prophylaxis. Nonimmune women can be vaccinated postpartum and breastfeeding is not a contraindication [104, 105]. Prophylaxis should be administered within 96 h of exposure. The recommended prophylactic agent is varicella zoster immunoglobulin (VZIG). If unavailable, intravenous immunoglobulin (IVIG) may be considered as an alternative [106–108].

14.2.6 Zika Virus

Zika virus was declared by the WHO in 2016 as a significant public health emergency [109]. Zika virus infection during pregnancy presents with similar symptoms to nonpregnant individuals and is usually a mild illness. However, severe complications such as microcephaly and Guillain–Barré syndrome have also been reported [110–113].

The primary mode of transmission is through the bite of infected mosquitoes in tropical regions. Nevertheless, there is evidence suggesting that Zika virus can also be transmitted via sexual contact, bites from infected animals, intrauterine transmission, blood transfusion, and even breastfeeding [114–118]. Studies have shown that Zika virus infection during pregnancy is associated with fetal loss, miscarriage, fetal growth restriction due to placental dysfunction, fetal hydrops, microcephaly, and cerebral calcifications [119–121]. Congenital Zika syndrome (CZS) is characterized by five distinguishing features: cerebral development anomalies (such as microcephaly and cerebral calcifications), ocular findings in the retina, congenital contractures, limb anomalies, and hypertonia [122]. Currently, no specific treatment exists for Zika virus infection. Management is primarily based on clinical supportive care and monitoring of the fetus for possible complications. It is recommended to maintain adequate hydration, and acetaminophen may be used to relieve fever or pain [123].

14.2.7 West Nile Virus

West Nile virus (WNV) is a mosquito-borne flavivirus that was first identified in Uganda in 1937. Since then, it has spread to various parts of the world, including the America, Asia, Europe, and Africa [124]. The clinical presentation of the disease varies from asymptomatic infection to severe neurological illness. However, severe neuroinvasive disease, characterized by fever with encephalitis, meningitis, flaccid paralysis, or a combination of symptoms, occurs in less than 1% of infected individuals. Diagnosis is made by detecting virus-specific antibodies in serum or cerebrospinal fluid [125–127].

During pregnancy, the main concern regarding WNV infection is the potential for teratogenic effects and poor pregnancy outcomes. Although a few cases have described fetuses with chorioretinitis and cerebral abnormalities, the overall body of evidence does not demonstrate a significant increase in congenital anomalies, adverse neonatal outcomes, spontaneous abortion, preterm delivery, or low birth weight when compared with the general population [128, 129].

To prevent infection, pregnant women are advised to avoid traveling to high-risk areas, and those living in or visiting such regions, particularly during summer and early autumn, should take precautions against mosquito bites, including wearing protective clothing and avoiding mosquitoes [130].

14.2.8 Coxsackie Virus

Coxsackie virus group B is an enterovirus belonging to the Picornavirus family. Enteroviruses are RNA viruses that spread through the gastrointestinal tract [131]. Group B coxsackie viruses are associated with neuronal tissue degeneration and focal muscle damage, leading to spastic paralysis. Additionally, these viruses can cause conditions like pleuritis, myocarditis, pericarditis, and hepatitis in organs such as the heart, pleura, pancreas, and liver. These viruses are also one of the potentially most fatal systemic neonatal infections due to their ability to affect multiple organs [132–134].

Transmission of enteroviruses from mother to baby typically occurs during vaginal delivery, when the newborn comes into contact with maternal secretions. Although less common, transplacental transmission has been reported and is associated with more severe and fatal outcomes [135–138]. The most specific test for diagnosis is the detection of viral RNA through PCR in serum, nasopharyngeal samples, cerebrospinal fluid, or amniotic fluid [139]. Fetal ultrasonography may reveal abnormalities such as cerebral ventriculomegaly, cardiomyopathy with ventricular dysfunction, polyhydramnios accompanied by ascites, and the presence of pericardial or pleural effusions [140, 141].

In newborns, clinical signs may include myocarditis, meningoencephalitis, hepatitis, disseminated intravascular coagulation, sepsis-like syndrome, pneumonia, gastrointestinal symptoms, pancreatitis, cutaneous exanthems, and seizures. Especially, coagulopathy and cardiomyopathy are being particularly linked to mortality. Additionally, it has been reported that congenital infections could be related to childhood type 1 diabetes [142–144].

The empiric treatment for enterovirus-infected neonates involves a combination of intravenous gamma globulin or hyperimmune globulin and leukocyte interferon. However, these treatments are not recommended for in utero therapy, and there is no evidence to suggest that they can prevent fatal outcomes of the disease. Antiviral agents such as pleconaril have shown potential efficacy in the management of meningitis and other severe infections caused by Coxsackie B virus. However, to date, no licensed vaccine or definitive antiviral therapy for Coxsackie B virus has been established in the literature. Therefore, pregnant women should primarily avoid contact with suspected individuals to prevent severe neonatal illness and perinatal complications [142, 145–148].

14.2.9 Epstein Barr Virus

Epstein–Barr virus (EBV), a member of the *Herpesviridae* family, is among the most prevalent viruses infecting humans. In the adult population, the worldwide EBV positivity rate is about 90% [149]. While EBV typically remains asymptomatic, it can also cause infectious mononucleosis. Additionally, the virus can remain latent in immune system cells, leading to conditions such as Burkitt lymphoma or nasopharyngeal carcinoma [150]. Diagnosis is made through tests detecting IgM and IgG antibodies against the viral capsid antigen and the identification of EBV nuclear antigens (EBNA) [149].

Primary EBV infection during pregnancy is rare. Generally, EBV reactivation due to immune system suppression during pregnancy leads to infection [151]. EBV infection during pregnancy can result in transplacental transmission, causing placental infection. A review of the literature suggests that, in most cases, the infection does not have serious effects on pregnancy outcomes. However, in some cases, it has been associated with severe congenital anomalies, although no specific syndrome has been identified [150].

14.2.10 Covid-19 and Influenza Viruses

Influenza is a highly contagious respiratory illness that contributes significantly to global morbidity and mortality. Each year, seasonal influenza epidemics are estimated to cause 3 to 5 million cases of severe illness and approximately 250,000 to 500,000 deaths worldwide [152]. The influenza virus generally has a self-limiting prognosis, but in specific conditions like pregnancy, the risk of complications is increased. This was particularly highlighted during the A/H1N1 pandemic, where pregnant women were found to be at a higher risk of experiencing more severe influenza infections [153–155]. During pregnancy, physiological changes in the immune and cardiopulmonary systems increase susceptibility to influenza infection [156]. Suppression of immunity for the purpose of increasing tolerability to fetal antigens is associated with more severe infection in pregnant women, prolonged hospitalization, and an increased likelihood of intensive care admission, especially as the gestational week increases [157].

The primary approach during the prenatal period is prevention of influenza infection. Vaccination is the most effective method to protect both the mother and newborn [158]. Inactivated influenza vaccines can be administered throughout the year during pregnancy. Live attenuated influenza vaccines are not recommended during pregnancy [158, 159]. For infected pregnant women, the decision to use antiviral medications should be made after evaluating the risk-benefit ratio. Antiviral agents can shorten the duration of symptoms and prevent serious complications, such as pneumonia, respiratory failure, the need for intensive care, and death, while reducing the inflammatory response [160–162]. Neuraminidase inhibitors like oseltamivir and zanamivir are recommended as the first-line antiviral treatment. However, vaccination remains the primary method to protect both mother and newborn [163].

COVID-19 is a severe respiratory illness caused by the SARS-CoV-2 virus, which carries the potential for life-threatening complications. Conditions such as diabetes, heart and liver diseases, and immune suppression are risk factors for increased disease severity. Pregnancy is also identified as a risk factor by the Centers for Disease Control and Prevention (CDC). Research has demonstrated that pregnant women infected with COVID-19 face an elevated risk of developing adverse maternal and perinatal outcomes [164, 165]. While transplacental transmission is rare during pregnancy, the virus can negatively affect pregnancy outcomes. Pregnant women with COVID-19 infection are at a heightened risk of developing preeclampsia or eclampsia, as well as experiencing adverse outcomes such as preterm birth and stillbirth [166, 167]. Negative outcomes for the newborn are often a result of the deterioration of the maternal condition due to the infection [168]. Fetal distress and neonatal respiratory distress syndrome have been identified as the most frequently reported clinical conditions associated with prematurity and admission to neonatal intensive care units [169]. The treatment of COVID-19 during pregnancy is similar to that of nonpregnant individuals. If the disease worsens, antiviral treatment and dexamethasone therapy are recommended. In addition, supportive care and close monitoring are suggested [170]. Moreover, while more studies are needed, current research has not shown any negative outcomes for the newborn or mother associated with vaccination. Therefore, vaccination should be considered as an effective preventive measure [171].

14.3 Protozoal Infections

14.3.1 Toxoplasma Infection

Toxoplasma Gondii infection, when contracted during pregnancy, can pass to the fetus, causing a tragic but preventable disease in the newborn. In the United States, an average of 500–5000 newborns are born with congenital toxoplasmosis each year. Although most of these newborns appear healthy at birth, long-term effects may emerge over months or years [172, 173]. Transmission to humans most frequently occurs through the consumption of raw or undercooked meat harboring viable tissue cysts. However, soil, water, and food can also become contaminated [174].

The first diagnostic method used to detect active or past infection is serological testing. IgM and IgG antibodies in maternal serum are screened. IgM and IgG titration tests are also used to distinguish between acute and chronic infections [175]. Women whose test positive on serological tests are recommended to undergo amniocentesis. A definitive diagnosis is made if the parasite is detected in the amniotic fluid. Additionally, ultrasound findings are highly significant in the diagnosis. Hydrocephalus, ventriculomegaly, intraserebral calcifications, splenomegaly, congenital nephrosis, and ascites are markers that may be associated with toxoplasmosis on ultrasound [176, 177]. If the test is positive, treatment should be initiated to prevent vertical transmission. If the infection is detected within the first 18 weeks or immediately before conception, spiramycin is recommended as the medical treatment. If infection occurs after the 18th week, the recommended treatment is pyrimethamine, sulfadiazine, and folinic acid. If the patient is already receiving spiramycin, it is recommended to continue spiramycin in combination with these agents [177, 178]. In conclusion, toxoplasma infection is a disease that affects many women and newborns, but with early diagnosis and appropriate treatment, it is preventable.

14.3.2 Malaria

Malaria remains a major global public health concern, accounting for approximately 247 million cases and an estimated 619,000 deaths annually in endemic regions. Pregnant women are particularly at risk due to the accumulation of *Plasmodium falciparum*-infected erythrocytes in the placenta [179, 180]. It is primarily transmitted to humans through the bite of female *Anopheles* mosquitoes infected with *Plasmodium* parasites. Additionally, there are other transmission routes, including intrauterine or perinatal vertical transmission, blood transfusion, organ transplant, or the use of infected needles [181].

The clinical presentation of malaria is often nonspecific, typically characterized by headache, fever, myalgia, chills, cough, and diarrhea. Paroxysmal fever is rare. In mild cases, laboratory investigations may reveal anemia, thrombocytopenia, hyperbilirubinemia, and elevated liver transaminase levels. Prompt diagnosis and timely initiation of treatment are crucial to prevent disease progression. Severe cases typically involve dysfunction of vital organs [182, 183].

Pregnant women with malaria infection are predisposed to more severe disease and unfavorable maternal outcomes. Anemia—resulting from impaired erythropoiesis, rupture of parasitized erythrocytes, and hemolysis of uninfected red cells—is a frequent complication that heightens the risk of both maternal and fetal morbidity. Placental malaria has also been linked to an increased incidence of preeclampsia and maternal anemia [182, 184]. Furthermore, placental malaria can lead to low birth weight, preterm birth, and stillbirth [182]. Congenital malaria may be associated with fever, lethargy, loss of appetite, irritability, and sepsis [185]. For rapid diagnosis, it is recommended that laboratory personnel perform thin and thick peripheral blood smears [186]. Treatment depends on whether the disease is mild or severe. For uncomplicated cases, chloroquine or hydroxychloroquine is recommended. If chloroquine resistance is present, artemether-lumefantrine is recommended [182]. In severe cases, parenteral artesunate treatment is recommended [187].

14.4 Fungal Infections

Fungal infections can cause fetal infections through ascending pathways or systemically. However, systemic mycoses are quite rare during pregnancy, except in cases involving travel to endemic regions or in immunosuppressed individuals [188].

Vaginal candidiasis is relatively common during pregnancy, but systemic disease is very rare. In cases of systemic infection, the infection is generally limited to the placenta, amniotic membrane, umbilical cord, and fetal skin. Placental and fetal infections are thought to occur through an ascending route. Chorioamnionitis is commonly seen and fetal infection can be associated with premature birth and fetal death. Nonspecific findings can be observed on ultrasound [188–193].

Pulmonary mycoses have been rarely reported during pregnancy. The relationship between pregnancy and blastomycosis has been documented in several case reports. Since the disease poses risks to both maternal and fetal health, antifungal treatment is crucial [194–197]. Blastomycosis is a systemic fungal infection that can involve multiple organ systems; however, the lungs are the most frequently affected site in the general population [198]. Since the clinical and radiological findings of blastomycosis are nonspecific, the gold standard for diagnosis is the demonstration of yeast forms in tissue and the growth of fungus in culture [199]. The treatment of blastomycosis requires a multidisciplinary approach. In pregnant women, intravenous liposomal amphotericin B is initiated, and oral itraconazole is used postpartum. Due to the small number of reported cases, no recommendations can be made regarding the mode of delivery. Although maternal death has not been reported, there have been two infant deaths after vaginal delivery. However, these infants did not have a diagnosis of blastomycosis and did not receive antifungal treatment before birth. In other reported infants, no disease burden or teratogenic effects have been reported [200].

Coccidioidomycosis is an infection endemic to the northwestern Mexico, United States, and select areas of South and Central America. Transmission occurs through inhalation of airborne arthroconidia, with approximately one-third of exposed individuals developing symptomatic disease. The clinical presentation can range from a mild flu-like illness to pneumonia and disseminated disease [201]. Although it can cause placental infection, fetal intrauterine infection is very rare [202]. Maternal mortality is correlated with delayed diagnosis and late initiation of antifungal therapy. In women diagnosed in the third trimester, the survival rate is even lower. Survival rates have significantly improved with effective antifungal treatment [203].

14.5 Bacterial Infections

14.5.1 Tuberculosis

The true prevalence of tuberculosis during pregnancy remains unclear, but according to data from 2011, it is estimated that there are approximately 216,500 cases worldwide [204]. Tuberculosis during pregnancy is associated with a sixfold increase in perinatal mortality and a twofold rise in preterm delivery and low birth weight. When coexisting with HIV infection, maternal and fetal morbidity and mortality rates increase by up to 400% [205]. Studies on the impact of tuberculosis on pregnancy outcomes have found that it is associated with stillbirth, severe preeclampsia, emergency cesarean sections, and low birth weight [206].

Due to the potential teratogenic effects of tuberculosis and drug-resistant tuberculosis treatments, these treatments further increase the risk in pregnancies that are already in high-risk. According to the U.S. Food and Drug Administration (FDA), both first- and second-line antituberculosis agents are classified as category C or D when used during pregnancy [207]. For drug-sensitive tuberculosis, first-line medications—including isoniazid, rifampin, pyrazinamide, and ethambutol—are designated as category C by the FDA. However, it is still recommended that pregnant women begin treatment as early as possible, with the risk-benefit ratio carefully evaluated [207–211]. Drug-resistant tuberculosis occurs in about 10% of cases, and due to its toxic and prolonged treatment, it has harmful effects on health and survival. Additionally, it can fail in 44% of cases. Second-line treatment agents are also generally classified as category C and category D. These drugs should be used on a case-by-case basis, considering the risk-benefit ratio, especially in cases of advanced disease, and the decision should be made by clinicians [207, 212].

14.5.2 Listeriosis

Listeriosis is an infection typically associated with Listeria microorganisms, usually transmitted through food, and primarily affects immunocompromised individuals, newborns, the elders, and pregnant women [213, 214]. Perinatal listeriosis exhibits a markedly different clinical course from that observed in the general population and is strongly associated with adverse perinatal outcomes. While maternal manifestations are typically mild or nonspecific, the infection poses significant risks to the fetus and newborn, including miscarriage, preterm delivery, stillbirth, intrauterine demise, and long-term neonatal complications. The fetal and neonatal mortality rates are around 20–35% [215]. The American College of Obstetricians and Gynecologists (ACOG) recommends administering high-dose ampicillin therapy (a minimum of 6 gm per day) for pregnant patients presenting with symptomatic or febrile perinatal listeriosis [216]. It has been shown that gestational age is related to fetal and neonatal survival, and as gestational age increases, fetal and neonatal survival rates also improve [217, 218].

14.5.3 Lyme Disease

In the United States, Lyme disease—caused by the spirochete *Borrelia burgdorferi*—is among the most common vector-borne diseases [219]. The diagnosis can be made based on clinical findings if erythema migrans is present. In the early stages, laboratory findings are generally negative. If the clinical course is uncertain, serological tests are necessary for confirmation. The enzyme-linked immunosorbent assay (ELISA) test is commonly used as a serological test [220]. Exposure to the causative agent during pregnancy or at birth can affect the health of both the fetus and the pregnant woman. There are scientific opinions suggesting that Borrelia burgdorferi may cause a congenital syndrome in the fetus and placenta similar to syphilis through vertical transmission [221–224]. The effect on the developing fetus can depend on various factors, such as the gestational age at the time of exposure, the structure of the fetomaternal interface, the immune response, and the severity of symptoms. When congenital infection is suspected, a neurological evaluation is very important. Cognitive functions, movement, and communication problems may be affected due to antenatal infection [225].

Although the treatment approach for pregnant women has not been clearly established, the general consensus is that the same treatment applied to nonpregnant individuals should be used. However, doxycycline, the primary treatment option, is not suitable for pregnant women, so amoxicillin and third-generation cephalosporins are preferred [226]. Early diagnosis and treatment can help reduce the short- and long-term effects of Lyme disease [227].

14.5.4 Group-A and Group-B Streptococci

Group A Streptococci are known as "flesh-eating bacteria"and, although their incidence decreased with the discovery of antibiotics, recent increases have been observed due to antibiotic resistance [228]. In recent years, an increase in Group A Streptococcus (GAS) infections during pregnancy and the postpartum period has been noted. These infections progress rapidly in pregnant women and are associated with high maternal and fetal mortality rates [229]. The most significant risk factor for postpartum infections, including Group A Streptococcus, is cesarean delivery. Other risk factors include invasive procedures, regional anesthesia, intravenous catheter placement, and catheter interventions. After vaginal delivery, vaginal tears, cervical dilation, and rupture of membranes can disrupt the vaginal mucosal barrier due to changes in pH levels. Additionally, the postpartum uterus, due to blood and necrotic decidual tissue, creates a suitable environment for bacterial growth [230]. Group A Streptococcus (GAS) is a gram-positive, beta-hemolytic bacterium that can cause a wide range of diseases, from mild pharyngitis to severe invasive pneumonia, meningitis, and endometritis [231]. The urogenital tract is generally not colonized by GAS. It is typically believed that self-contamination occurs after a history of previous GAS pharyngitis [232]. GAS infections can develop at any stage of pregnancy but usually manifest within 24 h postpartum, becoming fulminant within 48–96 h [233–235]. Early diagnosis and intervention for sepsis and septic shock are crucial in reducing morbidity and mortality. Management should be multidisciplinary [236].

Group B Streptococcus (GBS) is a gram-positive, beta-hemolytic bacterium [237]. GBS can colonize a woman's vagina, intestines, and urethral tissues during pregnancy, and newborns can become infected directly through the maternal genital tract during vaginal delivery. GBS infection can lead to a wide range of complications, including stillbirth, maternal infections, early- and late-onset neonatal sepsis, preterm birth, and hypoxic–ischemic encephalopathy [238]. The current treatment to prevent fetal GBS transmission is the use of antibiotics. However, due to antibiotic resistance, this intervention does not completely prevent the disease. To reduce the disease burden, interventions should be specifically planned with minimal harmful effects on the microbiome, aiming to prevent colonization and ascending infections, and thereby reduce vertical transmission [239–241]. Ampicillin and penicillin-derived antibiotics can be used for treatment and prevention. However, antibiotic resistance is a significant issue [242, 243]. Therefore, vaccination to immunize pregnant women would be the most effective method for maternal and fetal protection [244–247].

14.6 Sexually Transmitted Infections

14.6.1 Chlamydia Infection

Chlamydial infection during pregnancy can be associated with fetal loss, low birth weight, premature rupture of membranes, and preterm labor and birth. Studies have shown an increased risk association between chlamydial infection and preterm labor, low birth weight and perinatal death [248–254]. Screening in early pregnancy aims to prevent poor pregnancy outcomes. However, chlamydia screening has not yet become a standard practice globally in terms of cost-effectiveness and effect size [255, 256]. Nevertheless, since chlamydia is a treatable infection, recognizing and treating infected mothers through antenatal screening programs can help prevent neonatal and pregnancy complications. Current clinical guidelines recommend a single dose of azithromycin as the first-line therapy, while amoxicillin or erythromycin may be used as alternative treatment options [257, 258].

14.6.2 Gonorrhea Infection

Neisseria gonorrhoeae infection can be asymptomatic in up to 45% of infected women. However, it can lead to symptoms such as endocervicitis and urethritis, or it may spread hematogenously to other organs, causing disseminated infection. Gonorrhea infection during pregnancy has been linked to adverse obstetric outcomes, including premature rupture of membranes, postpartum endometritis, neonatal infections, preterm delivery, and low-birth-weight infants [259–261]. A woman at risk for gonorrhea infection should be screened in the early weeks of pregnancy, and if the risk persists, repeat screening tests should be done during the third trimester. Several antibiotic classes with similar effectiveness are available for the treatment of gonorrhea. Ceftriaxone, cefixime, amoxicillin + probenecid, and spectinomycin are antibiotics that can be used for gonorrhea treatment. Typically, a 250 mg intramuscular dose of ceftriaxone or a 400 mg oral dose of cefixime is recommended [262–264]. Early diagnosis and intervention help reduce fetal and maternal morbidity and mortality [265].

14.6.3 Syphilis

Syphilis is a chronic systemic infection caused by the spirochete *Treponema pallidum*. Risk factors for maternal transmission during pregnancy include African American or Hispanic ethnicity, younger maternal age, low socioeconomic and educational status, inadequate prenatal care, engagement in sex work, and substance use [266]. Congenital syphilis results from vertical transmission of *Treponema pallidum* from an infected mother to the fetus during pregnancy [267]. Its clinical manifestations may include stillbirth, nonimmune hydrops fetalis, and neonatal death [266]. The likelihood of congenital infection is closely associated with the degree of maternal spirochetemia and the duration of primary or secondary syphilis [266, 268]. In symptomatic neonates, signs may include hepatobiliary dysfunction, thrombocytopenia, anemia, bullous or mucocutaneous lesions, osteochondritis, or periostitis. The "moth-eaten" appearance in long bones is pathognomonic. Neonates presenting with symptoms suggestive of syphilis should be evaluated for neurosyphilis and treated [269–273]. Serological diagnostic tests are performed in the same way for pregnant and nonpregnant women [269]. The traditional syphilis screening algorithm involves screening with non-treponemal tests, followed by confirmation with treponemal tests [269]. Early congenital syphilis may present with maculopapular rashes that can progress to desquamation, osteochondritis, hepatosplenomegaly, iritis, and flu-like syndrome. In untreated or inadequately treated fetuses, the triad of Hutchinson teeth, eighth nerve deafness, and interstitial keratitis may be observed [274]. The most reliable and effective treatment during pregnancy is parenteral benzathine penicillin G, depending on the stage of the disease. If alternative treatment regimens were used during pregnancy, the newborn should be treated for potential congenital infection [269].

14.6.4 Human Insufficiency Virus

Mother-to-child transmission of human immunodeficiency virus (HIV) can be controlled through large-scale interventions, including a combination of antiretroviral therapy, infant prophylaxis, and the prevention of breastfeeding. In developed countries, the rate of mother-to-child HIV transmission decreased from 6.8% in 2001 to 1.1% in 2016 [275]. Complications such as preterm birth, ectopic pregnancy, spontaneous abortion, and fetal death are commonly observed in HIV-positive pregnancies. Studies have shown that the likelihood of poor pregnancy outcomes is significantly higher in HIV-positive women [276, 277]. The second and third trimesters of pregnancy and the first 6 months postpartum are identified as the highest-risk periods for HIV transmission [278]. The most effective way to prevent transmission in seroconvert pregnant women is to prevent them from becoming infected in the first place [279]. Several risk factors for vertical transmission have been identified, including the mother's health status, mode of delivery, duration of membrane rupture, obstetric complications such as maternal hemorrhage or infection, and perinatal feeding methods. It is generally believed that this risk is multifactorial. Vertical transmission has been most commonly associated with vaginal delivery [280]. HIV-positive pregnant women should start antiretroviral therapy as soon as possible, and their CD4 count should be maintained at high levels. Additionally, HIV-positive pregnant women who receive antiretroviral treatment in the first trimester should be closely monitored, as they have a higher risk of poor pregnancy outcomes [281]. Methods for preventing vertical transmission include administering antiretroviral therapy during pregnancy, labor, delivery, and the postnatal period for the infant, and planning elective cesarean delivery before the membranes rupture in cases where HIV viral load is detectable in late pregnancy [282]. Breastfeeding may be discontinued if conditions for providing adequate and healthy nutrition are met. However, if appropriate and sufficient conditions for infant feeding are not provided, breastfeeding should not be discontinued. If breastfeeding continues, infant antiretroviral prophylaxis regimens must also be started [283, 284].

14.6.5 Herpes Simplex Virus

Herpes simplex virus (HSV) infection continues to be associated with significant mortality and long-term morbidity despite advancements in prevention, diagnosis, and treatment. In industrialized nations, the incidence of neonatal herpes simplex virus (HSV) infection is estimated at approximately 10 cases per 100,000 live births, corresponding to around 14,000 cases annually, with a mortality rate of 0.82 per 100,000 births [285, 286]. Maternal HSV infection during pregnancy can be effectively managed with antiviral therapy, often leading to favorable maternal and neonatal outcomes. Primary maternal infection acquired in late pregnancy (25–50%) carries a higher risk of transmission to the newborn compared to recurrent genital infections (<3%) [287–289]. In utero infections are rare and account for 5% of neonatal HSV infections. Most neonatal HSV infections are acquired during birth (85%), with 10% acquired due to postpartum close contact. Vertical transmission usually occurs due to asymptomatic viral shedding. When symptomatic, cesarean delivery reduces the risk significantly [288, 290, 291]. Congenital HSV-1 and HSV-2 infections in neonates are rare but cause devastating outcomes [285]. The clinical spectrum of neonatal herpes simplex virus (HSV) infection is categorized into three forms: (1) skin, eye, and mouth (SEM) disease; (2) localized central nervous system (CNS) infection; and (3) disseminated systemic disease. Symptoms usually appear within the first 4 weeks postpartum [291]. The diagnosis of disseminated disease can be delayed until the second week due to the expected bacterial sepsis results. In treated neonates, the mortality rate is 40–50%, whereas untreated cases have a mortality rate of 80% [292]. The current treatment for neonatal HSV involves high-dose acyclovir (60 mg/kg/day). Acyclovir therapy has been shown to reduce neonatal mortality [293]. Asymptomatic neonates born to women with active herpetic lesions should always be tested for HSV. In cases of maternal primary infection, prophylaxis must be administered to the newborn. In cases of maternal recurrent infection, prophylaxis is not required until test results are obtained. However, the newborn should continue to be closely monitored [294]. If an infection occurs in the first or second trimester of pregnancy, oral acyclovir should be administered for 5 days. If the infection begins in the third trimester, the same treatment should be started immediately and continued until delivery [295]. To date, there have been no reports of adverse effects on the fetus from antiviral treatment during pregnancy [296].

14.6.6 Human Papillomavirus

Human papillomavirus (HPV) is a group of viruses responsible for the most common sexually transmitted infection. It is often self-limiting and asymptomatic, but it can also be associated with oropharyngeal and anogenital malignancies. HPV is a DNA virus from the Papillomaviridae family [297–300]. HPV infection during pregnancy has been linked to unfavorable obstetric outcomes. Studies have demonstrated links between HPV infection and complications such as preterm birth, spontaneous abortion, intrauterine growth restriction, preeclampsia, premature rupture of membranes, and fetal demise [301]. Therefore, primary prevention and vaccination are important. However, HPV vaccination during pregnancy is not recommended [302, 303].

References

1. Auruti C, De Rose DU, Santisi A, Martini L, Piersigilli F, Bersani I, Ronchetti MP, Caforio L. Pregnancy and viral infections; mechanisms of foetal damage, diagnosis, and prevention of neonatal adverse outcomes from cytomegalovirus to SARS-CoV-2 and Zika virus. Biochim Biophys Acta (BBA) Mol Basis Dis. 2021;1867:166198.
2. Simon, N.P. What Is a Congenital Infection? Emory University School of Medicine. 2023. Available online: https://med.emory.edu/departments/pediatrics/divisions/neonatology/dpc/conginf.html. Accessed on 6 Dec 2023.
3. Nelson NP, Weng MK, Hofmeister MG, et al. Prevention of Hepatitis A Virus Infection in the United States: recommendations of the Advisory Committee on Immunization Practices, 2020. MMWR Recomm Rep. 2020;69(5):1–38.
4. Yan Seto MT, Cheung KW, Hung IFN. Management of viral hepatitis A, C, D and E in pregnancy. Best Pract Res Clin Obstet Gynaecol. 2020. https://doi.org/10.1016/j.bpobgyn.2020.03.009.
5. World Health Organization [WHO]. Hepatitis A. World Heal Organ n.d. https://www.who.int/news-room/fact-sheets/detail/hepatitis-a. Accessed 11 Sept 2020.
6. Hamburg-Shields E., Prasad M., Infectious hepatitis in pregnancy. 2019.
7. Jiang W, et al. Sofosbuvir inhibits hepatitis A virüs replication in vitro assessed by a cell-based fluorescent reporter system. Antivir Res. 2018;154:51–7.
8. Dionne-Odom J, Cozzi GD, Franco RA, Njei B, Tita ATN. Treatment and prevention of viral hepatitis in pregnancy. Am J Obstet Gynecol. 2022;226(3):335–46.
9. World Health Organization. Media centre: hepatitis B. 2013. Available at: factsheets/fs204/en/. Accessed June 20, 2017.
10. Lozano R, Naghavi M, Foreman K, et al. Global and regional mortality from 235 causes of death for 20 age groups in 1990 and 2010: a systematic analysis for the Global Burden of Disease Study 2010. Lancet. 2012;380:2095–128.
11. Euler GL, Wooten KG, Baughman AL, et al. Hepatitis B surface antigen prevalence among pregnant women in urban areas: implications for testing, reporting, and preventing perinatal transmission. Pediatrics. 2003;111:1192–7.
12. WHO. Progress report on HIV, viral hepatitis and sexually transmitted infections. WHO; 2019.
13. Terrault NA, Levy MT, Cheung KW, Jourdain G. Viral hepatitis and pregnancy. Nat Rev Gastroenterol Hepatol. 2021;18(2):117–30.
14. Dionne-Odom J, Tita AT, Silverman NS. #38: hepatitis B in pregnancy screening, treatment, and prevention of vertical transmission. Am J Obstet Gynecol. 2016;214(1):6–14.

15. Su WJ. The impact of universal infant hepatitis B immunization on reducing the hepatitis B carrier rate in pregnant women. J Infect Dis. 2019;220
16. Goldstein ST. A mathematical model to estimate global hepatitis B disease burden and vaccination impact. Int J Epidemiol. 2005;34
17. Prevention of mother-to-child transmission of hepatitis B virus: guidelines on antiviral prophylaxis in pregnancy. World Health Organization; 2020.
18. Visvanathan K, Dusheiko G, Giles M, Wong ML, Phung N, Walker S, et al. Managing HBV in pregnancy. Prevention, prophylaxis, treatment and follow-up: position paper produced by Australian, UK and New Zealand key opinion leaders. Gut. 2016;65:340.
19. Wang C. et al. Protective effect of an improved immunization practice of mother- to-infant transmission of hepatitis B virus and risk factors associated with imm.
20. Kang W, et al. Risk factors associated with immunoprophylaxis failure against mother to child transmission of hepatitis B virus and hepatitis B vaccination status in Yunnan province, China. Vaccine. 2014;32:3362–6.
21. World Health Organization. Global hepatitis report, 2017 (WHO, 2017).
22. Schillie S, et al. Update: shortened interval for postvaccination serologic testing of infants born to hepatitis B- infected mothers. Morb Mortal Wkly Rep. 2015;64:1118–20.
23. Younossi ZM, Wong G, Anstee QM, et al. The global burden of liver disease. Clin Gastroenterol Hepatol. 2023;21(8):1978–91.
24. Dugan E, Blach S, Biondi M, et al. Global prevalence of hepatitis C virus in women of childbearing age in 2019: a modelling study. Lancet Gastroenterol Hepatol. 2021;6(3):169–84.
25. Carey I, Christiana M, Marie-Ange M, et al. Universal versus targeted screening for HCV infection in pregnancy in a diverse, multi-ethnic population: universal screening is more comprehensive. J Viral Hepat. 2022;29(12):1079–88.
26. Hachicha-Maalej N, Collins IJ, Ades AE, et al. Modelling the potential effectiveness of hepatitis C screening and treatment strategies during pregnancy in Egypt and Ukraine. J Hepatol. 2023;78(5):937–46.
27. Tang J, Zhao H, Zhou YH. Screening for viral hepatitis carriage. Best Pract Res Clin Obstet Gynaecol. 2024;96:102523.
28. Connell LE, Salihu HM, Salemi JL, August EM, Weldeselasse H, Mbah AK. Maternal hepatitis B and hepatitis C carrier status and perinatal outcomes. Liver Int. 2011;31:1163–70.
29. Benova L, Mohamoud YA, Calvert C, Abu-Raddad LJ. Vertical transmission of hepatitis C virus: systematic review and meta-analysis. Clin Infect Dis. 2014;59:765–73.
30. Azzari C, Moriondo M, Indolfi G, Betti L, Gambineri E, De Martino M, et al. Higher risk of hepatitis C virus perinatal transmission from drug user mothers is mediated by peripheral blood mononuclear cell infection. J Med Virol. 2008;80:65–71.
31. Chilakaa VN, Konje JC. Viral hepatitis in pregnancy. Eur J Obstet Gynecol Reprod Biol. 2021;256:287–96.
32. Dunkelberg JC, Berkley EMF, Thiel KW, Leslie KK. Hepatitis B and C in pregnancy: a review and recommendations for care. J Perinatol. 2014;34:882.
33. Zanetti AR, Tanzi E, Newell ML. Mother-to-infant transmission of hepatitis C virus. J Hepatol. 1999;31(Suppl 1):96–100.
34. Pisano MB, Giadans CG, Flichman DM, Ré VE, Preciado MV, Valva P. Viral hepatitis update: progress and perspectives. World J Gastroenterol. 2021;27(26):4018–44.
35. Aggarwal R. Diagnosis of hepatitis E. Nat Rev Gastroenterol Hepatol. 2013;10:24–33.
36. Jin H, Zhao Y, Zhang X, Wang B, Liu P. Case-fatality risk of pregnant women with acute viral hepatitis type E: a systematic review and meta-analysis. Epidemiol Infect. 2016;144:2098–106.
37. Seifoleslami M. An update of the incidence of fulminant hepatitis due to viral agents during pregnancy. Interv Med Appl Sci. 2018;10:210–2.
38. El Sayed Zaki M, El Razek MMA, El Razek HMA. Maternal- fetal hepatitis E transmission: is it underestimated? J Clin Transl Hepatol. 2014;2(2):117–23.

39. Gurley ES, et al. Estimating the burden of maternal and neonatal deaths associated with jaundice in Bangladesh: possible role of hepatitis E infection. Am J Public Health. 2012;102:2248–54.
40. Sharma S, et al. Risk factors for vertical transmission of hepatitis E virus infection. J Viral Hepat. 2017;24:1067–75.
41. Nishiyama T, et al. Screening of novel drugs for inhibiting hepatitis E virus replication. J Virol Methods. 2019;270:1–11.
42. Bertuzzo VR, et al. Pregnant woman saved with liver transplantation from acute liver failure due to hepatitis E virus. Transpl Int. 2014;27:87–9.
43. Li SW, et al. The development of a recombinant hepatitis E vaccine HEV 239. Hum Vaccin Immunother. 2015;11:908–14.
44. Levy R, Weissman A, Blomberg G, Hagay ZJ. Infection by parvovirus B19 during pregnancy: a review. Obstet Gynecol Surv. 1997;52(4):254–9.
45. Crane J. Parvovirus B19 infection in pregnancy. J Obstet Gynaecol Can. 2002;24(9):727–43.
46. Corcoran A, Doyle S. Advances in the biology, diagnosis and host-pathogen interactions parvovirus B19. J Med Microbiol. 2004;53:459–75.
47. Lamont RF, Sobel JD, Vaisbuch E, Kusanovic JP, Mazaki-Tovi S, Kim SK, Uldbjerg N, Romero R. Parvovirus B19 infection in human pregnancy. BJOG Int J Obstet Gynaecol. 2011;118:175–86.
48. Bascietto F, Liberati M, Murgano D, Buca D, Iacovelli A, Flacco ME, Manzoli L, Familiari A, Scambia G, D'Antonio F. Outcome of fetuses with congenital parvovirus B19 infection: systematic review and meta-analysis. Ultrasound Obstet Gynecol. 2018;52:569–76.
49. Yaegashi N. Pathogenesis of nonimmune hydrops fetalis caused by intrauterine B19 infection. Tohoku J Exp Med. 2000;190:65–82.
50. Hichijo A, Morine M. A case of fetal parvovirus B19 myocarditis that caused terminal heart failure. Case Rep Obstet Gynecol. 2014;2014:463571.
51. Cosmi E, Mari G, Delle Chiaie L, Detti L, Akiyama M, Murphy J, Stefos T, Ferguson JE, Hunter D, Hsu CD, Abuhamad A, Bahado-Singh R. Noninvasive diagnosis by Doppler ultrasonography of fetal anemia resulting from parvovirus infection. Am J Obstet Gynecol. 2002;187:1290–3.
52. Giorgio E, De Oronzo MA, Iozza I, Di Natale A, Cianci S, Garofalo G, Giacobbe AM, Politi S. Parvovirus B19 during pregnancy: a review. J Prenat Med. 2010;4:63–6.
53. Dollard SC, Grosse SD, Ross DS. New estimates of the prevalence of neurological and sensory sequelae and mortality associated with congenital cytomegalovirus infection. Rev Med Virol. 2007;17(5):355–63.
54. Britt W. Controversies in the natural history of congenital human cytomega-lovirus infection: the paradox of infection and disease in offspring of women with immunity prior to pregnancy. Med Microbiol Immunol. 2015;204(3):263–71.
55. Kimberlin DW, Jester PM, Sánchez PJ, Ahmed A, Arav-Boger R, Michaels MG, et al. Valganciclovir for symptomatic congenital cytomegalovirus disease. N Engl J Med. 2015;372(10):933–43.
56. Walker SP, Palma-Dias R, Wood EM, Shekleton P, Giles ML. Cytomegalovirus in pregnancy: to screen or not to screen. BMC Pregnancy Childbirth. 2013;13:96.
57. NICE. Antenatal Care CG62. Guidance#Lifestyle-Considerations 2008.
58. Picone O, Vauloup-Fellous C, Cordier AG, Parent Du Châtelet I, Senat MV, Frydman R, et al. A 2-year study on cytomegalovirus infection during pregnancy in a French hospital. BJOG. 2009;116(6):818–23.
59. Ahlfors K, Ivarsson SA, Harris S, Boppana S, Fowler KB. Secondary maternal cytomegalovirus infection-A significant cause of congenital disease [1] (multiple letters). Pediatrics. 2001;107(5)
60. Hamilton ST, Van Zuylen W, Shand A, et al. Prevention of congenital cytomegalovirus complications by maternal and neonatal treatments: a systematic review. Rev Med Virol. 2014;24:420–33.

61. Enders G, Daiminger A, Bader U, et al. Intrauterine transmission and clinical outcome of 248 pregnancies with primary cytomegalovirus infection in relation to gestational age. J Clin Virol. 2011;52:244–6.
62. Grangeot- Keros L, Mayaux MJ, Lebon P, Freymuth F, Eugene G, Stricker R, et al. Value of cytomegalovirus (CMV) IgG avidity index for the diagnosis of primary CMV infection in pregnant women. J Infect Dis. 1997;175(4):944–6.
63. Guerra B, Simonazzi G, Puccetti C, Lanari M, Farina A, Lazzarotto T, et al. Ultrasound prediction of symptomatic congenital cytomegalovirus infection. Am J Obstet Gynecol. 2008;198(4):380.e1–7.
64. Benoist G, Salomon LJ, Jacquemard F, Daffos F, Ville Y. The prognostic value of ultrasound abnormalities and biological parameters in blood of fetuses infected with cytomegalovirus. BJOG. 2008;115(7):823–9.
65. Lipitz S, Achiron R, Zalel Y, Mendelson E, Tepperberg M, Gamzu R. Outcome of pregnancies with vertical transmission of primary cytomegalovirus infection. Obstet Gynecol. 2002;100(3):428–33.
66. Revello MG, Gerna G. Diagnosis and management of human cytomegalovirus infection in the mother, fetus, and newborn infant. Clin Microbiol Rev. 2002;15(4):680–715.
67. Lazzarotto T, Guerra B, Gabrielli L, Lanari M, Landini MP. Update on the prevention, diagnosis and management of cytomegalovirus infection during pregnancy. Clin Microbiol Infect. 2011;17(9):1285–93.
68. Enders G, Bäder U, Lindemann L, Schalasta G, Daiminger A. Prenatal diagnosis of congenital cytomegalovirus infection in 189 pregnancies with known outcome. Prenat Diagn. 2001;21(5):362–77.
69. Leruez-Ville M, Foulon I, Pass R, Ville Y. Cytomegalovirus infection during pregnancy: state of the science. Am J Obstet Gynecol. 2020;223(3):330–49.
70. Navti OB, Al-Belushi FM, Konje JC, FRCOG. Cytomegalovirus infection in pregnancy–an update. Eur J Obstet Gynecol Reprod Biol. 2020;258:216–22.
71. Luck SE, Wieringa JW, Blázquez-Gamero D, et al. Congenital cytomegalovirus: a European expert consensus statement on diagnosis and management. Ped Infect Dis J. 2017;36(12):1205–13.
72. Centers for Disease Control and Prevention (CDC). Measles. In: Atkinson W, Wolfe S, Hamborsky J, editors. Epidemiology and prevention of vaccine-preventable diseases. 12th ed. Washington, DC: Public Health Foundation; 2011. p. 173–92.
73. Center for Disease Control and Prevention (CDC). Mumps. In: Atkinson W, Wolfe S, Hamborsky J, editors. Epidemiology and prevention of vaccine-preventable diseases. 12th ed. Washington, DC: Public Health Foundation; 2011. p. 205–14.
74. Center for Disease Control and Prevention (CDC). Rubella. In: Atkinson W, Wolfe S, Hamborsky J, editors. Epidemiology and prevention of vaccine-preventable diseases. 12th ed. Washington, DC: Public Health Foundation; 2011. p. 275–90.
75. Watson JC, Hadler SC, Dykewicz CA, et al. Measles, mumps, and rubella--vaccine use and strategies for elimination of measles, rubella, and congenital rubella syndrome and control of mumps: recommendations of the Advisory Committee on Immunization Practices (ACIP). MMWR Recomm Rep. 1998;47:1–57.
76. Gershon AA. Chickenpox, measles, and mumps. In: Remington JS, Klein JO, Wilson CB, et al., editors. Infectious diseases of the fetus and newborn infant. 7th ed. Philadelphia: Elsevier; 2011. p. 661–705.
77. Plotkin SA, Reef SE, Cooper LZ, et al. Rubella. In: Remington JS, Klein JO, Wilson CB, et al., editors. Infectious diseases of the fetus and newborn infant. 7th ed. Philadelphia: Elsevier. 2011. p. 861–98.
78. American Academy of Pediatrics (AAP) Committee on Fetus and Newborn and the American College of Obstetrics and Gynecology (ACOG) Committee on Obstetric Practice. Guide to perinatal care. 6th ed. Washington, DC; 2007. Perinatal Infections. p. 303–48.

79. Ornoy A, Tenenbaum A. Pregnancy outcome following infections by coxsackie, echo, measles, mumps, hepatitis, polio and encephalitis viruses. Reprod Toxicol. 2006;21:446–57.
80. Eberhart-Phillips JE, Frederick PD, Baron RC, et al. Measles in pregnancy: a descriptive study of 58 cases. Obstet Gynecol. 1993;82:797–801.
81. Centers for Disease Control and Prevention: Rubella. Epidemiology and prevention of vaccine preventable diseases. 13th ed; 2015.
82. Menser MA, Reye RD. The pathology of congenital rubella: a review written by request. Pathology. 1974;6:215–22.
83. Chantler J, Wolinsky JS, Tingle A. Rubella virus. 4th ed; 2001.
84. Best JM, Enders G. Chapter 3 Laboratory diagnosis of rubella and congenital rubella. Perspect Med Virol. 2006;15:39–77.
85. Manual for the laboratory diagnosis of measles and rubella virus infection, 2nd ed. Geneva: World Health Organization (WHO). 2007.
86. Dudgeon JA. Congenital rubella. J Pediatr. 1975;87:1078–86.
87. Ueda K, Nishda Y, Oshima K, et al. Congenital rubella syndrome: correlation of gestational age at time of maternal rubella with type of defect. J Pediatr. 1979;94:763–5.
88. Cooper LZ, Alford CA Jr. Chapter 28—rubella. In: Infectious diseases of the fetus and newborn infant. 6th ed. Philadelphia: W.B. Saunders; 2006. p. 893–926.
89. Oster ME, Riehle-Colarusso T, Correa A. An update on cardiovascular malformations in congenital rubella syndrome. Birth Defects Res A Clin Mol Teratol. 2010;88:1–8.
90. Givens KT, Lee DA, Jones T, et al. Congenital rubella syndrome: ophthalmic manifestations and associated systemic disorders. Br J Ophthalmol. 1993;77:358–63.
91. Macé M, Cointe D, Six C, et al. Diagnostic value of reverse transcription- PCR of amniotic fluid for prenatal diagnosis of congenital rubella infection in pregnant women with confirmed primary rubella infection. J Clin Microbiol. 2004;42:4818–20.
92. Bouthry E, Picone O, Hamdi G, Grangeot-Keros L, Ayoubi JM, Vauloup-Fellous C. Rubella and pregnancy: diagnosis, management and outcomes. Prenat Diagn. 2014;34:1246–53.
93. Bester JC. Measles and measles vaccination: a review. JAMA Pediatr. 2016;170(12):1209–15.
94. Rasmussen SA, Jamieson DJ. What obstetric health care providers need to know about measles and pregnancy. Obstet Gynecol. 2015;126(1):163–70.
95. McLean HQ, Fiebelkorn AP, Temte JL, Wallace GS. Centers for Disease Control and Prevention. Prevention of measles, rubella, congenital rubella syndrome, and mumps, 2013: summary recommendations of the Advisory Committee on Immunization Practices (ACIP). MMR Morb Mortal Wkly Rep. 2013;62(4):1–34.
96. Siegel M, Fuerst HT, Perres NS. Comparative fetal mortality in maternal virus diseases. A prospective study on rubella, measles, mumps, chickenpox and hepatitis. N Engl J Med. 1966;274:768–71.
97. Hyatt HW. Relationship of maternal mumps to congenital defects and fetal deaths and to maternal morbidity and mortality. Am Pract. 1961;12:359–63.
98. Siegel M. Congenital malformations following chickenpox, measles, mumps, and hepatitis. Results of a cohort study. JAMA. 1973;226(13):1521–4.
99. Noren GR, Adams P Jr, Anderson RC. Positive skin reactivity to mumps virus antigen in endocardial fibroelastosis. J Pediatr. 1963;62:604–6.
100. Shone JD, Armas SM, Manning JA, Keith JD. The mumps antigen skin test in endocardial fibroelastosis. Pediatrics. 1966;37:423–9.
101. Pastuszak AL, Levy M, Schick B, et al. Outcome after maternal varicella infection in the first 20 weeks of pregnancy. New Eng J Med. 1994;330:901–5.
102. Alkalay AL, Pomerance JJ, Rimoin DL. Fetal varicella syndrome. J Paediatr. 1987;111(3):320–3.
103. Blair RJ. Varicella–zoster virus. Pediatr Rev. 2019;40(7):375–7.
104. Bohlke K, Galil K, Jackson LA, et al. Postpartum varicella vaccination: is the vaccine virus excreted in breast milk? Obstet Gynaecol. 2003;102:970–7.

105. Watson B, Civen R, Reynolds M, et al. Validity of self-reported varicella disease history in pregnant women attending prenatal clinics. Public Health Rep. 2007;122(4):499–506.
106. Smith CK, Arvin AM. Varicella in the fetus and newborn. Semin Fetal Neonatal Med. 2009;14(4):209–17.
107. Centers for Disease Control and Prevention (CDC). A new product (VariZIG) for postexposure prophylaxis of varicella available under an investigational new drug application expanded access protocol. MMWR Morb Mortal Wkly Rep 2006;55(8):209–210.
108. Marin M, Guris D, Chaves SS, et al. Prevention of varicella: recommendations of the Advisory Committee on Immunization Practices (ACIP). MMWR Recomm Rep. 2007;56(RR-4):1–40.
109. World Health Organization. WHO statement on the first meeting of the International Health Regulations (2005) (IHR 2005) Emergency Committee on Zika virus and observed increase in neurological disorders and neonatal malformations. 2016. Available at: http://www.who.int/mediacentre/news/statements/2016/1st-emergency-committee-zika/en/. Accessed 14 Aug 2017.
110. Duffy MR, Chen TH, Hancock WT, et al. Zika virus outbreak on Yap Island, Federated States of Micronesia. N Engl J Med. 2009;360:2536–43.
111. Mallet HP, Vial AL, Musso D. Bilan de l'epidemie a virus Zika en Polynesie Francaise. 2013–2014. Bises Bulletin d'Informaion Sanitaires, Epidemiologiques et Statistiques. 2015;13:1–8.
112. Zika virus infection: global update on epidemiology and potentially associated clinical manifestation. Wkly Epidemiol Rec. 2016;91:73–81.
113. Reyna-Villasmil E, López-Sánchez G, Santos-Bolívar J. Guillain-Barre syndrome due to Zika virus during pregnancy. Med Clin (Barc). 2016;146:331–2.
114. Plourde AR, Bloch EM. A literature review of Zika virus. Emerg Infect Dis J. 2016;22:1185–92.
115. De Carvalho NS, De Carvalho BF, Fugaça CA, Dóris B, Biscaia ES. Zika virus infection during pregnancy and microcephaly occurrence: a review of literature and Brazilian data. Braz J Infect Dis. 2016;20:282–9.
116. Musso D, Roche C, Robin E, Nhan T, Teissier A, Cao-Lormeau VM. Potenial sexual transmission of Zika virus. Emerg Infect Dis. 2015;21:359–61.
117. Leung GHY, Baird RW, Druce J, Anstey NM. Zika virus infection in Australia following a monkey bike in Indonesia. Southeast Asian J Trop Med Public Health. 2015;46:460–4.
118. de Noronha L, Zanluca C, Azevedo MLV, Luz KG, dos Santos CND. Zika virus damages the human placental barrier and presents marked fetal neurotropism. Mem Inst Oswaldo Cruz. 2016;111:287–93.
119. Brasil P, Pereira JP Jr, Moreira ME, et al. Zika virus infection in pregnant women in Rio de Janeiro. N Engl J Med. 2016;375:2321–34.
120. Buathong R, Hermann L, Thaisomboonsuk B, et al. Detection of Zika virus infection in Thailand, 2012–2014. Am J Trop Med Hyg. 2015;93:380–3.
121. Sarno M, Sacramento GA, Khouri R, et al. Zika virus infection and stillbirths: a case of hydrops fetalis, hydranencephaly and fetal demise. PLoS Negl Trop Dis. 2016;10:e0004517.
122. Moore CA, Staples JE, Dobyns WB, et al. Characterizing the pattern of anomalies in congenital Zika syndrome for pediatric clinicians. JAMA Pediatr. 2017;171:288–95.
123. Possible Association Between Zika Virus Infection and Microcephaly—Brazil, 2015. [Internet]. 2016. wr/mm6529e1.htm?s_cid=mm6529e1_e. Accessed October 18, 2016.
124. Campbell GL, Marfin AA, Lanciotti RS, Gubler DJ. West Nile virus. Lancet Infect Dis. 2002;2:519–29.
125. Sejvar JJ. Clinical manifestations and outcomes ofWest Nile virus infection. Viruses. 2014;6:606–23.
126. Patel H, Sander B, Nelder MP. Long-term sequelae ofWest Nile virus-related illness: a systematic review. Lancet Infect Dis. 2015;15:951–9.

127. Roehrig JT, Nash D, Maldin B, Labowitz A, Martin DA, Lanciotti RS, Campbell GL. Persistence of virus-reactive serum immunoglobulin m antibody in confirmed West Nile virus encephalitis cases. Emerg Infect Dis. 2003;9:376–9.
128. Nguyen Q, Morrow C, Novick L, et al. Intrauterine West Nile virus infection-New York, 2002. MMWR Morb Mortal Wkly Rep. 51(50):1135–6.
129. O'Leary DR, Kuhn S, Kniss KL, et al. Birth outcomes following West Nile virus infection of pregnant women in the United States: 2003–2004. Pediatrics. 2006;117(3):e537–45.
130. CDC. 2015. Available at: http://www.cdc.gov/westnile/faq/repellent.html. Accessed 20 May 2015.
131. Kuhl U, Pauschinger M, Noutsias M, Seeberg B, Bock T, Lassner D, Poller W, Kandolf R, Schultheiss HP. High prevalence of viral genomes and multiple viral infections in the myocardium of adults with "idiopathic" left ventricular dysfunction. Circulation. 2005;111:887–93.
132. Lim B, Ju E, Lao DH, Yun S, Lee Y, Kim D, Jeon E. Development of a enterovirus diagnostic assay system for diagnosis of viral myocarditis in humans. Microbiol Immunol. 2013;57:281–7.
133. Muehlenbachs A, Bhatnagar J, Zaki SR. Tissue tropism, pathology and pathogenesis of enterovirus infection. J Pathol. 2014;235:217–28.
134. Increased Detections and Severe Neonatal Disease Associated with Coxsackievirus B1 Infection—United States. 2007. Available online: https://www.cdc.gov/mmwr/preview/mmwrhtml/mm5720a4.htm. Accessed on 14 July 2024.
135. Bryant PA, Tingay D, Dargaville PA, Starr M, Curtis N. Neonatal coxsackie B virus infection—a treatable disease? Eur J Pediatr. 2004;163:223–8.
136. Theodoridou M, Kakourou T, Laina I, Mostrou G, Tsakris A. Vesiculopapular rash as a single presentation in intrauterine cox-sackie virus infection. Eur J Pediatr. 2002;161:412–3.
137. Callen J, Paes BA. A case report of a premature infant with coxsackie B1 meningitis. Adv Neonatal Care. 2007;7:238–47.
138. Schneider C, Menticoglou S, Herath J, Del Bigio MR, Hunt JC. Antenatal and postnatal diagnosis of coxsackie b4 infection: case series. Am J Perinatol Rep. 2011;2:1–6.
139. Bendig JW, Franklin OM, Hebden AK, Backhouse PJ, Clewley JP, Goldman AP, Piggott N. Coxsackievirus B3 sequences in the blood of a neonate with congenital myocarditis, plus serological evidence of maternal infection. J Med Virol. 2003;70:606–9.
140. Dommergues M, Petitjean J, Aubry M, Delezoide A, Narcy F, Fallet-Bianco C, Freymuth F, Dumez Y, Lebon P. Fetal enteroviral infection with cerebral ventriculomegaly and cardiomyopathy. Fetal Diagn Ther. 1994;9:77–8.
141. Krivega M, Geens M, Van de Velde H. CAR expression in human embryos and hESC illustrates its role in pluripotency and tight junctions. Reproduction. 2014;148:531–44.
142. Longo C, Saito M, Castro PT, Traina E, Werner H, Júnior JE, Júnior EA. Coxsackievirus group B infections during pregnancy: an updated literature review. J Clin Med. 2024;13(16):4922.
143. Dahlquist G, Frisk G, Ivarsson S, Svanberg L, Forsgren M, Diderholm H. Indications that maternal coxsackie B virüs infection during pregnancy is a risk factor for childhood-onset IDDM. Diabetologia. 1995;38:1371–3.
144. Tracy S, Gauntt C. Group B Coxsackievirus virulence. Curr Top Microbiolo Immunol. 2008;323:49–63.
145. Kaplan MH, Klein SW, McPhee J, Harper RG. Group B coxsackievirus infections in infants younger than three months of age: a serious childhood illness. Clin Infect Dis. 1983;5:1019–32.
146. Ouellet A, Sherlock R, Toye B, Fung KFK. Antenatal diagnosis of intrauterine infection with coxsackievirus B3 associated with live birth. Infect Dis Obstet Gynecol. 2000;12:23–6.
147. Abzug MJ, Keyserling HL, Lee ML, Levin MJ, Rotbart HA. Neonatal enterovirus infection: virology, serology, and effects of intravenous immune globulin. Clin Infect Dis. 1995;20:1201–6.

148. Hyoty H, Leon F, Knip M. Developing a vaccine for type 1 diabetes by targeting coxsackievirus B. Expert Rev Vaccines. 2018;17:1071–83.
149. Behrman RE, Kliegman RM, Arvin AM. Nelson textbook of pediatrics. 15th ed. W.B. Saunders Co.; 1996. p. 897–901.
150. Avgil M, Ornoy A. Herpes simplex virus and Epstein-Barr virus infections in pregnancy: consequences of neonatal or intrauterine infection. Reprod Toxicol. 2006;21:436–45.
151. Purtilo DT, Sakamoto K. Reactivation of Epstein-Barr virus in pregnant women: social factors, and immune competence as determinants of lymphoproliferative diseases — a hypothesis. Med Hypotheses. 1982;8(4):401–8.
152. Influenza vaccination of women during pregnancy. http://www.who.int/vaccinesafety/topics/influenza/pregnancy/en/index.html. Published 2008. Accessed 8 June 2008.
153. Falagas ME, Cholevas NV, Kapaskelis AM, Vouloumanou EK, Michalopoulos A, Rafailidis PI. Epidemiological aspects of 2009 H1N1 influenza: the accumulating experience from the northern hemisphere. Eur J Clin Microbiol Infect Dis. 2010;29:1327–47.
154. Falagas ME, Koletsi PK, Baskouta E, Rafailidis PI, Dimopoulos G, Karageorgopoulos DE. Pandemic A (H1N1) 2009 influenza: review of the southern hemisphere experience. Epidemiol Infect. 2011;139:27–40.
155. Van Kerkhove MD, Vandemaele KA, Shinde V, Jaramillo Gutierrez G, Koukounari A, Donnelly CA, et al. Risk factors for severe outcomes following 2009 influenza A (H1N1) infection: a global pooled analysis. PLoS Med. 2011;8:e1001053.
156. Shahab SZ, Glezen WP. Influenza virus. In: Gonik B, editor. Vi ral diseases in pregnancy. New York: Springer; 1994. p. 215–23.
157. Yuen CYS, Tarrant M. A comprehensive review of influenza and influenza vaccination during pregnancy. J Perinat Neonatal Nurs. 28(4):261–70.
158. Centers for Disease Control and Prevention. Letter to providers: Influenza vaccination of pregnant women. Feb 2014, Atlanta: Department of Health & Human Services. Available from: http://www.cdc.gov/flu/pdf/protect/pregnancy-letter-2014.pdf
159. Lim B, Mahmood T. Pandemic H1N1 2009 (swine flu) and pregnancy. J Obstet Gynaecol India. 2011;61(4):386–93.
160. Siston AM, Rasmussen SA, Honein MA, Fry AM, Seib K, Callaghan WM, et al. Pandemic 2009 influenza A(H1N1) virus illness among pregnant women in the United States. JAMA. 2010;303(15):1517–25.
161. Rasmussen S, Jamieson D, Uyeki T. Effects of influenza on pregnant women and infants. Am J Obstet Gynecol. 2012;207(3 Suppl):3–8.
162. Saito S, Minakami H, Nakai A, Unno N, Kubo T, Yoshimura Y. Outcomesofinfantsexposed tooseltamivir or zanamivir in utero during pandemic (H1N1) 2009. Am J Obstet Gynecol. 2013;209(2):130.e1–9.
163. World Health Organization. Vaccines against influenza WHOposition paper—November2012. Wkly Epidemiol Rec. 2012;87:461–76.
164. Ellington S, Strid P, Tong VT, et al. Characteristics of women of reproductive age with laboratory-confirmed SARS-CoV-2 infection by pregnancy status – United States, January 22 June 7, 2020. MMWR Morb Mortal Wkly Rep. 2020;69:769–75.
165. Zambrano LD, Ellington S, Strid P, et al. Update: characteristics of symptomatic women of reproductive age with laboratory-confirmed SARS-CoV-2 infection by pregnancy status – United States, January 22-October 3, 2020. MMWR Morb Mortal Wkly Rep. 2020;69:1641–7.
166. Wei SQ, Bilodeau-Bertrand M, Liu S, Auger N. The impact of COVID-19 on pregnancy outcomes: a systematic review and meta-analysis. CMAJ. 2021;193:E540–8.
167. Villar J, Ariff S, Gunier RB, et al. Maternal and neonatal morbidity and mortality among pregnant women with and without COVID-19 infection: the INTERCOVID multinational cohort study. JAMA Pediatr. 2021;175:817–26.
168. Angelidou A, Sullivan K, Melvin PR, et al. Association of maternal perinatal SARS-CoV-2 infection with neonatal outcomes during the COVID-19 pandemic in Massachusetts. JAMA Netw Open. 2021;4:e217523.

169. Ciapponi A, Bardach A, Comandé D, et al. COVID-19 and pregnancy: an umbrella review of clinical presentation, vertical transmission, and maternal and perinatal outcomes. PLoS One. 2021;16:e0253974.
170. Jamieson DJ, Rasmussen SA. An update on COVID-19 and pregnancy. Am J Obstet Gynecol. 2022;226(2):177–86.
171. Lindsay L, Calvert C, Shi T, Carruthers J, Denny C, Donaghy J, Hopcroft LEM, Hopkins L, Goulding A, McLaughlin T, Moore E, Taylor B, Bhaskaran K, Katikireddi SV, McCabe R, McCowan C, Simpson CR, Robertson C, Sheikh A, Wood R, Stock SJ. Neonatal and maternal outcomes following SARS-CoV-2 infection and COVID-19 vaccination: a population-based matched cohort study. Nat Commun. 2023;14:5275.
172. Remington JS, McLeod R, Thuilliez P, Desmonts G. Toxoplasmosis. In: Remington JS, Klein JO, Wilson CB, Baker C, editors. Infectious dis eases of the fetus and newborn infant. 6th ed. Philadelphia: Elsevier Saunders; 2006. p. 947–1091.
173. Roberts T, Frenkel JK. Estimating income losses and other preventable costs caused by congenital toxoplasmosis in people in the United States. J Am Vet Med Assoc. 1990;196:249–56.
174. Dubey JP, Hill DE, Jones JL, et al. Prevalence of viable Toxoplasma gondii in beef, chicken, and pork from retail meat stores in the United States: risk assessment to consumers. J Parasitol. 2005;91:1082–93.
175. Centers for Disease Control and Prevention. Parasites toxoplasmosis (Toxoplasma infection). http://www.cdc.gov/parasites/toxoplasmosis/health_professionals/index.html. Updated 14 Apr 2014. Accessed 23 Oct 2014.
176. Serranti D., Buonsenso D., Valentini P., Congenital toxoplasmosis treatment. Eur Rev Med Pharmacol Sci 2011; 15 (2): 193198.
177. Montoya JG, Remington JS. Management of toxoplasma gondii infection during pregnancy. Clin Infect Dis. 2008;47(4):554–66.
178. Gilbert R, Gras L. European Multicentre Study on Congenital Toxo plasmosis. Effect of timing and type of treatment on the risk of mother to child transmission of Toxoplasma gondii. BJOG. 2003;110:112–20.
179. World Health Organization. World malaria report 2022. https://www.who.int/teams/global-malaria-programme/reports/world-malaria-report-2022. Accessed 14 July 2023.
180. Mahamar A, Andemel N, Swihart B, et al. Malaria infection is common and associated with perinatal mortality and preterm delivery despite widespread use of chemoprevention in Mali: an observational study 2010 to. Clin Infect Dis. 2021;73:1355–61.
181. Ashley EA, Pyae Phyo A, Woodrow CJ. Malaria. Lancet. 2018;391:1608–21.
182. Rasmussen SA, Arguin PM, Jamieson DJ. Malaria and pregnancy. Obstet Gynecol. 2023;142:1303–9.
183. World Health Organization. Management of severe malaria: a practical handbook. https://apps.who.int/iris/bitstream/handle/10665/79317/9789241548526_eng.Pdf. Accessed 15 July 2023.
184. Felician EK, Ngoda OA, Jahanpour OF, Kahima J, Msuya SE, Lukambagire AH. Placental parasitic infections and pregnancy outcomes among women delivering at a tertiary hospital in northern Tanzania. East Afr Health Res J. 2022;6:141–6.
185. Harrington WE, Kakuru A, Jagannathan P. Malaria in pregnancy shapes the development of foetal and infant immunity. Parasite Immunol. 2019;41:e12573.
186. Dimaio MA, Pereira IT, George TI, Banaei N. Performance of BinaxNOW for diagnosis of malaria in a U.S. hospital. J Clin Microbiol. 2012;50:2877–80.
187. Centers for Disease Control and Prevention. Treatment of malaria: guidelines for clinicians (United States). https://www.cdc.gov/malaria/diagnosis_treatment/clini cians1.html#pregnant. Accessed 17 July 2023.
188. Bailao LA, Osborne NG, Rizzi MCS, Bonilla-Musoles F, Duarte G, Bailao TCRS. Ultrasound markers of fetal infection, Part 2: bacterial, parasitic, and fungal infections. Ultrasound Q. 2006;22(2):137–51.

189. Whyte RK, Hussain Z, de Sa D. Antenatal infections with Candida. Arch Dis Child. 1982;57:528.
190. Lopez E, Alterman K. Intrauterine infection by Candida. Am J Dis Child. 1968;115:663.
191. Albarracin NS, Pattereson WS, Haust MD. Candida albicans infection of the placenta and fetus. Obstet Gynecol. 1967;30:838.
192. Osborne NG, Bonilla-Musoles F, Raga F, et al. Umbilical cord cysts: color Doppler and three-dimensional ultrasound evaluation. Ultrasound Q. 2000;16:133Y139.
193. Kingdom JCP, Burrell SJ, Kaufmann P. Pathology and clinical implications of abnormal umbilical artery Doppler waveforms. Ultrasound Obstet Gynecol. 1997;9:271.
194. Catanzaro A. Pulmonary mycosis in pregnant women. Chest. 1984;86:14–8.
195. Purtilo DT. Opportunistic mycotic infections in pregnant women. Am J Obstet Gynecol. 1975;122:607–10.
196. Blotta MHSL, Altemani AM, Amaral E, et al. Placental involvement in paracoccidioidomycosis. J Med Vet Mycol. 1993;31:249–57.
197. Chapman SW, Bradsher RW Jr, Campbell GD Jr, et al. Practice guidelines for the management of patients with blastomycosis. Clin Infect Dis. 2000;30:679–83.
198. Chapman SW, Lin AC, Hendricks KA, Nolan RL, Currier MM, Morris KR, et al. Endemic blastomycosis in Mississippi: epidemiological and clinical studies. Semin Respir Infect. 1997;12(3):219–28.
199. Saccente M, Woods GL. Clinical and laboratory update on blastomycosis. Clin Microbiol Rev. 2010;23(2):367–81.
200. Baker T, Patel A, Halteh P, Toussi SS, DeLaMora P, Lipner S, Schuetz AN, Hartman B. Blastomycosis during pregnancy: a case report and review of the literature. Diagn Microbiol Infect Dis. 2017;88(2):145–51.
201. Einstein HE, Johnson RH. Coccidioidomycosis: new aspects of epidemiology and therapy. Clin Infect Dis. 1993;16:349–56.
202. Spinello IM, Johnson RH, Baqı S. Coccidioidomycosis and pregnancy a review. Ann N Y Acad Sci. 2007;1111:358–64.
203. Crum NF, Ballon-Landa G. Coccidioidomycosis in pregnancy: case report and review of the literature. Am J Med. 2006;119(993):e11–993.e17.
204. Sugarman J, Colvin C, Moran AC, et al. Tuberculosis in pregnancy: an estimate of the global burden of disease. Lancet Glob Health. 2014;2(12):e710–6.
205. World Health Organization. Tuberculosis in women [Internet], 2019. Available: https://www.who.int/tb/publications/tbwomenfactsheet.pdf?ua=1
206. Walles J, Winqvist N, Hansson SR, Sturegård E, Baqir H, Westman A, Kjerstadius T, Schön T, Björkman P. Pregnancy outcomes in women screened for tuberculosis infection in Swedish Antenatal Care. Clin Infect Dis. 2024;78(1):125–32.
207. Mathad JS, Gupta A. Tuberculosis in pregnant and postpartum women: epidemiology, management, and research gaps. Clin Infect Dis. 2012;55:1532–49.
208. Rifampicin. Depth Answers [database on the Internet]. Greenwood Village (CO): Truven Health Analytics (Subscription required to view). Available: www.micromedexsolutions.com
209. Ethambutol. Depth Answers [database on the Internet]. Greenwood Village (CO): Truven Health Analytics (Subscription required to view), 2020. Available: www.micromedexsolutions.com
210. Pyrazinamide. Depth Answers [database on the Internet]. Greenwood Village (CO): Truven Health Analytics (Subscription required to view), 2020. Available: www.micromedexsolutions.com
211. Isoniazid. Depth Answers [database on the Internet]. Greenwood Village (CO): Truven Health Analytics (Subscription required to view), 2020. Available: www.micromedexsolutions.com
212. World Health Organization. Global tuberculosis report 2019. Geneva: Switzerland; 2019.
213. Jamshidi A, Zeinali T. Significance and characteristics of Listeria monocytogenes in poultry products. Int J Food Sci. 2019;2019:1–7.

214. De Luca C, Donati L, D'oria L, Licameli A, Pellegrino M, De Santis M. Listeria infection in pregnancy: a review of literature. Open Infect Dis J. 2015;9(1):20–5.
215. Madjunkov M, Chaudhry S, Ito S. Listeriosis during pregnancy. Arch Gynecol Obstet. 2017;296:143–52.
216. Committee on Obstetric Practice, American College of Obstetricians and Gynecologists. Committee Opinion No. 614: management of pregnant women with presumptive exposure to Listeria monocytogenes. Obstet Gynecol. 2014;124:1241–4.
217. Elinav H, Hershko-Klement A, Valinsky L, et al. Pregnancy-associated listeriosis: clinical characteristics and geospatial analysis of a 10-year period in Israel. Clin Infect Dis. 2014;59:953–61.
218. Tai YL, Chi H, Chiu NC, et al. Clinical features of neonatal listeriosis in Taiwan: a hospital-based study. J Microbiol Immunol Infect. 2019;53(6):866–74.
219. Elliott DJ, Eppes SC, Klein JD. Teratogen update: Lyme disease. Teratology. 2001;64:276–81.
220. Sigal LH. Diagnosis of Lyme disease. September 2005. Available at http://www.uptodate.com. Accessed June 2006.
221. O'Kelly B, Lambert JS. Vector-borne diseases in pregnancy. Ther Adv Infect Dis. 2020;7:204993612094172.
222. Walsh CA, Mayer EW, Baxi LV. Lyme disease in pregnancy: case report and review of the literature. Obstet Gynecol Surv. 2007;62:41–50.
223. Silver HM. Lyme disease during pregnancy. Infect Dis Clin N Am. 1997;11:93–7.
224. Wilson CB, Nizet V, Maldonado Y, Remington JS, Klein JO. In: Wilson CB, Nizet V, Maldonado YA, Remington JS, Klein JO, editors. Remington and Klein's infectious diseases of the fetus and newborn infant. 8th ed. Philadelphia: Elsevier, Saunders; 2016. ISBN 978-0-323-24147-2.
225. Mulkey SB, Arroyave-Wessel M, Peyton C, Bulas DI, Fourzali Y, Jiang J, Russo S, McCarter R, Msall ME, du Plessis AJ, et al. Neurodevelopmental abnormalities in children with in utero Zika virus ExposureWithout congenital Zika syndrome. JAMA Pediatr. 2020;174:269.
226. Agger WA, Callister SM, Jobe DA. In vitro susceptibilities of Borrelia burgdorferi to five oral cephalosporins and ceftriaxone. Antimicrob Agents Chemother. 1992;36:1788–90.
227. Williams ME, Schwartz DA, DeBiasi RL, Mulkey SB. Examining infant and child neurodevelopmental outcomes after Lyme disease during pregnancy. Pathogens. 2024;13(12):1029.
228. Henningham A, Barnett TC, Maamary PG, Walker MJ. Pathogenesis of group A streptococcal infections. Discov Med. 2012;13:329–42.
229. Sherwood E, Vergnano S, Kakuchi I, Bruce MG, Chaurasia S, David S, Dramowski A, Georges S, Guy R, Lamagni T, Levy-Bruhl D, Lyytikainen O, Naus M, Okaro JO, Oppegaard O, Vestrheim DF, Zulz T, Steer AC, Van Beneden CA, Seale AC. Invasive group A streptococcal disease in pregnant women and young children: a systematic review and meta-analysis. Lancet Infect Dis. 2022;22:1076–88.
230. Cooper J, Cooper S, Wolk D, Tice A, Persing T, Esolen L. Postpartum Streptococcus pyogenes outbreak in the labor and deliveryunit of a quaternary referral center: a case studies series and review of the literature. Clin Microbiol Newsl. 2017;39(2):11–5.
231. Mason K, Aronoff D. Postpartum Group A Streptococcus sepsis and maternal immunology. Am J Reprod Immunol. 2012;67(2):91–100.
232. Nguyen M, Bendi V, Guduru M, Olson E, Vivekanandan R, Foral P, Velagapudi M. Postpartum invasive Group A streptococcal infection: case report and mini-review. Cureus. 2018;10(8):e3184.
233. Hamilton SH, Stevens DL, Bryant AE. Pregnancy-related Group A streptococcal infections: temporal relationships between bacterial acquisition, infection onset, clinical findings, and outcome. Clin Inf Dis. 2013;57(6):870–6.
234. Crum NF, Chun HM, Gaylord TG, Hale B. Group A streptococcal toxic shock syndrome developing in the third trimester of pregnancy. Infec Dis Obstet Gynecol. 2002;10:209–16.

235. Deutscher M, Lewis M, Zell ER, Taylor TH, Van Beneden C, Schrag S. Incidence and severity of invasive Streptococcus pneumoniae, group A streptococcus, and group B Streptococcus infections among pregnant and postpartum women. Clin Inf Dis. 2011;53(2):114–23.
236. Phillips C, Walsh E. Group A streptococcal infection during, pregnancy and the postpartum period. Nurs Womens Health. 2020;24(1):13–23.
237. Russell NJ, Seale AC, O'Driscoll M, O'Sullivan C, Bianchi-Jassir F, Gonzalez-Guarin J, Lawn JE, Baker CJ, Bartlett L, Cutland C, et al. Maternal colonization with group B streptococcus and serotype distribution worldwide: systematic review and meta-analyses. Clin Infect Dis. 2017;65(Suppl. S2):100–11.
238. Lawn JE, Bianchi-Jassir F, Russell NJ, Kohli-Lynch M, Tann CJ, Hall J, Madrid L, Baker CJ, Bartlett L, Cutland C, et al. Group B streptococcal disease worldwide for pregnant women, stillbirths, and children: why, what, and how to undertake estimates? Clin Infect Dis. 2017;65(Suppl. S2):89–99.
239. Castor ML, et al. Antibiotic resistance patterns in invasive group B streptococcal isolates. Infect Dis Obstet Gynecol. 2008;2008:727505.
240. Langdon A, Crook N, Dantas G. The effects of antibiotics on the microbiome throughout development and alternative approaches for therapeutic modulation. Genome Med. 2016;8(1):39.
241. Bokulich NA, et al. Antibiotics, birth mode, and diet shape microbiome maturation during early life. Sci Transl Med. 2016;8(343):343ra82.
242. Dhudasia MB, Flannery DD, Pfeifer MR, Puopolo KM. Updated guidance: prevention and management of perinatal group B streptococcus infection. NeoReviews. 2021;22(3):e177–88.
243. Di RGC, Melin P, Berardi A, et al. Intrapartum GBS screening and antibiotic prophylaxis: a European consensus conference. J Matern Fetal Neonatal Med. 2015;28(7):766–82.
244. Heath PT. Status of vaccine research and development of vaccines for GBS. Vaccine. 2016;34(26):2876–9.
245. Abu-Raya B, Maertens K. Protection of the newborn through vaccination in pregnancy. NeoReviews. 2021;22(1):e25–39.
246. Choi MJ, Noh JY, Jang AY, et al. Age-stratified analysis of serotype-specific baseline immunity against group B Streptococcus. Hum Vaccin Immunother. 2020;16(6):1338–44.
247. Kobayashi M, Schrag SJ, Alderson MR, et al. WHO consultation on group B Streptococcus vaccine development: report from a meeting held on 27–28 April 2016. Vaccine. 2019;37(50):7307–14.
248. World Health Organization. Global incidence and prevalence of selected curable sexually transmitted infections−2008. Geneva: World Health Organization; 2012.
249. Adachi K, Nielsen-Saines K, Klausner JD. Chlamydia trachomatis infection in pregnancy: the global challenge of preventing adverse pregnancy and infant outcomes in Sub-Saharan Africa and Asia. BioMed Res Inte. 2016;2016:9315757.
250. Silveira MF, Ghanem KG, Erbelding EJ, Burke AE, Johnson HL, Singh RH, et al. Chlamydia trachomatis infection during pregnancy and the risk of preterm birth: a case-control study. Int J STD AIDS. 2009;20:465–9.
251. Locksmith G, Duff P. Infection, antibiotics, and preterm delivery. Semin Perinatol. 2001;25:295–309.
252. Silva MJ, Florencio GL, Gabiatti JR, Amaral RL, Eleuterio JJ, Goncalves AK. Perinatal morbidity and mortality associated with chlamydial infection: a meta-analysis study. Brazil J Infect Dis. 2011;15:533–9.
253. Gravett MG, Nelson HP, De Rouen T, Critchlow C, Eschenbach DA, Holmes KK. Independent associations of bacterial vaginosis and chlamydia trachomatis infection with adverse pregnancy outcome. JAMA. 1986;256:1899–903.
254. Rours GI, Duijts L, Moll HA, Arends LR, de Groot R, Jaddoe VW, et al. Chlamydia trachomatis infection during pregnancy associated with preterm delivery: a population-based prospective cohort study. Eur J Epidemiol. 2011;26:493–502.

255. Tang W, Mao J, Li KT, Walker JS, Chou R, Fu R, et al. Pregnancy and fertility-related adverse outcomes associated with chlamydia trachomatis infection: a global systematic review and meta-analysis. Sex Transm Infect. 2020;96:322–9.
256. Chen XS. Adverse pregnancy outcomes due to chlamydia trachomatis. Lancet Infect Dis. 2018;18:499.
257. Workowski KA, Berman SM. Centers for disease control and prevention sexually transmitted disease treatment guidelines. Clin Infect Dis. 2011;53(Suppl. 3):59–63.
258. Workowski KA, Bolan GA. Sexually transmitted diseases treatment guidelines, 2015. MMWR Recomm Rep. 2015;64:1–137.
259. Mullick S, Watson-Jones D, Beksinska M, Mabey D. Sexually transmitted infections in pregnancy: prevalence, impact on pregnancy outcomes, and approach to treatment in developing countries. Sex Transm Infect. 2005;81:294–302.
260. Kampmeier RH. Identification of the gonococcus by Albert Neisser. 1879. Sex Transm Dis. 1978;5(2):71–2.
261. Heumann CL, Quilter LA, Eastment MC, Heffron R, Hawes SE. Adverse birth outcomes and maternal Neisseria gonorrhoeae infection: a population-based cohort study in Washington state. Sex Transm Dis. 2017;44(5):266–71.
262. World Health Organization. WHO guidelines for the treatment of Chlamydia trachomatis. 2016. https://apps.who.int/iris/bitstream/handle/10665/246165/9789241549714-eng.pdf;jsessionid=B-B11A44FD96B305A6DC2AD8955CD21EC?sequence=1. Accessed 10 May 2020.
263. Workowski KA, Berman SM, For the Centers for Disease Control and Prevention. Sexually transmitted diseases treatment guidelines. 2006 [Published correction appears in MMWR Recomm Rep 2006; 55: 997]. MMWR Recomm Rep. 2006;55(RR-11):1–94. http://www.cdc.gov/mmwr/ PDF/rr/rr5511.pdf. Accessed 16 Apr 2020
264. Brocklehurst P. Antibiotics for gonorrhoea in pregnancy. Cochrane Database Syst Rev. 2002;2:CD000098. https://doi.org/10.1002/14651858.
265. Olaleye AO, Babah OA, Osuagwu CS, Ogunsola FT, Afolabi BB. Sexually transmitted infections in pregnancy—an update on chlamydia trachomatis and Neisseria gonorrhoeae. Eur J Obstet Gynecol Reprod Biol. 2020;255:1–12.
266. Sheffield JS, Wendel GD. Syphilis in pregnancy. Clin Obstet Gynecol. 1999;42:97–106.
267. CDC. Increase in incidence of congenital syphilis-United States 2012–2014. MMWR Morb Mortal Wkly Rep. 2015;64:1241–5.
268. Fiumara NJ, Fleming WL, Downing JG, et al. The incidence of prenatal syphilis at the Boston City Hospital. N Engl J Med. 1952;247:48–52.
269. Centers for Disease Control and Prevention. Sexually transmitted infections (STI) treatment guidelines, 2021. https://www.cdc.gov/std/treatment-guidelines/default.htm
270. Sánchez PJ. Congenital syphilis. Adv Pediatr Infect Dis. 1992;7:161–80.
271. Rasool MN, Govender S. The skeletal manifestations of congenital syphilis: a review of 197 cases. J Bone Joint Surg Br. 1989;71:752–5.
272. David M, Hcini N, Mandelbrot L, Sibiude J, Picone O. Fetal and neonatal abnormalities due to congenital syphilis: a literature review. Prenat Diagn. 2022;42:643–55.
273. Medoro AK, Sánchez PJ. Syphilis in neonates and infants. Clin Perinatol. 2021;48:293–309.
274. Ingall D., Sanchez P.J., Bakes C.J., 2006, Syphilis: infectious diseases of the fetus and newborn infant. Philadelphia: Elsevier Saunders.
275. Marcus U. HIV infections and HIV testing during pregnancy, Germany, 1993 to 2016. Euro surveillance: bulletin Europeen sur les maladies transmissibles = European communicable disease bulletin. 2019;24(48):1900078.
276. Choi H, Kim MH, Lee SJ, Kim EJ, Lee W, Jeong W, Jung IY, Ahn JY, Jeong SJ, Ku NS, Baek JH, Choi YH, Kim HY, Kim JM, Choi JY. Pregnancy rates and outcomes of HIV-infected women in Korea. J Korean Med Sci. 2018;33(47):e296.

277. Rollins NC, Coovadia HM, Bland RM, Coutsoudis A, Bennish ML, Patel D, Newell ML. Pregnancy outcomes in HIV-infected and uninfected women in rural and urban South Africa. J Acquir Defic Syndr. 2007;44(3):321–8.
278. Thomson KA, Hughes J, Baeten JM, et al. Increased risk of female HIV-1 acquisition throughout pregnancy and postpartum: a prospective per-coital act analysis among women with HIV-1 infected partners. J Infect Dis. 2018;218:16–25.
279. Fatti G, Shaikh N, Jackson D, et al. Low HIV incidence in pregnant and postpartum women receiving a community- based combination HIV prevention intervention in a high HIV incidence setting in South Africa. PLoS One. 2017;12:e0181691.
280. European Collaborative Study. Risk factors for mother to child transmission of HIV-I. Lancet. 1992;339:1007–12.
281. Wu M, Yan Y, Zou S, Wu S, Feng L, Liu Y, Guo W, Tang W, Liang K. Adverse pregnancy outcomes among pregnant women living with HIV in Hubei province, China: prevalence and risk factors. AIDS Care. 2023;35(3):351–8.
282. Panel on Treatment of HIV-Infected Pregnant Women and Prevention of Perinatal Transmission. [3 May 2014] Recommendations for Use of Antiretroviral Drugs in Pregnant HIV-1-Infected Women for Maternal Health and Interventions to Reduce Perinatal HIV Transmission in the United States. Available at http://aidsinfo.nih.gov/contentfiles/lvguidelines/PerinatalGL.pdf [Current U.S. guidelines for preventing HIV infection in infants.]
283. World Health Organization. [7 March 2014] Consolidated guidelines on the use of antiretroviral drugs for treating and preventing HIV infection. Recommendations for a public health approach. Jun. 2013 http://www.who.int/hiv/pub/guidelines/arv2013/download/en/. [Current WHO guidelines for preventing HIV infection in infants.]
284. World Health Organization. [7 March 2014] Guidelines on HIV and infant feeding 2010. Principles and recommendations for infant feeding in the context of HIV and a summary of evidence. http://www.who.int/maternal_child_adolescent/documents/9789241599535/en/
285. Looker KJ, Magaret AS, May MT, et al. First estimates of the global and regional incidence of neonatal herpes infection. Lancet Glob Health. 2017;5:300–9.
286. Sampath A, Maduro G, Schillinger JA. Infant deaths due to herpes simplex virus, congenital syphilis, and HIV in New York City. Pediatrics. 2016;137:e20152387.
287. ACOG. Management of genital herpes in pregnancy: ACOG practice bulletin, number 220. Obstet Gynecol. 2020;135:e193.
288. Brown ZA, Wald A, Morrow RA, Selke S, Zeh J, Corey L. Effect of serologic status and cesarean delivery on transmission rates of herpes simplex virus from mother to infant. JAMA. 2003;289:203–9.
289. Corey L, Wald A. Maternal and neonatal herpes simplex virus infections. N Engl J Med. 2009;361:1376–85.
290. Brown ZA, Selke S, Zeh J, Kopelman J, Maslow A, Ashley RL, et al. The acquisition of herpes simplex virus during pregnancy. N Engl J Med. 1997;337:509–16.
291. Kimberlin DW. Herpes simplex virus infections of the newborn. Semin Perinatol. 2007;31:19–25.
292. Melvin AJ, Mohan KM, Vora SB, Selke S, Sullivan E, Wald A. Neonatal herpes simplex virus infection: epidemiology and outcomes in the modern era. J Pediatric Infect Dis Soc. 2022;11:94–101.
293. Kimberlin DW, Lin CY, Jacobs RF, et al. Natural history of neonatal herpes simplex virus infections in the acyclovir era. Pediatrics. 2001;108:223–9.
294. Umberto De Rose D, Bompard S, Maddaloni C, Bersani I, Martini L, Santisi A, Longo D, Ronchetti MP, Dotta A, Auriti C. Neonatal herpes simplex virus infection: from the maternal infection to the child outcome. J Med Virol. 2023;95:e29024.
295. Hammad WAB, Konje JC. Herpes simplex virus infection in pregnancy—an update. Eur J Obstet Gynecol Reprod Biol. 2021;259:38–45.

296. Hollier LM, Wendel GD. Third trimester antiviral prophylaxis for preventing maternal genital herpes simplex virus (HSV) recurrences and neonatal infection. Cochrane Database Syst Rev. 2008;1:CD004946.
297. McQuillan G, Kruszon-Moran D, Markowitz LE, Unger ER, Paulose-Ram R. Prevalence of HPV in adults aged 18–69: United States, 2011–2014; NCHS data brief. Atlanta: National Center for Health Statistics; 2017. p. 1–8.
298. Sehnal B, Zikan M, Nipcova M, Dusek L, Cibula D, Slama J. The association among cervical, anal, and oral HPV infections in high-risk and low-risk women. Eur J Obstet Gynecol Reprod Biol X. 2019;4:100061.
299. Otter S, Whitaker S, Chatterjee J, Stewart A. The human papillomavirus as a common pathogen in oropharyngeal, anal and cervical cancers. Clin Oncol. 2019;31:81–90.
300. Park E, Kim JY, Choi S, Kim DS, Oh YL. Carcinogenic risk of human papillomavirus (HPV) genotypes and potential effects of HPV vaccines in Korea. Sci Rep. 2019;9:12556.
301. Condrat CE, Filip L, Gherghe M, Cretoiu D, Suciu N. Maternal HPV infection: effects on pregnancy outcome. Viruses. 2021;13:2455.
302. Tan J, Xiong Y, He Q, Liu Y, Wang W, Chen M, Zou K, Liu X, Sun X. Peri-conceptional or pregnancy exposure of HPV vaccination and the risk of spontaneous abortion: a systematic review and meta-analysis. BMC Pregnancy Childbirth. 2019;19(1):302.
303. Faber MT, Duun-Henriksen AK, Dehlendorff C, Tatla MK, Munk C, Kjaer SK. Adverse pregnancy outcomes and infant mortality after quadrivalent HPV vaccination during pregnancy. Vaccine. 2019;37:265–71.

Chapter 15
Oral Health During Pregnancy

Ezgi Demir

15.1 Introduction

Pregnancy is associated with a variety of physiological changes that can impact oral health, increasing the susceptibility to several dental conditions. These changes, primarily hormonal and behavioral, can alter the immune response, salivary composition, and oral hygiene habits, thereby predisposing pregnant individuals to specific oral diseases [8].

15.2 Common Oral and Dental Conditions and Their Treatments in Pregnancy

15.2.1 Pregnancy Gingivitis and Periodontitis

The association between pregnancy and periodontal inflammation has been recognized for years. While awareness of this phenomenon has existed for a long time, it is only in recent decades that research has begun to uncover the underlying pathophysiological mechanisms and systemic implications of pregnancy-related periodontal changes [9].

Pregnancy gingivitis is a particularly prevalent condition, affecting an estimated 30% to 100% of pregnant individuals [10–12]. Clinically, it presents with classic

E. Demir (✉)
Ege University, Faculty of Dentistry, Department of Endodontics, Izmir, Turkey

© The Author(s), under exclusive license to Springer Nature Switzerland AG 2026

I. Karaca (ed.), *Managing Maternal Chronic Diseases for a Healthy Pregnancy*,
https://doi.org/10.1007/978-3-032-15221-3_15

signs of inflammation including gingival erythema, edema, hyperplasia, and an exaggerated tendency to bleed. Although the histopathological features are consistent with those of conventional gingivitis, the etiological factors during pregnancy differ. Hormonal fluctuations, especially increased levels of estrogen and progesterone, appear to modulate the host response to plaque, leading to heightened inflammatory reactions in the gingival tissues [9] (Fig. 15.1).

The severity of pregnancy gingivitis can vary widely. While some cases remain mild, others may progress to pronounced gingival hyperplasia accompanied by discomfort, spontaneous bleeding, and, in rare instances, pain or functional impairment. These manifestations underscore the importance of early detection and intervention to maintain periodontal stability throughout pregnancy [9] (Fig. 15.2).

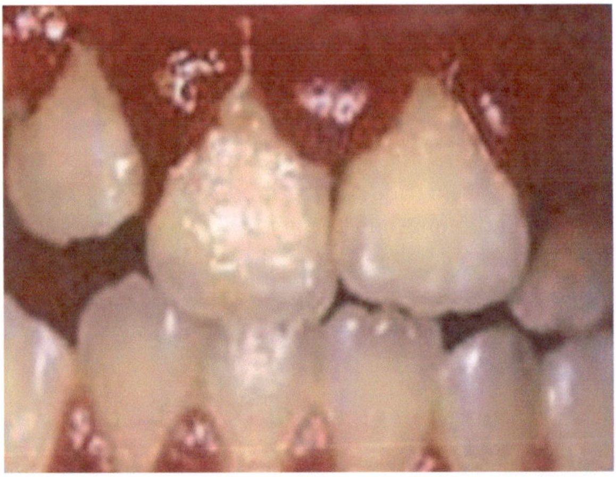

Fig. 15.1 Pregnancy gingivitis. (Reproduced from Babalola and Omole [13], published under Creative Commons license, CC-BY 3.0. [13])

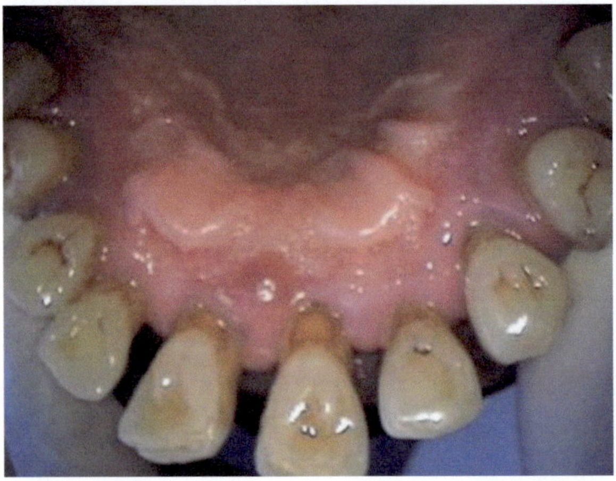

Fig. 15.2 Periodontal disease.. (Reproduced from Babalola and Omole [13], published under Creative Commons license, CC-BY 3.0. [13])

15.2.1.1 Treatment

Good oral hygiene remains the most effective way to reduce the impact of hormonal changes on the gums during pregnancy. Regular brushing, flossing, and professional cleanings help control plaque and prevent inflammation [14].

15.2.1.2 Mild cases

- *Brushing and flossing*: Brushing twice daily and flossing once a day are essential.
- *Saltwater rinse*: A rinse made with ½ teaspoon of salt in a glass of warm water can reduce gum swelling and should be used once or twice daily.
- *Alcohol-free mouthwash*: Helps reduce harmful bacteria without irritating sensitive tissue.
- *Baking soda rinse*: After vomiting, rinsing with a baking soda solution helps neutralize acids and protect the gums [14].

15.2.1.3 Severe Cases

If symptoms like persistent pain, bleeding, or swelling occur, dental care is necessary. Professional cleaning to remove plaque and calculus will reduce inflammation and restore gum health [15].

15.2.2 Pyogenic Granuloma (Granuloma Gravidarum)

Pyogenic granulomas, also known as pregnancy tumors or pregnancy epulis are benign vascular proliferations that may occur in pregnancies (Fig. 15.3). These lesions generally emerge during the second or third month and are clinically and histologically indistinguishable from those seen in nonpregnant individuals. Typically presenting as red to purplish-blue nodules, they may be pedunculated or sessile, often with surface ulceration and a tendency to bleed easily. The color of the lesion reflects its vascular content and degree of venous stasis [16].

Most frequently arising on the gingiva, particularly in interproximal areas of the anterior region, these lesions are associated with existing gingival inflammation and poor oral hygiene. Other intraoral sites may include the tongue, lips, buccal mucosa, and palate. Pregnancy-related changes such as increased mouth breathing especially during the third trimester due to pregnancy rhinitis can further exacerbate anterior site inflammation [9].

It is essential to rule out other soft tissue lesions with similar appearance, such as central giant cell granulomas or those related to systemic conditions. Pregnancy-related hormonal fluctuations, in combination with preexisting

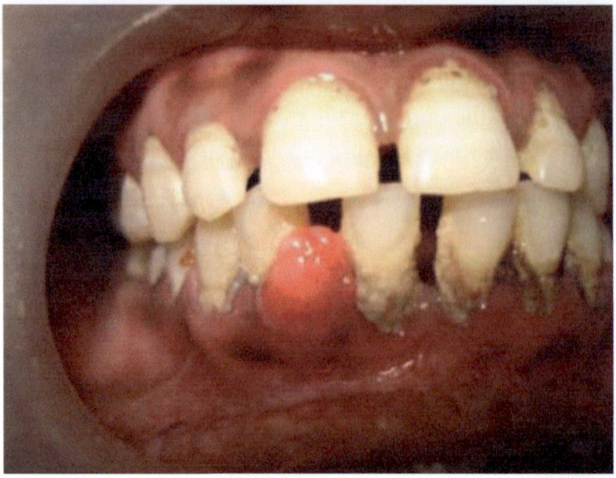

Fig. 15.3 Clinical appearance of a pyogenic granuloma located on the gingiva. (Reproduced from Verma et al. [17], published under Creative Commons license, CC-BY 4.0. https://opendentistryjournal.com/VOLUME/6/PAGE/153/ [17])

periodontal status, can influence the extent and severity of these growths. Increased tissue edema may contribute to transient tooth mobility and deeper periodontal pockets [12].

Although pyogenic granulomas appear alarming, they usually do not involve the underlying alveolar bone. Surgical excision, when indicated, generally heals well and without significant tissue loss [14].

15.2.2.1 Treatment

In most cases, pregnancy-related pyogenic granulomas regress spontaneously after delivery due to the reduction in capillary proliferation, earning them the nickname "vanishing tumors." However, if the lesion causes discomfort, it can be safely excised under local anesthesia during the second trimester or approximately 4 weeks postpartum. Postoperative care includes oral hygiene reinforcement and chlorhexidine rinses to support healing. Laser excision may also be considered as a minimally invasive alternative [18].

15.2.3 Dental Caries and Dental Erosion

Pregnancy is a period during which the risk of dental caries and erosion may increase due to a combination of physiological and behavioral factors [19]. While the long-standing myth that "the baby takes calcium from the mother's teeth" remains widespread, there is no scientific basis for this belief. The temporary changes observed in maternal teeth are not a result of fetal calcium demand, but rather of altered oral conditions during pregnancy [20] (Fig. 15.4).

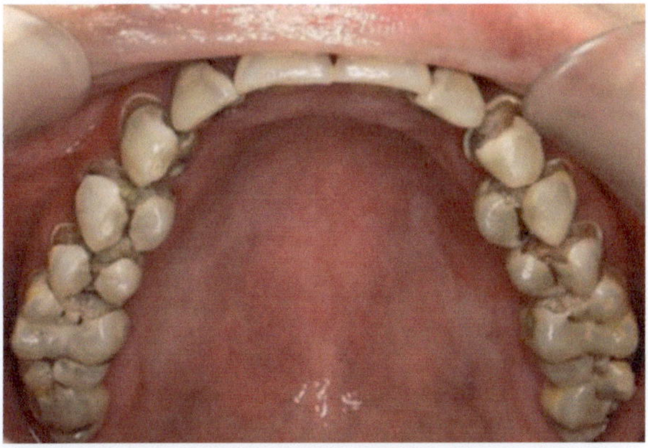

Fig. 15.4 Rampant dental caries lesions in permanent molars of a 14-year-old patient. (Reproduced from Chu et al. [22], published under Creative Commons license, CC-BY-2.0. https://doi.org/10.1186/1756-0500-7-3 [22])

The vertical transmission of *Streptococcus mutans* from mother to child may occur through maternal saliva and, to a lesser extent, breast milk. A recent study reported that although the presence of *S. mutans* in colostrum was infrequent, its detection was associated with the mother's oral hygiene habits and history of dental care during pregnancy [21]. These findings emphasize the importance of preventive oral care before and after childbirth to reduce the risk of early bacterial colonization in infants.

One of the main contributors to caries and erosion is nausea and vomiting, which affect up to 70% of pregnant women especially in the first trimester. Frequent vomiting can not only disrupt regular oral hygiene but also expose tooth surfaces to gastric acids, leading to enamel demineralization and erosion (Fig. 15.5). Despite a physiological drop in overall calcium concentration during pregnancy, the level of ionized calcium, the bioavailable form, remains stable. However, increased bone turnover and changes in saliva composition can still contribute to an acidic oral environment [1].

Several behavioral factors can further increase caries risk:

- Cravings for carbohydrate-rich foods during early pregnancy may lead to frequent snacking, often without subsequent tooth brushing [24].
- Heightened gingival sensitivity and bleeding caused by elevated estrogen and progesterone levels may discourage brushing, allowing plaque accumulation [25].
- Decreased salivary flow, common in pregnancy, limits the natural buffering and self-cleaning mechanisms of the oral cavity [26].
- Pregnant individuals may prioritize the baby's health over their own, leading to neglect of routine oral care [27].

If these habits persist, they contribute to a cariogenic environment that increases the risk of both enamel erosion and cavitated lesions. Preventive strategies such as frequent water intake, using fluoride toothpaste, avoiding brushing immediately after vomiting, and rinsing with a baking soda solution can help neutralize acids and protect dental structures [1].

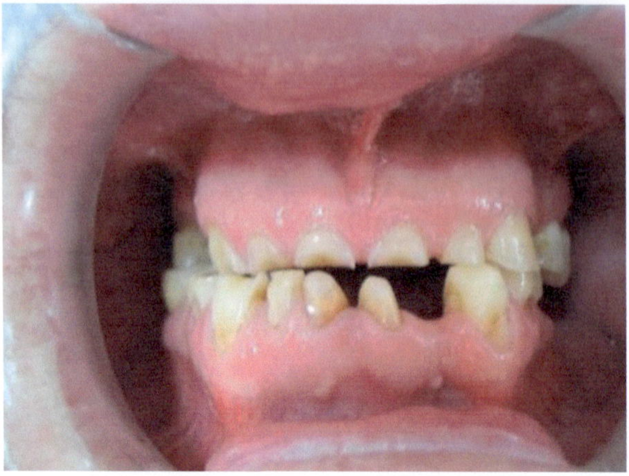

Fig. 15.5 Severe dental erosion affecting maxillary and mandibular teeth. (Reproduced from Cengiz et al. [23], published under Creative Commons license, CC-BY 2.0. https://doi.org/10.4076/1757-1626-2-8018 [23])

15.2.3.1 Treatment

Pregnancy-related vomiting and dietary changes can increase the risk of both caries and enamel erosion. To prevent erosion, patients should rinse with a sodium bicarbonate solution after vomiting to neutralize acids. Fluoride pastes and varnishes help remineralize enamel. Morning appointments should be avoided, and the dental chair should remain upright to reduce discomfort. Caries can be safely treated during pregnancy. While elective procedures may be delayed, active decay should be addressed as needed. Brushing twice daily with fluoride toothpaste and limiting sugar intake are essential preventive measures [15].

15.2.4 Tooth Mobility and Tooth Loss

Hormonal changes and alterations in the oral microbiome during pregnancy can affect the supporting structures of the teeth, such as the lamina dura and periodontal ligament, leading to increased tooth mobility [18] (Fig. 15.6). This condition is typically transient and resolves after childbirth without causing permanent damage. While the mobility is rarely severe enough to result in tooth loss, contributing factors such as vitamin C deficiency may exacerbate the situation. Therefore, appropriate nutritional counseling should be part of antenatal oral care recommendations [15].

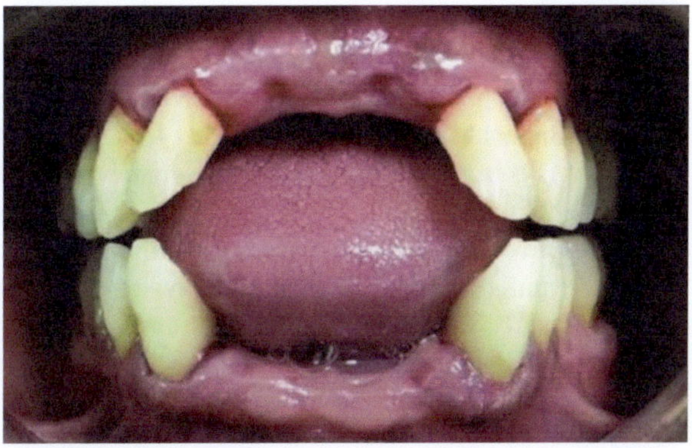

Fig. 15.6 Tooth loss. (Reproduced from Haralur and Al-Qahtani [28], published under Creative Commons license, CC-BY 3.0. https://onlinelibrary.wiley.com/doi/10.1155/2013/759162 [28])

15.3 Supine Hypotensive Syndrome in Dental Practice

Supine hypotensive syndrome (SHS) is a condition that can occur in pregnant women, particularly during the third trimester, due to the compression of the inferior vena cava by the enlarged uterus when the patient is in a supine position.This compression can lead to decreased venous return to the heart, resulting in hypotension, dizziness, nausea, and even syncope. To mitigate these risks during dental procedures, it is recommended to position pregnant patients in a semi-reclined position with a left lateral tilt of approximately 15 degrees or by elevating the right hip by 10–12 cm. This positioning helps alleviate the pressure on the vena cava, ensuring better hemodynamic stability during dental treatments [29–32].

15.4 Dental Radiography During Pregnancy

Dental radiography is considered safe for pregnant patients at all stages of pregnancy when protective measures such as abdominal and thyroid shielding are applied. The radiation dose received during dental imaging is minimal, and with appropriate precautions, exposure to the fetus remains extremely low. According to the American Dental Association, dental professionals who are pregnant should notify their employer in writing and use personal dosimetry badges to ensure occupational exposure does not exceed 0.5 mSv per month [33].

The general guideline for radiographic imaging in pregnant individuals aligns with the ALARA principle "as low as reasonably achievable" to minimize exposure while still achieving diagnostic efficacy [34]. Kelaranta et al. reported that fetal radiation dose levels without lead shielding were less than 1% of the annual 1 mSv public dose limit. While traditional lead shielding has been used to reduce perceived risks of breast and fetal radiation-induced cancers, their findings suggest that the actual reduction is minimal, rendering shielding largely unnecessary from a scientific standpoint [35]. However, its use may still offer psychological reassurance to patients.

Importantly, pregnancy should not be viewed as a reason to delay essential dental imaging. Bahanan et al. emphasized that the public often holds exaggerated fears about the risks of radiography during pregnancy, which can lead to treatment avoidance. Their findings highlight the need for community-level education initiatives aimed at correcting misinformation and improving awareness regarding radiation safety. Dental professionals should play an active role in reassuring pregnant patients, clearly explaining the benefits and minimal risks associated with dental radiographs during pregnancy [36].

15.5 Medication and Anesthesia Use During Pregnancy

The use of medications during pregnancy requires careful consideration due to potential teratogenicity, altered pharmacokinetics, and fetal vulnerability. Although pregnancy is not a contraindication to dental treatment, clinicians must modify treatment planning accordingly to ensure maternal and fetal safety [37].

15.5.1 Drug Classification and FDA Labeling System

Historically, the U.S. Food and Drug Administration (FDA) categorized medications used during pregnancy into five risk groups (A, B, C, D, X). Although phased out for prescription drugs in 2015 and replaced with a narrative-based system that includes summaries of risks and data for use during pregnancy and lactation, the alphabetical system continues to apply to over-the-counter (OTC) medications [38, 39]. For example:

- *Category A*: Controlled studies show no risk.
- *Category B*: No risk in humans despite adverse findings in animals.
- *Category C*: Risk cannot be ruled out.
- *Category D*: Positive evidence of risk exists, but benefits may outweigh risks in some cases.
- *Category X*: Contraindicated in pregnancy; risk outweighs any potential benefit.

Clinicians are encouraged to consult updated labeling, current literature, and when necessary the patient's obstetrician when prescribing medications during pregnancy [38, 40].

15.5.2 Medications Considered Safe for Use in Pregnancy

Ideally, the use of medications should be minimized during pregnancy, particularly in the first trimester. When treatment is necessary, clinicians are advised to consult current evidence and collaborate with the patient's physician to ensure safe and informed decision-making [37]. According to both ADA and evidence-based clinical literature, the following drugs are generally considered compatible with pregnancy and breastfeeding when used appropriately:

- *Local anesthetics*: lidocaine, prilocaine, etidocaine (FDA Category B) [37, 41, 42]
- *Antibiotics*: penicillins, cephalosporins, clindamycin, azithromycin, metronidazole [37, 42]
- *Analgesics*: acetaminophen remains the analgesic of choice, though recent studies suggest possible links between second/third trimester use and childhood asthma, which should be discussed with patients [37].

Other safe medications include antifungals such as nystatin and fluconazole, prednisone, and antivirals like acyclovir [37].

15.5.3 Medications Requiring Caution or Avoidance

Ibuprofen is generally not recommended during pregnancy, particularly after the 20th week of gestation, unless specifically advised by a healthcare provider. This caution is due to its potential effects on fetal circulation and kidney development. In certain cases, a short course of ibuprofen (up to 3 days) may be considered appropriate in earlier stages of pregnancy, depending on the clinical context and gestational age. However, alternative pain management options are often preferred. Therefore, it is essential that pregnant individuals consult a physician or pharmacist before using ibuprofen to carefully weigh its potential risks and benefits [37, 43].

Paracetamol (acetaminophen) remains the first-line analgesic during pregnancy, as it has a more established safety profile when used appropriately [43].

Tetracyclines, aminoglycosides (e.g., gentamicin), and long-term or high-dose opioids also carry known teratogenic or fetotoxic risks and should be avoided unless absolutely necessary [44, 45].

15.5.4 Timing of Dental Care and Drug Administration

Routine dental care is best performed during the second trimester, which poses the least risk to the developing fetus. Elective treatments should be postponed during the first trimester due to organogenesis and the potential for teratogenic effects. More complex procedures are ideally delayed until after delivery [46]. For lactating patients, clinicians may suggest timed feeding, milk banking, or temporary formula use if prescribed medications are known to pass into breast milk [37].

15.6 Recommendations

Pregnancy is a unique physiological state that introduces systemic, immunological, and hormonal changes, many of which directly impact oral health. Increased susceptibility to gingivitis, periodontal inflammation, dental caries, and erosion is frequently observed during gestation. Despite common misconceptions, preventive, diagnostic, and therapeutic dental procedures including radiographs and local anesthesia are considered safe during pregnancy when appropriate precautions are taken.

In light of the growing evidence base, oral health professionals are encouraged to:

- Educate pregnant patients on the importance of maintaining oral hygiene and seeking timely care.
- Reassure patients about the safety of dental radiographs and anesthesia when indicated.
- Collaborate with obstetricians in complex or medically compromised cases to determine individualized treatment plans.
- Avoid delaying necessary treatments based solely on pregnancy status.
- Consider the timing of care, favoring the second trimester for elective procedures and minimizing invasive interventions during the first trimester.

Finally, raising public awareness about the safety of dental interventions during pregnancy can help reduce unwarranted fear, prevent care avoidance, and contribute to improved maternal and fetal outcomes.

References

1. Yenen Z, Ataçağ T. Oral care in pregnancy. J Turk Ger Gynecol Assoc [Internet]. 2019 [cited 2025 May 4];20(4):264. Available from: https://pmc.ncbi.nlm.nih.gov/articles/PMC6883753/
2. Pascual ZN, Langaker MD. Physiology, Pregnancy. StatPearls [Internet]. 2023 May 16 [cited 2025 May 4]; Available from: https://www.ncbi.nlm.nih.gov/books/NBK559304/
3. Liu PP, Wen W, Yu KF, Gao X, Mei Wong MC. Dental care-seeking and information acquisition during pregnancy: a qualitative study. Int J Environ Res Public Health [Internet] 2019 [cited 2025 May 4];16(14):2621. Available from: https://pmc.ncbi.nlm.nih.gov/articles/PMC6679345/
4. Sachelarie L, El Haj Iman A, Romina MV, Huniadi A, Hurjui LL. Impact of Hormones and lifestyle on oral health during pregnancy: a prospective observational regression-based study. Medicina (B Aires) [Internet]. 2024 [cited 2025 May 4];60(11):1773. Available from: https://pmc.ncbi.nlm.nih.gov/articles/PMC11596282/

5. Islam NAB, Haque A. Pregnancy-related dental problems: a review. Heliyon [Internet]. 2024 [cited 2025 May 4];10(3):e24259. Available from: https://pmc.ncbi.nlm.nih.gov/articles/PMC10845246/
6. Tsikouras P, Oikonomou E, Nikolettos K, Andreou S, Kyriakou D, Damaskos C, et al. The impact of periodontal disease on preterm birth and preeclampsia. J Pers Med [Internet]. 2024 [cited 2025 May 4];14(4):345. Available from: https://pmc.ncbi.nlm.nih.gov/articles/PMC11051368/
7. Committee Opinion No. 569. Obstetrics & Gynecology [Internet]. 2013 [cited 2025 May 4];122(2):417–22. Available from: https://journals.lww.com/greenjournal/fulltext/2013/08000/committee_opinion_no__569__oral_health_care_during.47.aspx
8. Skouteris CA. Dental management of the pregnant patient. Dental Management of the Pregnant Patient [Internet]. 2018 [cited 2025 May 4];1–175. Available from: https://onlinelibrary.wiley.com/doi/book/10.1002/9781119286592
9. Newman, Perry R. Klokkevold, Satheesh Elangovan, Yvonne Kapila, Fermin A. Carranza HT. Newman and Carranza's clinical periodontology and implantology, 14th ed. Elsevier St Louis, Missouri [Internet]. 2023 [cited 2025 May 4];1048. Available from: https://www.nobelkitabevi.com.tr/periodontoloji/22267-newman-and-carranza-s-clinical-periodontology-and-implantology-14th-edition-9780323878876.html
10. Samant A, Malik CP, Chabra SK, Devi PK. Gingivitis and periodontal disease in pregnancy. J Periodontol [Internet] 1976 [cited 2025 May 4];47(7):415–418. Available from: https://pubmed.ncbi.nlm.nih.gov/1065739/
11. Löe H, Silness J. Periodontal disease in pregnancy. I. Prevalence and severity. Acta Odontol Scand [Internet]. 1963 [cited 2025 May 4];21(6):533–51. Available from: https://pubmed.ncbi.nlm.nih.gov/14121956/
12. Lieff S, Boggess KA, Murtha AP, Jared H, Madianos PN, Moss K, et al. The oral conditions and pregnancy study: periodontal status of a cohort of pregnant women. J Periodontol [Internet]. 2004 [cited 2025 May 4];75(1):116–126. Available from: https://pubmed.ncbi.nlm.nih.gov/15025223/
13. Babalola DA, Omole F. Periodontal disease and pregnancy outcomes. J Pregnancy [Internet] 2010 [cited 2025 May 4];2010(1):293439. Available from: https://onlinelibrary.wiley.com/doi/full/10.1155/2010/293439
14. Steinberg BJ, Hilton IV, Iada H, Samelson R. Oral health and dental care during pregnancy. Dent Clin N Am. 2013;57(2):195–210.
15. Mehta S, Grover A. Infections and pregnancy infections and pregnancy. Springer; 2022. p. 1–685.
16. Pecci-Lloret MP, Linares-Pérez C, Pecci-Lloret MR, Rodríguez-Lozano FJ, Oñate-Sánchez RE. Oral manifestations in pregnant women: a systematic review. J Clin Med. 2024;13(3):707 [Internet]. 2024 [cited 2025 May 4]. Available from: https://www.mdpi.com/2077-0383/13/3/707/htm
17. Verma PK, Srivastava R, Baranwal H, Chaturvedi T, Gautam A, Singh A. Pyogenic granuloma – hyperplastic lesion of the gingiva: case reports." Open Dent J [Internet] 2012 [cited 2025 May 4];6(1):153. Available from: https://pmc.ncbi.nlm.nih.gov/articles/PMC3474946/
18. Flynn TR, Susarla SM. Oral and maxillofacial surgery for the pregnant patient. Oral Maxillofac Surg Clin North Am [Internet]. 2007 May [cited 2025 May 4];19(2):207–21. Available from: https://pubmed.ncbi.nlm.nih.gov/18088879/
19. Best Practices: Perinatal and Infant OHC 262 the Reference Manual of Pediatric Dentistry Latest Revision Perinatal and Infant Oral Health Care.
20. Al Habashneh R, Guthmiller JM, Levy S, Johnson GK, Squier C, Dawson D V., et al. Factors related to utilization of dental services during pregnancy. J Clin Periodontol [Internet] 2005 [cited 2025 May 4];32(7):815–821. Available from: https://www.researchgate.net/publication/7776320_Factors_related_to_utilization_of_dental_services_during_pregnancy
21. da Silva CB, Mendes MM, Rodrigues BR, Pereira TL, Rodrigues DBR, Rodrigues Junior V, et al. *Streptococcus mutans* detection in saliva and colostrum samples. Einstein [Internet].

2019 [cited 2025 May 11];17(1):eAO4515. Available from: https://pmc.ncbi.nlm.nih.gov/articles/PMC6438671/
22. Chu CH, Lee AHC, Zheng L, Mei ML, Chan GCF. Arresting rampant dental caries with silver diamine fluoride in a young teenager suffering from chronic oral graft versus host disease post-bone marrow transplantation: a case report. BMC Res Notes [Internet] 2014 [cited 2025 Jun 20];7(1):3. Available from: https://pmc.ncbi.nlm.nih.gov/articles/PMC3880541/
23. Cengiz S, Cengiz MI, Saraç YŞ. Dental erosion caused by gastroesophageal reflux disease: a case report. Cases J [Internet]. 2009 [cited 2025 Jun 20];2(7):8018. Available from: https://pmc.ncbi.nlm.nih.gov/articles/PMC2740145/
24. Mobley C, Marshall TA, Milgrom P, Coldwell SE. The contribution of dietary factors to dental caries and disparities in caries. Acad Pediatr [Internet]. 2009 [cited 2025 May 4];9(6):410. Available from: https://pmc.ncbi.nlm.nih.gov/articles/PMC2862385/
25. Dörtbudak O, Eberhardt R, Ulm M, Persson GR. Periodontitis, a marker of risk in pregnancy for preterm birth. J Clin Periodontol [Internet]. 2005 [cited 2025 May 4];32(1):45–52. Available from: https://pubmed.ncbi.nlm.nih.gov/15642058/
26. Yilmaz F, Carti Dorterler O, Eren Halici S, Kasap B, Demirbas A. The effects of pregnancy on oral health, salivary ph and flow rate. BMC Oral Health [Internet] 2024 [cited 2025 May 4];24(1):1286. Available from: https://bmcoralhealth.biomedcentral.com/articles/10.1186/s12903-024-05057-0
27. George A, Dahlen HG, Reath J, Ajwani S, Bhole S, Korda A, et al. What do antenatal care providers understand and do about oral health care during pregnancy: a cross-sectional survey in New South Wales, Australia. BMC Pregnancy Childbirth [Internet]. 2016 [cited 2025 May 4];16(1). Available from: https://pubmed.ncbi.nlm.nih.gov/27903257/
28. Haralur SB, Al-Qahtani AS. Replacement of missing anterior teeth in a patient with chronic mouth breathing and tongue thrusting. Case Rep Dent [Internet]. 2013 [cited 2025 May 4];2013:759162. Available from: https://pmc.ncbi.nlm.nih.gov/articles/PMC3891747/
29. Skouteris CA. Dental management of the pregnant patient. Dental Management of the Pregnant Patient [Internet]. 2018 [cited 2025 May 11];1–175. Available from: https://onlinelibrary.wiley.com/doi/book/10.1002/9781119286592
30. Naseem M, Khurshid Z, Khan HA, Niazi F, Zohaib S, Zafar MS. Oral health challenges in pregnant women: recommendations for dental care professionals. Saudi J Dental Res. 2016;7(2):138–46.
31. Fagoni TG, de Vasconcelos RA, Cardoso PE, Gomes APM, Camargo CHR, Gonçalves SHF. Dental treatment for the pregnant patient. Braz Dent Sci [Internet] 2014 [cited 2025 May 11];17(3):3–10. Available from: https://www.researchgate.net/publication/276510677_Dental_Treatment_for_the_Pregnant_Patient
32. Giglio JA, Lanni SM, Laskin DM. Oral health care for the pregnant patient. 2009 [cited 2025 May 11];75(4). Available from: www.cda-adc.ca/jcda
33. Pregnancy | American Dental Association [Internet]. [cited 2025 May 11]. Available from: https://www.ada.org/resources/ada-library/oral-health-topics/pregnancy
34. Radiation protection of pregnant women in dental radiology | IAEA [Internet]. [cited 2025 May 11]. Available from: https://www.iaea.org/resources/rpop/health-professionals/dentistry/pregnant-women
35. Kelaranta A, Ekholm M, Toroi P, Kortesniemi M. Radiation exposure to foetus and breasts from dental X-ray examinations: effect of lead shields. Dentomaxillofac Radiol [Internet]. 2016 [cited 2025 May 11];45(1). Available from: https://pubmed.ncbi.nlm.nih.gov/26313308/
36. Bahanan L, Tehsin A, Mousa R, Albadi M, Barayan M, Khan E, et al. Women's awareness regarding the use of dental imaging during pregnancy. BMC Oral Health [Internet]. 2021 [cited 2025 May 11];21(1). Available from: https://pubmed.ncbi.nlm.nih.gov/34284764/
37. Berman LH, Hargreaves KM. Cohen's pathways of the pulp, Twelfth Edition. Angewandte Chemie Int Ed. 2021;6(11):951–2; 2.
38. Pregnancy and Lactation Labeling Resources | FDA [Internet]. [cited 2025 May 13]. Available from: https://www.fda.gov/drugs/labeling-information-drug-products/pregnancy-and-lactation-labeling-resources

39. Questions and Answers on the Pregnancy and Lactation Labeling Rule | FDA [Internet]. [cited 2025 May 13]. Available from: https://www.fda.gov/drugs/labeling-information-drug-products/questions-and-answers-pregnancy-and-lactation-labeling-rule
40. FDA Drug Safety Communication: FDA has reviewed possible risks of pain medicine use during pregnancy | FDA [Internet]. [cited 2025 May 13]. Available from: https://www.fda.gov/drugs/drug-safety-and-availability/fda-drug-safety-communication-fda-has-reviewed-possible-risks-pain-medicine-use-during-pregnancy
41. Manautou MA, Mayberry ME. Local anesthetics and pregnancy. A review of the evidence and why dentists should feel safe to treat pregnant people. J Evid Based Dent Pract [Internet]. 2023 [cited 2025 May 13];23(2). Available from: https://pubmed.ncbi.nlm.nih.gov/37201975/
42. Oral Health Care During Pregnancy: A National Consensus Statement. 2012.
43. Pregnancy, breastfeeding and fertility while taking or using ibuprofen – NHS [Internet]. [cited 2025 May 13]. Available from: https://www.nhs.uk/medicines/ibuprofen-for-adults/pregnancy-breastfeeding-and-fertility-while-taking-ibuprofen/
44. Schaefer C, Peters P, Miller RK, York N, Diego S. Drugs during pregnancy and lactation treatment options and risk assessment, 3rd ed. 2015 [cited 2025 May 13]; Available from: http://elsevier.com/locate/permissions,
45. Kuzekanani M. Latest concepts in endodontic management of pregnant patients. Int J Dent [Internet]. 2023 [cited 2025 May 13];2023. Available from: https://pubmed.ncbi.nlm.nih.gov/37899798/
46. Best Practices: Pregnant Adolescent Patient the Reference Manual of Pediatric Dentistry 333 Oral Health Care for the Pregnant Pediatric Dental Patient Latest Revision.

Chapter 16
Ocular Diseases in Pregnancy

Seda Karaca Adıyeke

16.1 Introduction

As a unique physiological condition, pregnancy involves a wide range of systemic modifications that facilitate maternal adaptation, ensure fetal protection, and prime the body for childbirth [1]. These changes span across multiple systems, including cardiovascular, pulmonary, renal, metabolic, hormonal, immunological, and hematological pathways.

The eye is among the organs most variably influenced by the physiological and pathological changes of pregnancy, thereby necessitating careful clinical evaluation [2]. During pregnancy, ocular changes are classified into physiological and pathological types. While the majority are mild, transient, and reversible, some have the potential to worsen underlying eye diseases or precipitate novel ocular pathologies [2].

The pathologic ocular changes during pregnancy can be further categorized into disorders that occur for the first time during gestation, preexisting ocular diseases that undergo modification, and secondary ocular complications resulting from systemic conditions [3–5]. Importantly, the need to avoid teratogenic medications and invasive diagnostics imposes limitations on management, necessitating early and cautious ophthalmologic assessment to prevent sight-threatening outcomes.

While most ocular manifestations of pregnancy are transient and benign, early identification and appropriate intervention are crucial for preventing permanent visual impairment and for elucidating the systemic conditions underlying these symptoms [5]. This chapter seeks to provide an overview of the principal physiological and pathological ocular changes associated with pregnancy.

S. K. Adıyeke (✉)
Izmir Bakircay University, Faculty of Medicine, Department of Ophthalmology, Izmir, Turkey
e-mail: seda.karacaadiyeke@bakircay.edu.tr

© The Author(s), under exclusive license to Springer Nature Switzerland AG 2026

I. Karaca (ed.), *Managing Maternal Chronic Diseases for a Healthy Pregnancy*,
https://doi.org/10.1007/978-3-032-15221-3_16

16.2 Physiological Changes in the Eye During Pregnancy

16.2.1 Eyelids

Melasma, often referred to as chloasma or the "mask of pregnancy," represents one of the most frequent physiological manifestations encountered during pregnancy [6]. Clinically, it manifests as increased pigmentation around the eyes, with possible extension to the eyelids and malar areas [4]. This condition is primarily driven by elevated levels of oestrogen, progesterone, and melanocyte-stimulating hormone, which stimulate melanogenesis and lead to enhanced melanin production [7]. The severity of melasma is influenced by individual skin type, sunlight exposure, and genetic predisposition [6]. In most cases, pregnancy-associated melasma is transient and tends to resolve spontaneously in the postpartum period, although depigmenting agents may be used when necessary [8].

16.2.2 Corneal and Ocular Surface Changes

During pregnancy, systemic hormonal, cardiovascular, and metabolic changes induce a variety of physiological alterations in the eye, particularly affecting the cornea, conjunctiva, eyelids, and tear production mechanisms [9, 10]. Fluid retention, in particular, has the potential to induce corneal edema, resulting in central corneal thickening of up to 16 microns and an approximate 1-diopter increase in corneal curvature [5]. These changes are believed to result from elevated levels of estrogen, progesterone, and relaxin, which stimulate collagen degradation and enhance matrix metalloproteinase activity, ultimately weakening the biomechanical structure of the cornea [5].

While these refractive changes are typically short-lived and regress in the postpartum period, they can nevertheless result in marked refractive fluctuations during gestation. Consequently, laser refractive procedures are contraindicated during this period and should be deferred until after childbirth and lactation [6]. Hormonal factors, particularly elevated estrogen, relaxin, and cortisol levels, have also been implicated in the progression of keratoconus and the development of corneal ectasia [7, 8]. Additionally, in the later stages of pregnancy, corneal sensitivity may decrease, possibly due to edema-induced thickening of the cornea [11].

Despite these changes, studies have not demonstrated significant alterations in average keratometric values or in anterior and posterior corneal biomechanical parameters throughout pregnancy. All parameters have been shown to return to baseline levels within 1 year postpartum [12]. Pregnancy has additionally been associated with a reduction in meibomian gland function and a subtle decline in tear film stability, most likely secondary to hormonal variations and gestational physiological changes.

Tear film quality and quantity are also affected during pregnancy. Altered tear composition has the potential to impair the structural stability of the tear film, contributing to the development of dry eye disease (DED) [13]. This condition is considered to result from heightened immunoreactivity of prolactin, epidermal growth factor, and transforming growth factor-β1 in ductal cells, which may impair lacrimal acinar function [13]. Beyond the classic symptoms of dry eye disease (DED)—including irritation, blurred vision, and a foreign body sensation—tear film instability may increase susceptibility of the ocular surface to infections, inflammatory processes, and mechanical injuries such as corneal abrasions [2].

Moreover, conjunctival vascular changes, including increased granularity due to decreased blood flow, can be observed during pregnancy [2]. Subconjunctival hemorrhage is another benign and self-limiting condition seen in approximately 10% of pregnant or postpartum women, generally requiring no treatment beyond blood pressure monitoring [2].

Increased corneal thickness, reduced sensitivity, and alterations in tear production and lid physiology can also lead to contact lens intolerance during pregnancy. Therefore, temporary discontinuation of lens wear and regular ophthalmologic monitoring are recommended throughout gestation [6].

Changes in intraocular pressure (IOP) pregnancy is associated with a gradual decline in IOP, typically around 10%, with the most notable reduction observed between weeks 12 and 18, particularly in ocular hypertensive patients [14]. This decline progresses from the first through the third trimester and may persist into the postpartum period [14, 15]. Diurnal IOP fluctuations also diminish during pregnancy compared to prepregnancy levels [16]. The decrease is mainly attributed to enhanced uveoscleral outflow and reduced episcleral venous pressure, both associated with lowered systemic venous pressure. These physiological changes often lead to an improvement in preexisting glaucoma during pregnancy [4].

16.2.3 Changes in Visual Field

With respect to visual field alterations, both bitemporal contraction and concentric constriction have been documented during pregnancy [17]. Several theories have been proposed regarding the mechanisms and severity of these changes. Akar et al. reported a significant rise in visual field mean threshold sensitivity among healthy pregnant women in the third trimester, with all asymptomatic visual field changes fully resolving after childbirth [18].

Normal pituitary enlargement is a recognized physiological change in pregnancy; however, in the absence of structural abnormalities involving the optic chiasm, this process generally does not cause visual field defects [19].

16.3 Preexisting Eye Conditions Altered During Pregnancy

16.3.1 Glaucoma

Increased intraocular pressure (IOP) is a principal risk factor for both the development and progression of glaucoma. During pregnancy, physiological adaptations—principally mediated by increased progesterone levels—enhance uveoscleral outflow and reduce episcleral venous pressure, resulting in a physiological decline in IOP of approximately 2–3 mmHg [20, 21]. Elevated relaxin levels may further facilitate aqueous humor drainage, while fluctuations in sex hormones may confer neuroprotective effects on the optic nerve [22, 23]. Notably, IOP tends to decline progressively with advancing gestational age and typically returns to baseline within 3 months postpartum [24, 25]. Consequently, many pregnant patients with preexisting glaucoma may experience a decreased requirement for topical IOP-lowering therapy during gestation.

Despite these general trends, considerable interindividual variability has been observed. A retrospective analysis of 28 eyes from 15 pregnant women with glaucoma revealed that 36% experienced either increased intraocular pressure or progressive visual field loss during pregnancy [23]. The investigators partially attributed these findings to medication noncompliance, frequently driven by patient apprehensions regarding potential teratogenic effects of antiglaucoma agents [23]. Moreover, 87% of participants required continued or modified treatment to maintain adequate IOP control, underscoring the necessity of rigorous monitoring throughout pregnancy to prevent irreversible visual impairment [23, 26]. Therefore, preconception counseling is essential for women of reproductive age who have a confirmed diagnosis of glaucoma.

The teratogenic potential of antiglaucoma medications limits their use during pregnancy, as most agents fall under FDA pregnancy categories B or C. Brimonidine, classified as Category B, is generally regarded as safe for use during the first and second trimesters; however, it should be discontinued before delivery because of the potential risk of neonatal apnea [26]. Beta-adrenergic antagonists, while effective, readily cross the placenta and have been linked to fetal bradycardia and cardiac arrhythmias [27, 28]. Carbonic anhydrase inhibitors may be used with caution during the second and third trimesters, whereas prostaglandin analogues are generally contraindicated due to their potential to trigger uterine contractions and miscarriage [26, 29].

In cases where pharmacological therapy proves inadequate, laser trabeculoplasty is regarded as a safe and effective option both prior to and during pregnancy [30]. In addition, cyclophotocoagulation and minimally invasive glaucoma procedures, including Xen gel stent implantation, have been successfully performed during pregnancy [31–33]. For women anticipating pregnancy, early surgical interventions—including laser trabeculoplasty, trabeculectomy, or shunt tube procedures—may optimize IOP control during gestation [23, 34]. Nevertheless, traditional glaucoma surgeries present particular challenges in pregnant patients, notably anesthesia-related risks, limitations in postoperative pharmacotherapy, and the need for prolonged supine positioning.

16.3.2 Uveitis

With an annual prevalence of about 115 per 100,000 individuals, the management of uveitis during pregnancy presents significant clinical challenges [35]. Elevated levels of estrogen, progesterone, and cortisol during pregnancy suppress Th1-mediated immunity and enhance Th2 responses, leading to improvement in autoimmune diseases such as uveitis [36–38]. Alpha-fetoprotein (AFP), synthesized by the yolk sac and fetal liver, supports immune tolerance by suppressing lymphocyte activity and enhancing anti-inflammatory responses [39, 40].

Clinically, uveitis activity commonly persists or worsens in the first trimester but generally improves during the second and third trimesters, with disease flares frequently observed in the postpartum period [36, 41, 42]. In mild cases, topical corticosteroids (Category C) are generally regarded as safe, whereas moderate to severe disease may necessitate low-dose oral prednisolone, azathioprine, cyclosporine, tacrolimus, or anti-TNF therapy [43]. Teratogenic agents such as methotrexate (Category X) and mycophenolate mofetil (Category D) should be avoided, and patients should be counseled about fertility and pregnancy-related risks when initiating immunosuppressive therapies [43].

Toxoplasmic chorioretinitis, which accounts for roughly 7% of posterior uveitis cases, may reactivate during pregnancy, although it usually does not present with a more severe clinical course [44–46]. Management consists of spiramycin in the first trimester, while in later stages clindamycin or sulfadiazine combined with pyrimethamine and corticosteroids may be employed; intravitreal therapy can also be considered [47]. Fortunately, reactivation does not pose an increased risk of fetal transmission due to maternal immunity.

16.3.3 Diabetes Mellitus

Diabetic retinopathy (DR) represents the most common ocular pathology influenced by pregnancy, carrying an increased risk of both onset and progression, especially in women with type 1 diabetes mellitus [48–50]. Although progression of diabetic retinopathy may also be observed in type 2 diabetes, it is considerably more frequent and severe in patients with type 1 disease [51].

Several factors contribute to the progression of diabetic retinopathy during pregnancy, including longer disease duration, poor glycemic control reflected by elevated HbA1c levels, greater baseline severity of retinopathy at conception—considered the most important predictor—and the coexistence of comorbidities such as hypertension or diabetic macular edema [52]. Moreover, the progression of diabetic retinopathy has been associated with alterations in retinal blood flow during pregnancy. While some studies report reduced retinal venous diameter and diminished blood flow leading to ischemia, others suggest enhanced retinal perfusion that may induce endothelial injury and exert stress on already compromised retinal vessels [53, 54]. Additionally, hormonal influences such as progesterone-induced local production of VEGF and angiopoietin factors may exacerbate DR [50].

Patients with minimal or no preexisting DR generally experience stable disease during pregnancy, with mild worsening observed in 10–20% of cases [55]. In women with moderately severe nonproliferative diabetic retinopathy (NPDR), the risk of progression is substantially elevated, with proliferative disease developing in as many as one-third of cases [2]. Severe NPDR or proliferative DR (PDR) should prompt a delay in conception until the retinopathy is adequately treated [56]. Preconception laser photocoagulation is advised for women with severe NPDR or early PDR to reduce the likelihood of rapid disease progression [57] (Fig. 16.1).

Clinical guidelines recommend that all women with preexisting diabetes receive a comprehensive dilated fundus examination before conception and undergo repeat evaluation during the first trimester [58]. Follow-up is tailored to the severity of retinopathy, with women who have moderate to severe NPDR or PDR undergoing monthly ophthalmic evaluations during the second and third trimesters [59]. For high-risk patients, close multidisciplinary monitoring involving ophthalmologists, endocrinologists, and perinatologists is essential [60].

Management of DR during pregnancy aligns with that in nonpregnant patients, emphasizing timely laser photocoagulation or vitrectomy if needed [50]. Diabetic macular edema (DME) that develops during pregnancy may regress spontaneously after delivery, rendering observation an appropriate management option in selected cases [61]. While anti-VEGF therapies are effective in nonpregnant populations,

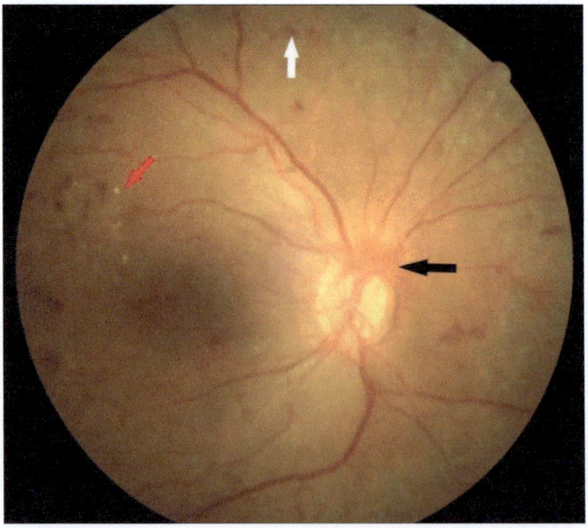

Fig. 16.1 Fundus photography of a case diagnosed with proliferative diabetic retinopathy, demonstrating optic disc neovascularization (black arrow), hard exudates (red arrow), and retinal hemorrhages (white arrow)

their use during pregnancy is discouraged due to uncertain fetal safety [51]. Intravitreal corticosteroids may serve as a safer alternative for managing DME [61].

Surgical intervention for diabetic retinopathy during pregnancy is uncommon and is generally limited to complications such as non-resolving vitreous hemorrhage, neovascular glaucoma, or tractional retinal detachment [62]. Due to increased perioperative risks during pregnancy, stabilization of diabetic retinopathy prior to conception is highly recommended [62].

Although progression may occur during gestation, pregnancy does not appear to adversely affect the long-term prognosis of diabetic retinopathy [63]. Interestingly, DR that emerges during pregnancy often regresses postpartum, with studies reporting complete or partial resolution in a significant proportion of cases [64].

16.4 Ocular Disorders That Initially Manifest During Pregnancy

16.4.1 Central Serous Chorioretinopathy

Central serous chorioretinopathy (CSCR) is a retinal disorder defined by serous detachment of the neurosensory retina, resulting from focal defects in the retinal pigment epithelium (Fig. 16.2). Although traditionally more prevalent in males, pregnancy represents a distinct physiological state that predisposes women to CSCR, particularly during the third trimester [65]. Clinical manifestations include reduced visual acuity, metamorphopsia, central scotoma, and perception of halos.

The pathophysiology of CSCR in pregnancy is multifactorial, encompassing elevated endogenous cortisol levels, hormonal fluctuations, hypercoagulability, increased vascular permeability, reduced colloidal osmotic pressure, and prostaglandin-mediated vascular alterations [65, 66]. The presence of white subretinal exudates adjacent to areas of pigment epithelial detachment is a frequent ancillary finding.

Because of the potential teratogenic risks linked to fluorescein angiography, optical coherence tomography (OCT) is the preferred noninvasive modality for diagnosing and longitudinally monitoring CSCR during pregnancy [67]. The condition

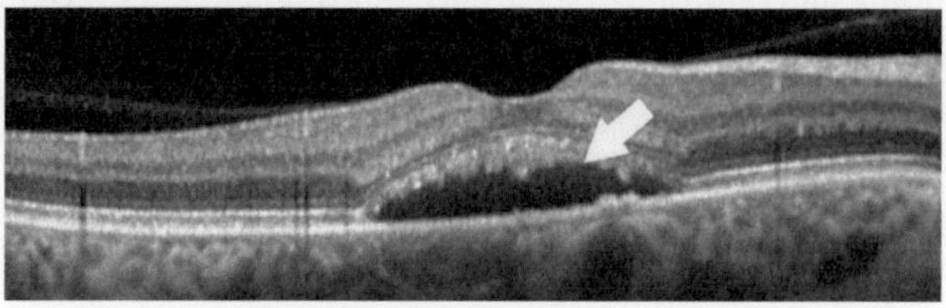

Fig. 16.2 Optical coherence tomography (OCT) of a patient with central serous chorioretinopathy showing serous detachment of the neurosensory retina (white arrow)

typically resolves spontaneously by late gestation or within a few weeks after delivery, although recurrences in subsequent pregnancies have been documented [66].

16.4.2 *Hypertensive Disorders of Pregnancy and Ocular Manifestations*

Hypertension during pregnancy may either represent a worsening of preexisting disease or arise de novo in a previously normotensive individual [68]. Among hypertensive disorders of pregnancy, preeclampsia is a major complication defined by the onset of hypertension and proteinuria after 20 weeks of gestation. Risk factors include extremes of maternal age, multifetal gestation, diabetes mellitus, chronic hypertension, and underlying renal disease. Eclampsia denotes the development of seizures in a patient with preeclampsia, signifying progression of the hypertensive disorder [69].

Ocular involvement is frequently observed in preeclampsia and eclampsia, with visual disturbances occurring in up to 25% of patients with severe preeclampsia and in approximately 50% of those with eclampsia [70, 71]. Typical symptoms include blurred vision, photopsia, transient scotomas, diplopia, and sudden difficulty with focusing [71]. Notably, these visual symptoms may precede the onset of seizures, especially in the postpartum period, underscoring the importance of vigilant monitoring. Funduscopic examination, although valuable for detecting retinal vascular changes mirroring systemic involvement, should be undertaken cautiously, as light stimuli may precipitate seizures.

Fundus findings associated with preeclampsia include focal arteriolar spasm, generalized narrowing of retinal arterioles, arteriolar attenuation, retinal hemorrhages, optic nerve swelling, and vascular tortuosity. Soft exudates, retinal edema, and papilledema may also be observed in more advanced cases [66]. These retinal changes are typically transient and tend to resolve postpartum, although rare cases of permanent damage, such as proliferative retinopathy secondary to peripheral microvascular thrombosis, have been reported.

Severe hypertensive states in pregnancy can also result in cortical blindness or serous retinal detachment (SRD). Cortical blindness—characterized by vision loss despite a normal fundus and preserved pupillary reflexes—arises from vasogenic edema secondary to increased capillary permeability. It may precede seizure activity by several hours and represent the earliest neurological manifestation of impending eclampsia [69]. Serous retinal detachment (SRD), defined as the separation of the neurosensory retina from the retinal pigment epithelium, is believed to result from choroidal ischemia secondary to severe hypertension. Although SRD generally resolves with postpartum recovery, a subset of patients may experience residual and permanent visual dysfunction.

Importantly, the severity of maternal retinopathy has been shown to correlate inversely with fetal birth weight and positively with both maternal blood pressure and fetal mortality, emphasizing the critical role of early ophthalmologic and systemic evaluation in patients with preeclampsia [4, 70].

16.4.3 Retinal Vascular Occlusive Disease

Retinal vascular occlusive diseases during pregnancy encompass both arterial and venous events. Purtscher-like retinopathy is a rare, vision-threatening condition typically observed within 24 h postpartum. It is characterized by multifocal retinal infarctions, often involving the macula, and can result in profound, irreversible bilateral vision loss [68]. Funduscopic evaluation often demonstrates multiple white retinal lesions consistent with confluent cotton-wool spots, particularly clustered around the optic nerve head, frequently accompanied by superficial retinal hemorrhages [68]. The majority of cases occur in the setting of complicated pregnancies. At present, no effective treatment exists for Purtscher-like retinopathy, as retinal ischemic injury is typically established by the time visual symptoms become apparent.

Pregnancy creates a hypercoagulable state that predisposes individuals to retinal venous occlusive events, including branch and central retinal vein occlusion (Fig. 16.3). These events most commonly arise in the third trimester or early postpartum period, with reported incidence rates ranging from 0.05% to 1.8%. Importantly, the clinical presentation of venous occlusions in pregnant patients may differ from that seen in the nonpregnant population [50].

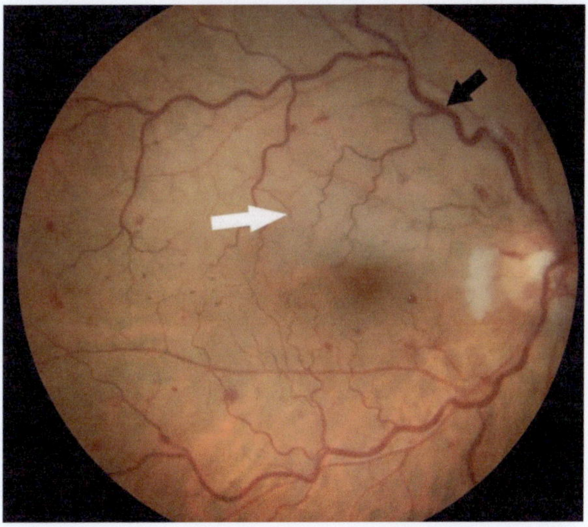

Fig. 16.3 Fundus photography of a case diagnosed with combined retinal artery and vein occlusion, demonstrating venous dilatation (black arrow) and retinal whitening secondary to arterial occlusion–related edema (white arrow)

16.4.4 *Spontaneous Orbital Hemorrhage*

Spontaneous orbital hemorrhage may develop during the first trimester, particularly in association with severe episodes of nausea and vomiting, or may occur during labor [72]. Clinical manifestations typically include acute onset of proptosis, diplopia, and orbital pain. Anticoagulant therapy has been recognized as an important predisposing factor for spontaneous orbital hemorrhage [73]. Diagnosis is confirmed through orbital imaging modalities. In most cases, no specific treatment is required, as the hemorrhage tends to resolve spontaneously without intervention [74].

16.5 Ophthalmic Manifestations of Pregnancy-Related Complications

16.5.1 *Disseminated Intravascular Coagulation and Ocular Manifestations*

Disseminated intravascular coagulation (DIC) is an acquired, life-threatening disorder marked by systemic activation of the coagulation cascade. It is frequently associated with obstetric complications, including acute peripartum hemorrhage, placental abruption, severe preeclampsia, eclampsia, HELLP syndrome, amniotic fluid embolism, septic abortion, intrauterine fetal demise, intrauterine infection, placenta praevia, acute fatty liver of pregnancy, and retained products of conception [75, 76].

The pathological process involves widespread microvascular thrombosis, leading to tissue ischemia and potential multiorgan failure. Paradoxically, consumption of platelets and coagulation factors can also result in uncontrollable hemorrhage [77]. Laboratory findings usually demonstrate prolonged prothrombin time, activated partial thromboplastin time, and thrombin clotting time, along with decreased platelet counts and reduced fibrinogen levels, indicative of excessive fibrinolytic activity [77].

Ophthalmic involvement in DIC, though uncommon, typically occurs at the choroidal level, where thrombotic capillary occlusions result in retinal pigment epithelium (RPE) atrophy and serous retinal detachment [78]. Clinically, patients may present with bilateral blurred vision, visual field defects, metamorphopsia, and transient reductions in visual acuity [79]. In certain cases, residual alterations of the retinal pigment epithelium (RPE) may persist despite resolution of the serous retinal detachment.

Moreover, coagulopathy associated with DIC can precipitate ischemia, retinal hemorrhage, massive edema, elevated episcleral venous pressure, and secondary increases in intraocular pressure. These events may culminate in central retinal artery occlusion, representing one of the most vision-threatening complications of DIC. Management is directed chiefly at treating the underlying obstetric condition, which usually results in resolution of the ocular manifestations [77].

16.5.2 Haemolysis, Elevated Liver Enzymes, and Low Platelets (HELLP) Syndrome

HELLP syndrome is a serious pregnancy-related condition defined by hemolysis, elevated liver enzyme levels, and thrombocytopenia, occurring in roughly 10% of women with preeclampsia or eclampsia [80]. Blurred vision is the most frequently reported visual symptom, whereas retinal arteriolar narrowing constitutes the most common ophthalmic finding. Retinal detachment, occurring in approximately 0.9% of patients with HELLP syndrome, is most often observed in the third trimester [81].

The pathogenesis of retinal detachment in HELLP syndrome is thought to arise from choroidal ischemia induced by severe arterial vasospasm, leading to disruption of the blood–retinal barrier [82]. Prompt obstetric management, including immediate delivery of the fetus, is crucial once HELLP syndrome is diagnosed. Additionally, early ophthalmologic assessment and intervention are recommended to address ocular involvement and minimize the risk of permanent visual impairment [80].

16.5.3 Thrombotic Thrombocytopenic Purpura

Thrombotic thrombocytopenic purpura (TTP) is a rare, acute, and potentially life-threatening disorder defined by thrombocytopenia and hemolytic anemia, often accompanied by systemic manifestations such as fever, renal dysfunction, and neurological symptoms [83]. Ocular involvement is observed in nearly 10% of cases and may present as retinal or vitreous hemorrhages, exudates, serous retinal detachment, arteriolar narrowing, papilledema, or optic disc neovascularization [84, 85]. In the setting of compromised optic nerve perfusion, additional manifestations such as subconjunctival hemorrhage, extraocular muscle paresis, scintillating scotoma, anisocoria, optic atrophy, and homonymous hemianopia have also been reported [4].

Management depends on disease severity, ranging from supportive care and fundus monitoring in mild cases to interventions such as photocoagulation, vitrectomy, or retinal reattachment surgery in more severe ocular involvement [84].

16.5.4 Antiphospholipid Antibody Syndrome

Antiphospholipid syndrome (APS) is an autoimmune condition linked to a prothrombotic state, defined by the presence of antiphospholipid antibodies, including anticardiolipin antibodies, lupus anticoagulant, and anti-β2 glycoprotein I antibodies [86, 87]. Patients commonly present with blurred vision, ocular redness, pain, or vision loss, and the diagnosis relies on the integration of clinical findings with serological confirmation.

Ocular involvement in APS can be classified into anterior segment, posterior segment, and neuro-ophthalmic manifestations. Anterior segment findings include episcleritis, scleritis, limbal or filamentary keratitis, iritis, and conjunctival telangiectasia or microaneurysms [86]. Posterior segment complications may include retinal vasculitis, vitritis, retinal detachment, posterior scleritis, cotton-wool spots, venous tortuosity, central serous chorioretinopathy, and retinal vascular occlusions, such as branch or central retinal vein occlusion, cilioretinal artery occlusion, and bilateral choroidal infarction [86, 88].

Neuro-ophthalmic manifestations may include transient monocular or bilateral vision loss, anterior ischemic optic neuropathy, progressive optic atrophy, and, in certain cases, involvement of the visual pathways or ocular motor nerves [4, 86]. APS requires multidisciplinary management involving haematology, ophthalmology, and obstetrics. Despite long-term anticoagulation therapy, pregnancy outcomes remain suboptimal, with up to 20% of pregnancies resulting in complications [89]. The prognosis for ocular manifestations of APS remains poorly defined [86].

16.5.5 Grave's Disease

Thyroid dysfunction is prevalent in women of reproductive age and may either manifest for the first time or exacerbate during pregnancy and the postpartum period [90]. Hyperthyroidism occurs in about 0.2% of pregnancies, most commonly as a result of Graves' disease [90]. Graves' disease results from antibodies that stimulate the thyroid-stimulating hormone receptor. Its diagnosis during pregnancy can be challenging, as nonspecific features such as increased appetite, fatigue, and heat intolerance may overlap with normal gestational changes, whereas findings like weight loss, hypertension, tachycardia, and tremor are more specific indicators [91].

Thyroid-associated orbitopathy represents the most common extrathyroidal manifestation, occurring or exacerbating in approximately 0.2–0.4% of pregnancies [92]. Pregnancy-associated hypervolemia may contribute to orbital tissue expansion. Clinical manifestations include proptosis, lid lag, periorbital edema, enlargement of the extraocular muscles, optic neuropathy, and lacrimal gland dysfunction [93].

Management involves anti-thyroid drugs as the primary treatment, despite potential teratogenic risks [94]. Surgical intervention is reserved for complicated cases. Multidisciplinary care and close postpartum monitoring are essential [91].

16.6 Ocular Pharmacotherapy During Pregnancy

The early stages of pregnancy constitute a critical window of fetal development, during which drug administration must be approached with caution. Nearly 50% of women may use medications before pregnancy is recognized. Topical ophthalmic agents, in particular, should be prescribed at the minimum effective dose and concentration, with patients advised to perform punctal occlusion and apply pressure over the nasolacrimal duct to limit systemic absorption. Despite these precautions, the safety of many ophthalmic medications during pregnancy has not been fully established.

Beta-blockers may be used with caution in the first trimester but are typically discontinued 2–3 days prior to delivery to avoid neonatal beta-blockade and bradycardia. Their administration is generally discouraged during lactation, as they are excreted in breast milk. Both topical and systemic carbonic anhydrase inhibitors are contraindicated in pregnancy due to their potential teratogenic effects and risk of hepatorenal toxicity [22]. Although studies in rodents have linked systemic acetazolamide exposure to limb malformations, data in humans are limited; acetazolamide may be considered if no safer alternatives are available. It is present in breast milk at low concentrations and is unlikely to pose a risk to the infant; however, monitoring of serum electrolyte levels may be considered if necessary [95]. Sympathomimetic agents such as brimonidine, clonidine, and dipivefrin lack sufficient safety data and should only be used when no alternative treatments exist. Prostaglandin analogues are contraindicated because they may induce labor and impair fetal perfusion. Miotics, however, are generally considered safe.

Systemic corticosteroids are best avoided during pregnancy due to their teratogenic potential and their possible association with the development of central serous chorioretinopathy (CSCR). In contrast, topical corticosteroids have not been associated with adverse fetal outcomes and are considered safe for use. Among antibiotics, chloramphenicol, tetracycline, and neomycin are not recommended, whereas tobramycin, erythromycin, polymyxin B, gentamicin, and quinolones may be used with caution. Topical antiviral agents should also be administered carefully due to uncertain safety profiles in pregnancy [96, 97].

Occasional use of mydriatic agents for retinal examination is regarded as safe in pregnancy. Similarly, topical mast cell stabilizers and antihistamines are considered safe throughout all trimesters. In patients with chronic open-angle glaucoma, laser trabeculoplasty serves as an effective non-pharmacologic approach to lowering intraocular pressure, particularly when the use of topical medications should be minimized.

Fluorescein angiography is an important tool for diagnosing and monitoring retinal disorders. Fluorescein has been shown to cross the placental barrier and may remain detectable in breast milk for up to 72 h following intravenous administration. Although no harmful fetal or neonatal effects have been documented to date, its use warrants caution [97]. When diagnostic imaging is required during pregnancy, noninvasive modalities such as optical coherence tomography (OCT) or OCT angiography are preferred to dye-based angiographic techniques.

16.7 Conclusion

In conclusion, pregnancy is associated with diverse physiological and pathological alterations that can substantially impact ocular health. While the majority of these changes are transient and reversible, some may pose a risk of permanent visual impairment or serious ophthalmic complications. Therefore, early recognition of ocular symptoms, regular ophthalmologic monitoring, and timely implementation of appropriate treatment strategies are essential. Pharmacologic interventions must be carefully planned, taking into account the potential effects on fetal development, and noninvasive diagnostic methods should be prioritized whenever possible. A multidisciplinary approach, with close collaboration between ophthalmologists, obstetricians, and other specialists, is crucial to safeguarding both maternal visual function and fetal well-being throughout pregnancy. These measures collectively contribute to optimizing both visual and systemic outcomes for the mother and the child.

References

1. Chandra M, Paray AA. Natural physiological changes during pregnancy. Yale J Biol Med. 2024;97(1):85–92. https://doi.org/10.59249/JTIV4138.
2. Morya AK, Gogia S, Gupta A, Prakash S, Solanki K, Naidu AD. Motherhood: what every ophthalmologist needs to know. Indian J Ophthalmol. 2020;68(8):1526–32. https://doi.org/10.4103/ijo.IJO_2033_19.
3. Kalogeropoulos D, Sung VC, Paschopoulos M, Moschos MM, Panidis P, Kalogeropoulos C. The physiologic and pathologic effects of pregnancy on the human visual system. J Obstet Gynaecol. 2019;39(8):1037–48. https://doi.org/10.1080/01443615.2019.1584891.
4. Chawla S, Chaudhary T, Aggarwal S, et al. Ophthalmic considerations in pregnancy. Med J Armed Forces India. 2013;69(3):278–84.
5. Samra KA. The eye and visual system in pregnancy, what to expect? An in-depth review. Oman J Ophthalmol. 2013;6(2):87–91.
6. Neagu N, Conforti C, Agozzino M, et al. Melasma treatment: a systematic review. J Dermatolog Treat. 2022;33(4):1816–37. https://doi.org/10.1080/09546634.2021.1914313.
7. Yenerel NM, Küçümen RB. Hamilelik ve Göz. Turk J Ophthalmol. 2015;45:213–9.
8. Ghasemiyeh P, Fazlinejad R, Kiafar MR, Rasekh S, Mokhtarzadegan M, Mohammadi-Samani S. Different therapeutic approaches in melasma: advances and limitations. Front Pharmacol. 2024;15:1337282. https://doi.org/10.3389/fphar.2024.1337282.

9. Asiedu K, Kyei S, Adanusa M, et al. Dry eye, its clinical subtypes and associated factors in healthy pregnancy: a cross-sectional study. PLoS One. 2021;16(10):e0258233. https://doi.org/10.1371/journal.pone.0258233.
10. Sarac O, Yesilirmak N, Caglayan M, et al. Dynamics of keratoconus progression after a previous successful accelerated crosslinking treatment during and after pregnancy. J Cataract Refract Surg. 2022;48(5):599–603. https://doi.org/10.1097/j.jcrs.0000000000000801.
11. Goldich Y, Cooper M, Barkana Y, et al. Ocular anterior segment changes in pregnancy. J Cataract Refract Surg. 2014;40(11):1868–71.
12. Naderan M, Jahanrad A. Topographic, tomographic and biomechanical corneal changes during pregnancy in patients with keratoconus: a cohort study. Acta Ophthalmol. 2017;95(4):e291–6.
13. Taradaj K, Ginda T, Maciejewicz P, et al. Pregnancy and the eye. Changes in morphology of the cornea and the anterior chamber of the eye in pregnant woman. Ginekol Pol. 2018;89(12):695–9. https://doi.org/10.5603/GP.a2018.0117.
14. Ibraheem WA, Ibraheem AB, Tjani AM, Oladejo S, Adepoju S, Folohunso B. Tear film functions and intraocular pressure changes in pregnancy. Afr J Reprod Health. 2015;19(4):118–22.
15. Uzun İ, Mutaf Ç, Reyhan AH, Yüksekyayla F, Colak E, Yolaçan M. Pregnancy-induced ocular changes: impacts on intraocular pressure, the cornea, and the anterior chamber. BMC Ophthalmol. 2025;25(1):298. https://doi.org/10.1186/s12886-025-04130-8.
16. Mathew S, Harris A, Ridenour CM, et al. Management of glaucoma in pregnancy. J Glaucoma. 2019;28(10):937–44. https://doi.org/10.1097/IJG.0000000000001324.
17. Kunduracı MS, Koçkar A, Helvacıoğlu Ç, Kırık F, Karakuş Hacıoğlu G, Akçay BİS. Evaluation of dry eye and meibomian gland function in pregnancy. Int Ophthalmol. 2023;43(11):4263–9. https://doi.org/10.1007/s10792-023-02836-6.
18. Akar Y, Yucel I, Akar ME, et al. Long-term fluctuation of retinal sensitivity during pregnancy. Can J Ophthalmol. 2005;40(4):487–91.
19. Yenerel NM, Küçümen RB. Pregnancy and the eye. Turk J Ophthalmol. 2015;45(5):213–9. https://doi.org/10.4274/tjo.43815.
20. Saylık M, Saylık SA. Not only pregnancy but also the number of fetuses in the uterus affects intraocular pressure. Indian J Ophthalmol. 2014;62(6):680–2.
21. Kumari R, Saha BC, Onlar A, et al. Management of glaucoma in pregnancy–balancing safety with efficacy. Ther Adv Ophthalmol. 2021;13:25158414211022876.
22. Kaufman AR, Ali Al-Djasim L, Rivkin AC, et al. Pregnancy outcomes in the medical management of glaucoma: an international multicenter descriptive survey. Eur J Ophthalmol. 2024;34(2):471–9. https://doi.org/10.1177/11206721231199774.
23. Razeghinejad MR, Nowroozzadeh MH. Anti-glaucoma medication exposure in pregnancy: an observational study and literature review. Clin Exp Optom. 2010;93(6):458–65. https://doi.org/10.1111/j.1444-0938.2010.00526.x.
24. Shrinkhal, Agrawal A, Bahadur A, et al. Intraocular pressure and tear production changes in pregnant women at term pregnancy and immediate post-partum: a pilot study. J Family Med Prim Care. 2020;9(9):5010–7. https://doi.org/10.4103/jfmpc.jfmpc_795_20.
25. Grant AD, Chung SM. The eye in pregnancy: ophthalmologic and neuro-ophthalmologic changes. Clin Obstet Gynecol. 2013;56(2):397–412.
26. Salim S. Glaucoma in pregnancy. Curr Opin Ophthalmol. 2014;25(2):93–7.
27. Pellegrino M, D'Oria L, De Luca C, et al. Glaucoma drug therapy in pregnancy: literature review and teratology information service (TIS) case series. Curr Drug Saf. 2018;13(1):3–11. https://doi.org/10.2174/1574886312666171030125804.
28. Wu P, Green M, Myers JE. Hypertensive disorders of pregnancy. BMJ. 2023;381:e071653. https://doi.org/10.1136/bmj-2022-071653.
29. Sethi HS, Naik M, Gupta VS. Management of glaucoma in pregnancy: risks or choices, a dilemma? Int J Ophthalmol. 2016;9(11):1684.
30. Hashimoto Y, Michihata N, Yamana H, et al. Intraocular pressure-lowering medications during pregnancy and risk of neonatal adverse outcomes: a propensity score analysis using a

large database. Br J Ophthalmol. 2021;105(10):1390–4. https://doi.org/10.1136/bjophthalmol-2020-316198.
31. Strelow B, Fleischman D. Glaucoma in pregnancy: an update. Curr Opin Ophthalmol. 2020;31(2):114–22.
32. Colas-Tomas T, Lopez Tizon E. Ex-PRESS mini-shunt implanted in a pregnant patient with iridocorneal endothelial syndrome. Eur J Ophthalmol. 2020;30(1):NP25–8.
33. Zehavi-Dorin T, Heinecke E, Nadkami S. Bilateral consecutive Xen gel stent surgery during pregnancy for uncontrolled early-onset primary open angle glaucoma. Am J Ophthalmol Case Rep. 2019;15:100510.
34. Razeghinejad MR, Masoumpour M, Eghbal MH, Myers JS, Moster MR. Glaucoma surgery in pregnancy: a case series and literature review. Iran J Med Sci. 2016;41(5):437–45.
35. Giorgiutti S, Jamilloux Y, Gerfaud-Valentin M, et al. The course of non-infectious uveitis in pregnancy: a retrospective study of 79 pregnancies. Graefes Arch Clin Exp Ophthalmol. 2023;261(5):1391–8. https://doi.org/10.1007/s00417-022-05949-3.
36. Chiam NPY, Lim LLP. Uveitis and gender: the course of uveitis in pregnancy. J Ophthalmol. 2014;2014(1):401915. https://doi.org/10.1155/2014/401915.
37. Ting MYL, Vega-Tapia F, Anguita R, et al. Non-infectious uveitis and pregnancy, is there an optimal treatment? Uveitis course and safety of uveitis treatment in pregnancy. Ocul Immunol Inflamm. 2024;32(8):1819–31. https://doi.org/10.1080/09273948.2023.2296030.
38. Elenkov IJ, Wilder RL, Bakalov VK, et al. IL-12, TNF-α, and hormonal changes during late pregnancy and early postpartum: implications for autoimmune disease activity during these times. J Clin Endocrinol Metabol. 2001;86(10):4933–8.
39. Magatti M, Stefani FR, Papait A, et al. Perinatal mesenchymal stromal cells and their possible contribution to fetal-maternal tolerance. Cells. 2019;8(11):1401. https://doi.org/10.3390/cells8111401.
40. Mizejewski GJ. Role of alpha-fetoprotein and derived peptides in remission of autoimmune diseases during pregnancy: a proposed mechanism of action. Ann Med Med Res. 2024;7:1081.
41. Xu X, Ray I, Tang E, Arnold BF, Acharya NR. Impact of pregnancy and the postpartum period on noninfectious uveitis flare-ups. Ocul Immunol Inflamm. 2025;33:2178–82. https://doi.org/10.1080/09273948.2025.2532826.
42. Chiam NPY, Hall AJH, Stawell RJ, et al. The course of uveitis in pregnancy and postpartum. Br J Ophthalmol. 2013;97(10):1284–8.
43. Grotting LA, Papaliodis GN. A review of the course and treatment of non-infectious uveitis during pregnancy. Semin Ophthalmol. 2017;32:75–81. Taylor & Francis.
44. Tsirouki T, Dastiridou A, Symeonidis C, et al. A focus on the epidemiology of uveitis. Ocul Immunol Inflamm. 2018;26(1):2–16. https://doi.org/10.1080/09273948.2016.1196713.
45. Artiaga JCM, Azarcon CP, Levina FD, Bromeo AJ, Mesina BVQ, Arcinue CA. Considerations in the management of ocular toxoplasmosis in pregnancy: a review of literature. Eye (Lond). 2024;38(7):1262–8. https://doi.org/10.1038/s41433-023-02916-y.
46. Reich M, Ruppenstein M, Becker MD, et al. Risk of recurrence of preexisting ocular toxoplasmosis during pregnancy. Ocul Immunol Inflamm. 2015;23(3):240–5.
47. Soheilian M, Ramazani A, Azimzadeh A, et al. Randomized trial of intravitreal clindamycin and dexamethasone versus pyrimethamine, sulfadiazine, and prednisolone in treatment of ocular toxoplasmosis. Ophthalmology. 2011;118(1):134–41.
48. Huang J, Liang C, Huang J, Liu L. Update on diabetic retinopathy during pregnancy. Eur J Ophthalmol. 2024;34(6):1695–706. https://doi.org/10.1177/11206721241248868.
49. Amoaku WM, Ghanchi F, Bailey C, et al. Diabetic retinopathy and diabetic macular oedema pathways and management: UK Consensus Working Group. Eye (Lond). 2020;34(Suppl 1):1–51. https://doi.org/10.1038/s41433-020-0961-6.
50. Errera MH, Kohly RP, Da Cruz L. Pregnancy-associated retinal diseases and their management. Surv Ophthalmol. 2013;58(2):127–42.
51. Chandrasekaran PR, Madanagopalan VG, Narayanan R. Diabetic retinopathy in pregnancy – a review. Indian J Ophthalmol. 2021;69(11):3015–25.

52. Bain SC, Klufas MA, Ho A, Matthews DR. Worsening of diabetic retinopathy with rapid improvement in systemic glucose control: a review. Diabetes Obes Metab. 2019;21(3):454–66. https://doi.org/10.1111/dom.13538.
53. Moreno A, Lozano M, Salinas P. Diabetic retinopathy. Nutr Hosp. 2013;28(Suppl 2):53–6. https://doi.org/10.3305/nh.2013.28.sup2.6714.
54. Sarvepalli SM, Bailey BA, D'Alessio D, et al. Risk factors for the development or progression of diabetic retinopathy in pregnancy: meta-analysis and systematic review. Clin Experiment Ophthalmol. 2023;51(3):195–204. https://doi.org/10.1111/ceo.14168.
55. Pomytkina NV, Sorokin EL. Investigation of diabetic retinopathy progression in women with diabetes mellitus during pregnancy. Vestn oftalmol. 2023;139(3):30–40. https://doi.org/10.17116/oftalma202313903130.
56. Toda J, Kato S, Sanaka M, Kitano S. The effect of pregnancy on the progression of diabetic retinopathy. Jpn J Ophthalmol. 2016;60(6):454–8. https://doi.org/10.1007/s10384-016-0464-y.
57. Feldman AZ, Brown FM. Management of type 1 diabetes in pregnancy. Curr Diab Rep. 2016;16(8):76. https://doi.org/10.1007/s11892-016-0765-z.
58. Feder RS, Olsen TW, Prum BE, et al. Comprehensive adult medical eye evaluation Preferred Practice Pattern® guidelines. Ophthalmology. 2016;123(1):P209–36.
59. Bourry J, Courteville H, Ramdane N, et al. Progression of diabetic retinopathy and predictors of its development and progression during pregnancy in patients with type 1 diabetes: a report of 499 pregnancies. Diabetes Care. 2021;44(1):181–7. https://doi.org/10.2337/dc20-0904.
60. Lee SC, Siebert E, Raja V, et al. Determinants of progression of diabetic retinopathy in pregnancy. Diabetes Res Clin Pract. 2024;214:111784. https://doi.org/10.1016/j.diabres.2024.111784.
61. Rosenthal JM, Johnson MW. Management of retinal diseases in pregnant patients. J Ophthalmic Vis Res. 2018;13(1):62.
62. Mohan S, Egan AM. Diagnosis and treatment of hyperglycemia in pregnancy: type 2 diabetes mellitus and gestational diabetes. Endocrinol Metab Clin N Am. 2024;53(3):335–47. https://doi.org/10.1016/j.ecl.2024.05.011.
63. Widyaputri F, Lim LL, Utami TP, et al. Prevalence of diabetes in pregnancy and microvascular complications in native Indonesian women: the Jogjakarta diabetic retinopathy initiatives in pregnancy (Jog-DRIP). PLoS One. 2022;17(6):e0267663. https://doi.org/10.1371/journal.pone.0267663.
64. Rathinavelu J, Sarvepalli SM, Bailey B, D'Alessio D, Hadziahmetovic M. The impact of pregnancy on diabetic retinopathy: a single-site study of clinical risk factors. Ophthalmic Res. 2023;66(1):1169–80. https://doi.org/10.1159/000533416.
65. Daruich A, Matet A, Dirani A, et al. Central serous chorioretinopathy: recent findings and new physiopathology hypothesis. Prog Retin Eye Res. 2015;48:82–118.
66. Morikawa M, Cho K, Kojima T, et al. Risk factors for central serous chorioretinopathy in pregnant Japanese women. J Obstet Gynaecol Res. 2017;43(5):866–72. https://doi.org/10.1111/jog.13289.
67. Yu J, Li L, Jiang C, Chang Q, Xu G. Clinical characteristics of pregnancy-associated central serous chorioretinopathy in the Chinese population. J Ophthalmol. 2021;2021:5580075. https://doi.org/10.1155/2021/5580075.
68. Leung M, Ostrovski I, Peng-Franklin M, Wyne A. Blinding lights: acute persistent vision loss in pregnancy. Obstet Med. 2025;18(1):57–9. https://doi.org/10.1177/1753495X231200658.
69. Samra KA. The eye and visual system in the preeclampsia/eclampsia syndrome: what to expect? Saudi J Ophthalmol. 2013;27(1):51–3.
70. Liu F, Yang L, Zheng Y, Zhang W, Zhi J. Effects and molecular mechanisms of AT1-AA in retinopathy of preeclampsia. Acta Biochim Biophys Sin Shanghai. 2019;51(1):51–8. https://doi.org/10.1093/abbs/gmy144.
71. Lee H, Yang SW, Kim Y, et al. Risk of retinopathy in women with pregnancy-induced hypertension: a nationwide population-based cohort study of 9-year follow-up after delivery. Am J Obstet Gynecol MFM. 2023;5(7):100985. https://doi.org/10.1016/j.ajogmf.2023.100985.

72. Sheth NT, Lee IT, Woodward JA, Dermarkarian CR. Nontraumatic orbital hematoma secondary to labor and childbirth: a case report and review of the literature. Int Ophthalmol. 2024;44(1):202. https://doi.org/10.1007/s10792-024-03149-y.
73. McNab AA. Nontraumatic orbital hemorrhage. Surv Ophthalmol. 2014;59(2):166–84. https://doi.org/10.1016/j.survophthal.2013.07.002.
74. Moss HE. Neuro-ophthalmology and pregnancy. Continuum (Minneap Minn). 2022;28(1):147–61. https://doi.org/10.1212/CON.0000000000001059.
75. Mayer-Pickel K, Mörti MG, Jetzl J, et al. Orbital hemorrhage as a primary manifestation of disseminated intravascular coagulation (DIC) associated with intrauterine fetal death and placental abruption. Case Rep Perinat Med. 2013;2(1–2):1–4.
76. Erez O, Mastrolia SA, Thachil J, et al. Disseminated intravascular coagulation in pregnancy: insights in pathophysiology, diagnosis and management. Am J Obstet Gynecol. 2015;213(4):452–63.
77. Levi M. Diagnosis and treatment of disseminated intravascular coagulation. Int J Lab Hematol. 2014;36(3):228–36.
78. Rabinovich A, Abdul-kadir R, Thachil J. DIC in obstetrics: diagnostic score, highlights in management, and international registry-communication from the DIC and Women's Health SSCs of the International Society of Thrombosis and Haemostasis. J Thromb Haemost. 2019;17(9):1562–6.
79. Lee IJ, Pulido JS, Regillo CD, Leys M. Multiple organ dysfuction syndrome and disseminated intravascular coagulation causing extensive multiple Amalrıc triangular choroidal infarctions. Retin Cases Brief Rep. 2024;18(2):251–4. https://doi.org/10.1097/ICB.0000000000001360.
80. Schönfeld CL. Bilateral exudative retinal detachment in HELLP syndrome. Case Rep Ophthalmol. 2012;3(1):35–7.
81. Pradeep A, Rao S, Kumar RR. Partial HELLP syndrome with unilateral exudative retinal detachment treated conservatively. Saudi J Ophthalmol. 2014;28(4):329–31.
82. Phang DSK, Ariffin N, Abd Aziz H, Vendargon FM, Sonny Teo KS. Bilateral serous retinal detachment in pregnancy. Cureus. 2022;14(10):e30019. https://doi.org/10.7759/cureus.30019.
83. Alsulmi E. Thrombotic thrombocytopenic purpura in pregnancy: a comprehensive review. J Perinat Med. 2025;53(6):727–32. https://doi.org/10.1515/jpm-2024-0527.
84. Yong PJ, Lim LY, Lim KY. Acute vision loss as an initial manifestation of thrombotic thrombocytopenic purpura in pregnancy: a case report. AME Med J. 2023;8:37.
85. Madike R, Cugati S, Qin Q, Chen C. Pregnancy and the eye: what do we need to watch out for? A review. Clin Exp Ophthalmol. 2024;52(2):234–47. https://doi.org/10.1111/ceo.14346.
86. Tsironi E, Gatselis N, Kotoula MG, et al. Ocular disorders as the prevailing manifestations of antiphospholipid syndrome: a case series. Cases J. 2009;2:1–6.
87. Vandevelde A, Devreese KMJ. Laboratory diagnosis of antiphospholipid syndrome: insights and hindrances. J Clin Med. 2022;11(8):2164.
88. Durrani OM, Gordon C, Murray PI. Primary anti-phospholipid antibody syndrome (APS): current concepts. Surv Ophthalmol. 2002;47(3):215–38.
89. Mezhov V, Segan JD, Tran H, et al. Antiphospholipid syndrome: a clinical review. Med J Aust. 2019;211(4):184–8.
90. Lazarus JH. Thyroid function in pregnancy. Br Med Bull. 2011;97(1):137–48.
91. Fitzpatrick DL, Russell MA. Diagnosis and management of thyroid disease in pregnancy. Obstet Gynecol Clin North Am. 2010;37(2):173–93.
92. Aranyosi JK, Deli T, Erdei A, et al. Unusual onset of thyroid associated orbitopathy during pregnancy: case report and review of literature. BMC Endocr Disord. 2020;20:1–5.
93. Burch HB, Cooper DS. Management of Graves disease: a review. JAMA. 2015;314(23):2544–54.
94. Nguyen CT, Sasso EB, Barton L, et al. Graves' hyperthyroidism in pregnancy: a clinical review. Clin Diabetes Endocrinol. 2018;4:1–9.
95. Lee AG, Pless M, Falardeau J, et al. The use of acetazolamide in idiopathic intracranial hypertension during pregnancy. Am J Ophthalmol. 2005;139(5):855–9.

96. Demarinis G, Tatti F, Taloni A, et al. Treatments for ocular diseases in pregnancy and breastfeeding: a narrative review. Pharmaceuticals (Basel). 2023;16(10):1433. https://doi.org/10.3390/ph16101433.
97. Ong AY, Kiire CA, de Silva SR, Frise C. Collaborative care for pregnant women with eye conditions. Clin Med (Lond). 2025;25(3):100314. https://doi.org/10.1016/j.clinme.2025.100314.

Chapter 17
Pregnancy and Rheumatological Diseases

Vedat Gerdan

17.1 Introduction

Pregnancy is a multilayered biological program that necessitates a marked recalibration of the immune system so that the semi-allogeneic fetus can be carried without rejection [1, 2]. The adaptations that enable fetal survival can also influence maternal autoimmunity—sometimes reducing activity, sometimes predisposing to flares. Despite advances in therapy, pregnancies complicated by SLE and/or antiphospholipid syndrome (APS) continue to carry higher risk than the obstetric background [3, 4]. This chapter summarizes the immunologic changes of pregnancy, their clinical reflections in rheumatic diseases, practical management principles, and the compatibility of frequently used antirheumatic drugs in pregnancy and lactation (Table 17.1).

17.2 Immunological Adaptations in Pregnancy and Clinical Implications

The immune system distinguishes self from non-self through the continuous interplay of innate and adaptive components. Because placental tissues bear paternal antigens, the feto-placental unit could, in principle, be perceived as an allograft; however, rather than global suppression, pregnancy is characterized by a recalibration that strengthens mutual tolerance between mother and fetus. The first trimester comprises an orderly inflammatory window orchestrated by macrophages, dendritic

V. Gerdan (✉)
Izmir Bakircay University, Faculty of Medicine, Department of Rheumatology, Izmir, Turkey
e-mail: vedat.gerdan@bakircay.edu.tr

© The Author(s), under exclusive license to Springer Nature Switzerland AG 2026

I. Karaca (ed.), *Managing Maternal Chronic Diseases for a Healthy Pregnancy*,
https://doi.org/10.1007/978-3-032-15221-3_17

Table 17.1 Antirheumatic drugs in pregnancy

Safe to use	May be used if needed	Severe or refractory cases only	Discontinue before conception	Avoid (insufficient data)
Hydroxychloroquine	IL-12/23i (ustekinumab)	IV methyl-prednisolone	Cyclophosphamide[a]	Apremilast
Sulfasalazine	IL-6i (tocilizumab, sarilumab)	IVIG	Mycophenolate[a]	Avacopan
Azathioprine	IL-1i (anakinra, canakinumab)	Sildenafil	Methotrexate	JAKi (tofacitinib, baricitinib, upadacitinib, filgotinib)
6-Mercaptopurine	IL-17i (secukinumab, ixekizumab)	C5i (eculizumab)		Voclosporin
Cyclosporine	Anti-T cell (abatacept)	IL-5i (mepolizumab)		Leflunomide (stop 5 half-lives preconception)
Tacrolimus	Anti-B cell (rituximab, belimumab)	IL-23i (guselkumab, risankizumab)		Bosentan
Colchicine	COX-2 inhibitors	IFNAR1i (anifrolumab)		
All TNFα inhibitors				
NSAIDs[b] (stop at 28 gestational week)				
Prednisone/ prednisolone (≤5 mg/day)				

This table is adapted from Rüegg et al. [48]. The original content has been reorganized and summarized by the author. Please refer to the original publication for full recommendations and detailed context

Anti-B cell B-cell-targeted therapy, *anti-T cell* T cell co-stimulation modulator, *C5i* complement protein C5 inhibitor, *COX2i* cyclooxygenase2 inhibitor, *CyC* GW, gestational week, *ILi* interleukin inhibitor, *IFNAR1i* interferonα/β receptor subunit 1 inhibitor, *IV* intravenous, *IVIG* intravenous immunoglobulin, *JAKi* kinase inhibitor, *NSAID* nonsteroidal anti-inflammatory drug, *TNFi* tumor necrosis factor inhibitor

[a]Can be considered in severe organ- or life-threatening disease during second and third trimester: cyclophosphamide, mycophenolate

[b]Restrictive use recommended: can be considered if needed to control disease activity

cells, NK cells, and neutrophils in the uterine microenvironment; thus, early pregnancy is not a period of immunosuppression [5].

The decidua contains a dense immune cell presence. In the first trimester, invasive trophoblasts are surrounded by dendritic cells, macrophages, and uterine NK cells that support trophoblast invasion. NK-cell deficiency disrupts vascular remodeling and can result in miscarriage [6]. Dendritic cells are required for decidualization and implantation [7]. Syncytiotrophoblasts lack classical MHC I/II expression and generally do not trigger maternal T-cell responses; HLA-G contributes to tolerance by limiting NK activity [7, 8].

A Th1 → Th2 inclination at the maternal–placental interface supports tolerance [9]. Th2 accumulation in the decidua and dendritic cell–mediated polarization of naïve T cells restrict excessive Th1 activity. Mediators such as progesterone, estradiol, PGD2, and leukemia inhibitory factor promote this profile [5]. Elevated Th2 cytokines (e.g., IL-4, IL-10) and monocyte colony-stimulating factor in blood and at the interface are associated with successful pregnancy [9]. IL-10, produced by cytotrophoblasts, macrophages, and Treg cells, strengthens tolerance to fetal alloantigens [10].

Regulatory T cells (Treg; CD4 + CD25+) are key players that curb autoimmunity via TGF-β and IL-10 [11]. Thymic-derived (tTreg) and peripherally induced (pTreg) populations increase in blood, lymph nodes, and thymus during pregnancy and return to baseline postpartum [9].

Across gestation, three immune phases are recognized [12]: an early inflammatory period that supports implantation and placentation, a predominantly anti-inflammatory mid-gestation that permits rapid fetal growth, and a late prepartum inflammatory rise that facilitates uterine contractions and placental separation.

17.3 Principles of Managing Rheumatic Diseases in Pregnancy

Because active disease adversely affects obstetric outcomes, maintaining control with pregnancy-compatible agents is essential. Some diseases abate in pregnancy while others flare [13]. Preconception counseling should therefore encompass timing conception for inactive disease, discussing how pregnancy may affect the disease and vice versa, and reviewing medication risk–benefit balances with the patient and family.

17.4 Pregnancy and Rheumatoid Arthritis (RA)

RA is common among women of reproductive age and poses management challenges before, during, and after pregnancy. Although roughly half of patients improve during gestation, postpartum flares are frequent [14]. When activity persists, choosing disease-modifying therapy that balances maternal control with fetal safety is critical.

17.4.1 Fertility

Fertility may be reduced in RA, prolonging time to pregnancy. Factors associated with delay include advanced age, nulliparity, high DAS28, preconception NSAID use, and daily prednisone >7.5 mg [15]. Smoking status, disease duration, RA antibody positivity, prior methotrexate use, and preconception sulfasalazine were not linked to longer time to pregnancy [15].

17.4.2 Disease Activity During Pregnancy and Postpartum

Prospective data show that universal remission does not occur in pregnancy: among those with moderate–high activity in the first trimester, only ~48% improved and ~25% reached remission by the third trimester; flares were uncommon in those without early activity [16]. Postpartum worsening occurs in ~39% [16]. A meta-analysis reported ~60% improvement in pregnancy and ~47% flares postpartum [17]. RF or anti-CCP positivity is associated with persistent activity [18]. Discontinuing TNF inhibitors after a positive pregnancy test increases flare risk; in one cohort, discontinuation was linked to CRP-associated flares, most of which abated after restarting TNFi or adding glucocorticoids [19].

17.4.3 Pregnancy Outcomes

Compared with the general population, women with active RA have increased risks of adverse obstetric outcomes, including lower birth weight and higher cesarean rates. High third-trimester activity is independently associated with reduced birth weight [20, 21]. Exposure during pregnancy to prednisone and to some permitted agents (e.g., sulfasalazine, hydroxychloroquine) has been associated with earlier delivery [21].

17.5 Pregnancy and Systemic Lupus Erythematosus (SLE)

SLE is a systemic autoimmune disease with a flare–remission pattern in women of reproductive age; fertility is usually preserved, although some treatments (e.g., cyclophosphamide) may impair it. Despite improved strategies, SLE pregnancies remain higher risk than the obstetric background [3]. Distinguishing physiological pregnancy changes and preeclampsia from SLE flares can be clinically challenging.

17.5.1 Preconception Planning and Education

Preconception counseling improves outcomes. Conception should be deferred in those with active disease until at least 6 months of stable control is achieved and, preferably, pregnancy- and breastfeeding-compatible medications are in place. Organ involvement and serologies (aPL, anti-Ro/SSA, anti-La/SSB) should be reassessed before conception.

17.5.2 Flares During Pregnancy and Postpartum

Active disease before or during pregnancy, shorter disease duration, a history of lupus nephritis, positive lupus anticoagulant (LAC), use of antihypertensives, and low platelet count have been reported as predictors of adverse pregnancy outcomes; flares occur in 25–70% across pregnancy and postpartum [22]. A meta-analysis of 2,751 pregnancies across 37 studies [23] reported maternal complications including flares (25.6%), hypertension (16.3%), nephritis (16.1%), preeclampsia (7.6%), and eclampsia (0.8%); fetal complications included spontaneous abortion (16.0%), stillbirth (3.6%), neonatal death (2.5%), and intrauterine growth restriction (12.7%); preterm birth was 39.4%. In the Hopkins cohort, flare rates increased during pregnancy and peaked in the first 3 postpartum months; hydroxychloroquine (HCQ) was protective and steroid-sparing [24]. High preconception activity consistently predicts adverse outcomes. A history of nephritis and SLEDAI ≥4 within 6 months of conception predict maternal adverse outcomes; flares during pregnancy predict fetal adverse outcomes. First-trimester hypocomplementemia and/or anti-dsDNA positivity, younger age, and primigravidity increase flare risk; nephritis flares may cluster postpartum [25]. A recent study [26] showed renal relapse rates of only ~11% in patients in renal remission prior to pregnancy, but as high as 72% in unplanned pregnancies or when full remission had not been achieved—underscoring the importance of planned conception during inactive disease.

17.5.3 Pregnancy Loss

Although pregnancy loss rates have declined over decades, they remain higher than background (recent cohorts ~10–25%) [27]. Risk increases with active disease, low complement, second-trimester anti-dsDNA positivity, APS overlap, proteinuria, thrombocytopenia, and hypertension [28]. Lupus anticoagulant is a strong predictor of first-trimester loss [29].

17.5.4 Fetal Growth Restriction (FGR) and Small for Gestational Age (SGA)

FGR is more frequent in SLE (about 5.3% vs 1.6% in the general population) and is associated with activity during pregnancy and up to six months prior to conception; HCQ use correlates with lower FGR [30–32]. SGA frequency is also increased.

17.5.5 Preeclampsia

Preeclampsia occurs in 9–25% of SLE pregnancies (vs ~5% generally). Predictors include renal involvement, aPL positivity, and thrombocytopenia. In the absence of renal disease and aPL, rates approach background (~6.1%) [22, 33].

17.5.6 Preterm Birth

Preterm birth (~30–40%) is associated with glucocorticoid exposure in pregnancy, active disease, and/or lupus nephritis [30, 33–35].

17.5.7 Differentiating SLE Flare from Preeclampsia

Lupus nephritis flares and preeclampsia can overlap clinically (proteinuria, hypertension, thrombocytopenia, renal dysfunction). Features favoring flare include prior LN, concomitant extrarenal activity, onset before 20 weeks, active urinary sediment, high anti-dsDNA and low complement, antiplatelet antibodies, and/or Coombs-positive cytopenia. Prior obstetric complications, first or multiple gestation, APS, and high uric acid favor preeclampsia; HELLP syndrome (thrombocytopenia, elevated liver enzymes, hemolysis) should be distinguished.

17.5.8 Neonatal Lupus

Passive transfer of maternal anti-Ro/SSA and anti-La/SSB antibodies can result in neonatal lupus with cutaneous and cardiac manifestations, most importantly congenital heart block (CHB). CHB risk is ~1% without a previously affected child but rises to ~17% in subsequent pregnancies after an affected child; live birth is ~80%, and many cases require pacemakers [36, 37].

17.5.9 Treating Flares and Preventing Complications

Treatment is individualized by severity and organ involvement and balanced against fetal safety. Those requiring immunosuppression should be transitioned to pregnancy-compatible agents (e.g., tacrolimus, azathioprine, cyclosporine) and observed for 4–6 months preconception. Because data on belimumab are limited, it is generally avoided; however, among ~300 first-trimester exposures, no increase in malformations has been detected [22]. Mild flares may be managed with the lowest effective doses of non-fluorinated glucocorticoids (≤20 mg prednisone equivalent, tapered to <10 mg); dexamethasone/betamethasone cross the placenta and are reserved for fetal indications. Azathioprine can be added for cutaneous/articular activity; sulfasalazine may help arthritis [38]. Moderate disease may require GC + azathioprine; refractory cases may warrant selected biologics (abatacept, anifrolumab, belimumab, rituximab) before active transplacental transfer begins. Severe flares may require higher-dose GC, IVIG, plasmapheresis, and calcineurin inhibitors; in life-threatening disease, continuation of biologics beyond the first trimester may be necessary. Cyclophosphamide is avoided in the first trimester and reserved for refractory, severe disease later in gestation [38]. HCQ should generally be continued—it is associated with lower risks of preeclampsia, FGR, preterm birth, aPL-related thrombosis, and recurrent fetal cardiac disease; particularly in SSA-positive patients, initiation by week 10 is advised [38, 39]. NSAIDs should be discontinued after 20 weeks (except for low-dose aspirin). Low-dose aspirin is recommended for SLE patients with prior preeclampsia, renal disease, or hypertension and for those with high-risk aPL profiles; LMWH is added based on APS history and risk. Vitamin D is recommended during pregnancy and lactation, particularly with GC/LMWH [22, 40].

17.6 Pregnancy and Spondyloarthritis (SpA)

SpA encompasses axial spondyloarthritis (radiographic and non-radiographic), psoriatic arthritis, reactive arthritis, and IBD-associated arthropathies. With ASAS classification and earlier imaging/serology (sacroiliac MRI, HLA-B27), recognition in women has increased. Meta-analyses report modestly increased preeclampsia and cesarean rates in axial SpA; there are tendencies toward lower birth weight, SGA, congenital anomalies, and NICU admission, but findings are not uniform [41]. A broad analysis of 21 studies showed increased preterm birth in axial SpA and PsA, and higher SGA and preeclampsia risk in axial SpA; postpartum flares are common in both groups [42, 43]. Some cohorts reported complication rates up to 48.5% in axial SpA, whereas the DESIR cohort reported a lower lifetime risk (~16.7%) [44–46]. Active disease at conception, high CRP, and discontinuation of TNF-alpha inhibitors after pregnancy confirmation or in mid-gestation increase risk; in selected cases, continuing into the third trimester may confer benefits that outweigh potential risks, with dosing adjusted to minimize placental transfer at delivery [19, 47].

17.7 Pharmacological Management in Pregnancy and Lactation

Given the unpredictability of individual disease courses, treatment adjustments should be guided by clinical activity, flare severity, and limited laboratory data, always weighing maternal benefit against fetal risk. The following summary is consistent with the 2024 EULAR recommendations [48].

17.7.1 Glucocorticoids

Non-fluorinated glucocorticoids (prednisone, prednisolone, hydrocortisone, methylprednisolone) undergo placental metabolism, keeping fetal exposure below ~10%, and are generally compatible with pregnancy and lactation. Use the lowest effective dose to limit risks of gestational diabetes, hypertension, and infection. Fluorinated glucocorticoids (dexamethasone, betamethasone) cross the placenta and are reserved for fetal indications.

17.7.2 Conventional Synthetic DMARDs (csDMARDs)

Teratogenic csDMARDs should be stopped preconception: methotrexate (3 months), mycophenolate mofetil (≥6 weeks), and cyclophosphamide (3 months). Because data on leflunomide are limited, cholestyramine or activated charcoal washout is recommended. Generally pregnancy- and lactation-compatible csDMARDs include hydroxychloroquine, colchicine, sulfasalazine, azathioprine, cyclosporine, and tacrolimus.

17.7.3 Targeted Synthetic DMARDs (tsDMARDs)

Apremilast and JAK inhibitors (tofacitinib, baricitinib, upadacitinib) are contraindicated in pregnancy and lactation; their short half-lives make discontinuation about one month before planned conception practical.

17.7.4 Biologic DMARDs (bDMARDs)

Anti-TNF agents are generally considered acceptable during pregnancy. When disease control requires it, selected non-TNF biologics (e.g., secukinumab, abatacept, anakinra, rituximab, belimumab, canakinumab, ixekizumab, ustekinumab, sarilumab, tocilizumab) may be considered on a case-by-case basis, taking placental transfer timing into account; agents with very limited data (anifrolumab, eculizumab, guselkumab, mepolizumab, risankizumab) should be reserved for refractory situations.

17.7.5 Biosimilars and Pregnancy

Although comprehensive pregnancy data remain limited, biosimilars share molecular targets and antibody structures with their reference products; thus, their use may be considered based on evidence for the originators.

17.7.6 Analgesics, Adjuvants, and Vaccines

Intermittent NSAID use is possible in early pregnancy, but guidelines recommend discontinuation between 20 and 28 weeks; short-half-life nonselective agents (e.g., ibuprofen) are preferred. NSAID cessation may be considered in subfertility. Codeine may be used short-term in pregnancy and warrants caution during lactation. Amitriptyline is acceptable; data for gabapentin and pregabalin in gestation are insufficient. Non-live vaccines are safe in infants with intrauterine biologic exposure; timing of live vaccines in the first 6 months depends on the specific drug and extent of transplacental transfer.

17.7.7 Special (Exceptional) Situations

In severe, refractory maternal disease, pulse intravenous methylprednisolone, IVIG, sildenafil, pregnancy-compatible conventional and/or biologic DMARDs, or—exceptionally—cyclophosphamide or mycophenolate mofetil may be considered in the second and third trimesters.

17.7.8 *Lactation*

Most agents compatible with pregnancy are also compatible with breastfeeding: hydroxychloroquine, colchicine, sulfasalazine, azathioprine, cyclosporine, tacrolimus; as well as prednisone/prednisolone, pulse methylprednisolone, IVIG, and non-selective NSAIDs. Many biologics (TNFi and selected non-TNFi) are also considered acceptable during lactation.

17.8 Conclusion

The best outcomes in pregnancies complicated by rheumatic disease are achieved through advance planning, trimester-specific monitoring, and balanced treatment using agents with acceptable maternal–fetal safety. Close collaboration between rheumatology and obstetrics (and nephrology/hematology when needed) is central to harmonizing maternal disease control with fetal well-being.

References

1. Abu-Raya B, Michalski C, Sadarangani M, Lavoie PM. Maternal immunological adaptation during normal pregnancy. Front Immunol. 2020;11:575197.
2. Mor G, Cardenas I, Abrahams V, Guller S. Inflammation and pregnancy: the role of the immune system at the implantation site. Ann N Y Acad Sci. 2011;1221:80–7.
3. Clowse ME. Pregnancy in women with lupus: we have come so far and have so far to go. Ann Intern Med. 2019;171(3):212–3.
4. Yelnik CM, Porter TF, Branch DW, et al. Brief report: changes in antiphospholipid antibody titers during pregnancy: effects on pregnancy outcomes. Arthritis Rheumatol. 2016;68(8):1964–9.
5. Orefice R. Immunology and the immunological response in pregnancy. Best Pract Res Clin Obstet Gynaecol. 2021;76:3–12.
6. Moffett A, Colucci F. Uterine NK cells: active regulators at the maternal-fetal interface. J Clin Invest. 2014;124:1872–9.
7. Tilburgs T, Evans JH, Crespo ÂC, Strominger JL. The HLA-G cycle provides for both NK tolerance and immunity at the maternal-fetal interface. Proc Natl Acad Sci USA. 2015;112:13312–7.
8. Ferreira LMR, Meissner TB, Tilburgs T, Strominger JL. HLA-G: at the interface of maternal-fetal tolerance. Trends Immunol. 2017;38:272–86.
9. Mor G, Cardenas I. The immune system in pregnancy: a unique complexity. Am J Reprod Immunol. 2010;63:425–33.
10. Chen SJ, Liu YL, Sytwu HK. Immunologic regulation in pregnancy: from mechanism to therapeutic strategy for immunomodulation. Clin Dev Immunol. 2010;64(4):231e44.
11. Chen T, Darrasse-Jeze G, Bergot AS, Courau T, Churland G, Valdivia K, et al. Self-specific memory regulatory T cells protect embryos at implantation in mice. J Immunol. 2013;191(5):2272e81.
12. Förger F, Villiger PM. Immunological adaptations in pregnancy that modulate rheumatoid arthritis disease activity. Nat Rev Rheumatol. 2020;16(2):113–22.
13. Andreoli L, et al. Disease activity assessment of rheumatic diseases during pregnancy: a comprehensive review of indices used in clinical studies. Autoimmun Rev. 2019;18(2):164–76.

14. Giles I, Yee CS, Gordon C. Stratifying management of rheumatic disease for pregnancy and breastfeeding. Nat Rev Rheumatol. 2019;15(7):391–402.
15. Littlejohn EA. Pregnancy and rheumatoid arthritis. Best Pract Res Clin Obstet Gynaecol. 2020;64:52–8.
16. de Man YA, Dolhain RJ, van de Geijn FE, Willemsen SP, Hazes JM. Disease activity of rheumatoid arthritis during pregnancy: results from a nationwide prospective study. Arthritis Rheum. 2008;59(9):1241e8.
17. Jethwa H, Lam S, Smith C, Giles I. Does rheumatoid arthritis really improve during pregnancy? A systematic review and metaanalysis. J Rheumatol. 2019;46(3):245e50.
18. Förger F, Vallbracht I, Helmke K, Villiger PM, Østensen M. Pregnancy mediated improvement of rheumatoid arthritis. Swiss Med Wkly. 2012;142
19. van den Brandt S, Zbinden A, Baeten D, Villiger PM, Østensen M, F€orger F. Risk factors for flare and treatment of disease flares during pregnancy in rheumatoid arthritis and axial spondyloarthritis patients. Arthritis Res Ther. 2017;19(1):64.
20. Keeling S, Bowker S, Savu A, Kaul P. A population level analysis of the differing impacts of rheumatoid arthritis and spondyloarthritis on peripartum outcomes. J Rheumatol. 2019:181320.
21. De Man YA, Hazes JMW, Van Der Heide H, Willemsen SP, de Groot CJ, Steegers EA, et al. Association of higher rheumatoid arthritis disease activity during pregnancy with lower birth weight: results of a national prospective study. Arthritis Rheum. 2009;60:3196e206.
22. Zucchi D, Fischer-Betz R, Tani C. Pregnancy in systemic lupus erythematosus. Best Pract Res Clin Rheumatol. 2023;37(4):101860.
23. Smyth A, Oliveira GH, Lahr BD, et al. A systematic review and meta-analysis of pregnancy outcomes in patients with systemic lupus erythematosus and lupus nephritis. Clin J Am Soc Nephrol. 2010;5(11):2060–8.
24. Cortes-Hernandez J, Ordi-Ros J, Paredes F, et al. Clinical predictors of fetal and maternal outcome in systemic lupus erythematosus: a prospective study of 103 pregnancies. Rheumatology. 2002;41(6):643–50.
25. Kwok LW, Tam LS, Zhu T, Leung YY, Li E. Predictors of maternal and fetal outcomes in pregnancies of patients with systemic lupus erythematosus. Lupus. 2011;20(8):829–36.
26. Chen Y, Li K, Zhang H, et al. Good pregnancy outcomes in lupus nephritis patients with complete renal remission. Nephrol Dial Transplant. 2022;37(10):1888–94.
27. Clark CA, Spitzer KA, Laskin CA. Decrease in pregnancy loss rates in patients with systemic lupus erythematosus over a 40-year period. J Rheumatol. 2005;32(9):1709–12.
28. Clowse ME, Magder LS, Witter F, et al. Early risk factors for pregnancy loss in lupus. Obstet Gynecol. 2006;107(2 Pt 1):293–9.
29. Mankee A, Petri M, Magder LS. Lupus anticoagulant, disease activity and low complement in the first trimester are predictive of pregnancy loss. Lupus Sci Med. 2015;2:e000095.
30. Chakravarty EF, Nelson L, Krishnan E. Obstetric hospitalizations in the United States for women with systemic lupus erythematosus and rheumatoid arthritis. Arthritis Rheum. 2006;54(3):899–907.
31. Canti V, Scarrone M, De Lorenzo R, et al. Low incidence of intrauterine growth restriction in pregnant patients with systemic lupus erythematosus taking hydroxychloroquine. Immunol Med. 2021;44(3):204–10. Clark CA, Spitzer KA, Nadler JN, et al. Preterm deliveries in women with systemic lupus erythematosus. J Rheumatol 2003;30(10):2127–32
32. Kim SY, Lee JH. Prognosis of neonates in pregnant women with systemic lupus erythematosus. Yonsei Med J. 2008;49(4):515–20.
33. Tani C, Zucchi D, Haase I, et al. Impact of low-dose acetylsalicylic acid on pregnancy outcome in systemic lupus erythematosus: results from a multicentre study. Lupus Sci Med. 2022;9(1)
34. Wei S, Lai K, Yang Z, et al. Systemic lupus erythematosus and risk of preterm birth: a systematic review and meta-analysis of observational studies. Lupus. 2017;26(6):563–71.
35. Skorpen CG, Lydersen S, Gilboe IM, et al. Influence of disease activity and medications on offspring birth weight, pre-eclampsia and preterm birth in systemic lupus erythematosus: a population-based study. Ann Rheum Dis. 2018;77(2):264–9.

36. Llanos C, Izmirly PM, Katholi M, et al. Recurrence rates of cardiac manifestations associated with neonatal lupus and maternal/fetal risk factors. Arthritis Rheum. 2009;60(10):3091–7.
37. Fredi M, Andreoli L, Bacco B, et al. First report of the Italian registry on immune-mediated congenital heart block (Lu.Ne registry). Front Cardiovasc Med. 2019;6:11.
38. Andreoli L, et al. EULAR recommendations for women's health and the management of family planning, assisted reproduction, pregnancy and menopause in patients with systemic lupus erythematosus and/or antiphospholipid syndrome. Ann Rheum Dis. 2017;76(3):476.
39. Sammaritano LR, Bermas BL, Chakravarty EE, et al. American college of rheumatology guideline for the management of reproductive health in rheumatic and musculoskeletal diseases. Arthritis Rheumatol. 2020;72(4):529–56.
40. Clark KEN, Giles I. Updates on the antiphospholipid syndrome. Medicine. 2024;52(12):778–85.
41. Maguire S, O'Dwyer T, Mockler D, O'Shea F, Wilson F. Pregnancy in axial spondyloarthropathy: a systematic review & meta-analysis. Semin Arthritis Rheum. 2020;50(6):1269–79.
42. Hamroun S, Hamroun A, Bigna JJ, Allado E, Förger F, Molto A. Fertility and pregnancy outcomes in women with spondyloarthritis: a systematic review and meta-analysis. Rheumatology (Oxford). 2022;61(4):1314–27.
43. Østensen M, Fuhrer L, Mathieu R, Seitz M, Villiger PM. A prospective study of pregnant patients with rheumatoid arthritis and ankylosing spondylitis using validated clinical instruments. Ann Rheum Dis. 2004;63:1212–7.
44. Maguire S, Wilson F, Gallagher P, Mohamed MM, Maher S, O'Shea F. What to expect when women with axial spondyloarthritis are expecting: prevalence of complications of pregnancies in women with axial spondyloarthritis. Semin Arthritis Rheum. 2022;54:151993.
45. Pons M, Dougados M, Costedoat-Chalumeau N, et al. Pregnancy rates and outcomes in early axial spondyloarthritis: an analysis of the DESIR cohort. Joint Bone Spine. 2021;88(2):105075.
46. Zbinden A, van den Brandt S, Østensen M, Villiger PM, Förger F. Risk for adverse pregnancy outcome in axial spondyloarthritis and rheumatoid arthritis: disease activity matters. Rheumatology (Oxford). 2018;57(7):1235–42.
47. Wright GC, Kaine J, Deodhar A. Understanding differences between men and women with axial spondyloarthritis. Semin Arthritis Rheum. 2020;50:687–94.
48. Rüegg L, et al. EULAR recommendations for use of antirheumatic drugs in reproduction, pregnancy, and lactation: 2024 update. Ann Rheum Dis. 2025 Jun;84(6):910–926. https://doi.org/10.1016/j.ard.2025.02.023. Epub 2025 Apr 26. PMID: 40287311.

Chapter 18
Neoplastic Diseases During Pregnancy

Mücahit Furkan Balcı

18.1 Introduction

Due to the increasing maternal age in developed countries, the coexistence of malignancies with pregnancy is reported at a rare frequency, occurring in approximately 1 in 1000 to 1 in 2000 pregnancies [1, 2]. Among the most frequently encountered benign neoplasms during pregnancy are uterine leiomyomas and ovarian cysts [3]. The most common malignancies diagnosed during pregnancy include breast neoplasms (1 in 5000 pregnancies), thyroid neoplasms (1 in 7000 pregnancies), and cervical neoplasms (1 in 8500 pregnancies) [4]. Together with lymphomas and melanomas, these malignancies account for approximately 65% of all cancer cases occurring during pregnancy [5]. In contrast, less frequently encountered but more prognostically unfavorable malignancies include lung and gastric cancers [6–8]. The incidence of malignancies diagnosed during pregnancy and within 12 months postpartum is summarized in Table 18.1 [4].

Pregnancy itself is not considered a predisposing factor for the development of malignancy [8, 9]. However, because certain clinical signs of malignancy may be attributed to normal pregnancy-related changes, diagnosis is often delayed [2]. This delay can lead to complex ethical, emotional, and therapeutic dilemmas for the obstetrician [9]. Therefore, treatment planning should be individualized, considering both maternal and fetal well-being, and should be conducted in collaboration with a multidisciplinary team (MDT). This team should include specialists such as a gynecologic oncologist, medical and clinical oncologist, radiologist, and perinatologist [1].

Decisions regarding pregnancy termination or iatrogenic preterm delivery are often highly complex and require comprehensive evaluation by a tumor board [6, 10]. The MDT must provide the parents with clear, informative guidance regarding

M. F. Balcı (✉)
Izmir Torbali State Hospital, Department of Obstetrics and Gynecology, Izmir, Turkey

© The Author(s), under exclusive license to Springer Nature Switzerland AG 2026

I. Karaca (ed.), *Managing Maternal Chronic Diseases for a Healthy Pregnancy*,
https://doi.org/10.1007/978-3-032-15221-3_18

Table 18.1 Distribution of malignancies diagnosed during pregnancy and within 12 months postpartum

Malignancy	Percentage (%)
Breast cancer	16.2
Cervical cancer	13.5
Lymphoma	12.1
Thyroid cancer	10.6
Ovarian cancer	10.5
Melanoma	9.6
Leukemia	7.1
Neural tumors	4.4
Gastrointestinal cancers	3.5

oncologic prognosis, the urgency of initiating treatment, and available therapeutic options [6, 10].

Physiological changes and common symptoms associated with pregnancy can prolong the interval between disease onset and the initiation of treatment [6]. Therefore, persistent fatigue, anemia, postcoital bleeding, abnormal vaginal discharge or bleeding, breast tenderness, or a palpable mass should be carefully assessed through thorough clinical examination [1]. A detailed medical history should be obtained at the onset of every pregnancy, with a focused physical examination to identify any genetic predisposition to malignancy (e.g., a strong family history of breast or ovarian cancer, BRCA1/BRCA2 mutations) or other risk factors [11]. Newly arising symptoms should be thoroughly investigated before attributing them solely to pregnancy [11]. When symptoms are present, the physical examination should include not only the breasts, genital tract, and uterus, but also the skin and peripheral lymph nodes [11].

Importantly, it has been demonstrated that prognosis and survival rates do not significantly differ between pregnant and nonpregnant patients when stratified by cancer stage [9]. To minimize fetal exposure to radiation or potentially harmful diagnostic procedures, unnecessary imaging and testing should be avoided. Diagnostic pathways should be optimized early in the evaluation process with close coordination by the MDT [12].

18.2 Principles of Cancer Treatment During Pregnancy

The management of women diagnosed with cancer during pregnancy requires a multidisciplinary and individualized approach that ensures both maternal health and fetal safety. Treatment strategies should be tailored based on cancer type and stage, gestational age, and the patient's preferences regarding continuation of pregnancy (Table 18.2) [7, 10].

Table 18.2 Trimester-based feasibility of cancer treatment modalities during pregnancy

Treatment modality	First trimester	Second–third trimester
Surgery	Risky; performed only if necessary	Generally feasible
Chemotherapy	Contraindicated	Selectively feasible
Radiotherapy	Contraindicated	Limited use with fetal shielding
Immunotherapy	Insufficient data	Use with caution
Targeted therapy	Generally not recommended	Consider only if strictly necessary

18.2.1 Surgical Management

Surgical procedures for diagnosis, staging, or treatment can often be performed safely during pregnancy. Interventions that do not directly involve gynecologic organs are generally well-tolerated by both mother and fetus. Although some surgeries are scheduled after 12–14 weeks of gestation to avoid the risk of miscarriage in the first trimester, surgery should not be delayed when maternal health is at risk, regardless of gestational age.

Both pregnancy and malignancy independently increase the risk of venous thromboembolism. Therefore, patients undergoing surgery should receive low-molecular-weight heparin along with mechanical thromboprophylaxis (e.g., compression stockings) [13].

18.2.2 Diagnostic Imaging

Imaging during pregnancy should be planned to minimize fetal exposure. Ultrasonography remains the first-line modality. When necessary, computed tomography (CT) with appropriate abdominal shielding may be used, particularly in the evaluation of extra-abdominal pathologies. The American College of Obstetricians and Gynecologists (ACOG) recommends that clinically indicated imaging should not be delayed if it would affect treatment decisions [14].

Magnetic resonance imaging (MRI) is preferred from the second trimester onward. Gadolinium-based contrast agents can cross the placenta and accumulate in the fetus; hence, their use is reserved for essential cases and avoided during the first trimester [15]. Positron emission tomography (PET) is contraindicated due to fetal radiation exposure.

18.2.3 Radiotherapy

Radiation therapy may cause severe fetal complications depending on dose, target site, and field size. The period of organogenesis (first trimester) is particularly sensitive, during which fetal cell death, growth restriction, microcephaly, and neurodevelopmental disorders may occur [16]. Radiotherapy to the abdominal region is contraindicated due to high fetal risk; however, with proper shielding, localized radiotherapy to thoracic or cervical regions may be feasible.

18.2.4 Chemotherapy

Most chemotherapeutic agents, particularly during organogenesis in the first trimester, are associated with an increased risk of major malformations. As such, chemotherapy is typically initiated after the first trimester [10]. Chemotherapy administered after organogenesis is not strongly associated with short-term severe fetal complications.

Chemotherapy is not recommended within 3 weeks of delivery due to increased risk of maternal neutropenia, infection, and postpartum hemorrhage. Moreover, as neonates have limited capacity to eliminate chemotherapy metabolites, breastfeeding is contraindicated during chemotherapy [17].

18.2.5 Molecular Therapies and Growth Factors

Limited but reassuring data exist on the use of colony-stimulating factors such as filgrastim (Neupogen) and pegfilgrastim (Neulasta) during pregnancy. Similarly, data support the safety of erythropoietic agents like epoetin alfa in pregnant patients [7].

18.2.6 Immunotherapy and Targeted Therapies

The use of targeted therapies such as monoclonal antibodies and tyrosine kinase inhibitors during pregnancy is based on limited evidence. Some of these agents have potential teratogenic effects; thus, their use should only be considered when the maternal benefit clearly outweighs the fetal risk [18].

Table 18.3 Key considerations in cancer treatment during pregnancy

Key topic	Critical points
Timing of diagnosis	Gestational age is crucial in planning diagnosis and treatment timing
Organogenesis period	Chemotherapy and radiotherapy are contraindicated
Surgery	May be performed regardless of gestational age if clinically indicated
Imaging	MRI and ultrasound are preferred; CT may be used with shielding
Chemotherapy	May be initiated after the second trimester; should be discontinued ≥3 weeks before delivery
Fetal monitoring	Serial assessments of fetal growth and anatomy are recommended
Fertility	Fertility preservation options should be discussed prior to treatment
Breastfeeding	Not recommended during chemotherapy

18.2.7 Fertility and Pregnancy After Cancer Treatment

Chemotherapy and radiotherapy—especially when administered at a young age—may have lasting effects on fertility. Oncofertility counseling should be offered prior to treatment, including options such as oocyte or embryo cryopreservation, ovarian transposition, or ovarian protection with GnRH analogs [19].

In women who have undergone pelvic radiotherapy, reduced uterine volume may lead to complications such as preterm birth, low birth weight, or postpartum hemorrhage [20]. Nonetheless, studies indicate that children born to women treated for cancer in childhood do not have a significantly increased risk of congenital malformations [21].

18.2.8 Placental Metastases

Placental metastasis is rare but has been reported in association with malignancies such as melanoma, leukemia, lymphoma, and breast cancer. In such cases, histopathologic examination of the placenta is recommended. Fetal metastasis is uncommon, with melanoma being the most frequently reported cause. When fetal metastases occur, they most commonly involve the liver and skin and are associated with high mortality [22] (Table 18.3) [14, 15].

18.3 Reproductive Tract Neoplasms

Benign neoplasms of the female reproductive system are frequently encountered, with uterine leiomyomas, ovarian tumors, and endocervical polyps being the most commonly identified. In contrast, malignancies of these organs constitute the most prevalent cancers diagnosed during pregnancy. Among gynecological cancers observed in pregnant women, cervical malignancies are the most dominant.

18.3.1 Endocervical Polyps

Benign, premalignant, and malignant cervical neoplasms are not uncommonly diagnosed during pregnancy. Endocervical polyps represent benign hyperplastic growths of the endocervical stroma, covered by epithelial tissue. They are often asymptomatic and incidentally discovered during the initial pelvic examination. However, some patients may present with intermenstrual or postcoital bleeding. These lesions typically manifest as red, smooth-surfaced, elongated, fleshy masses protruding from the endocervical canal. Although usually benign, they may be associated with cytological abnormalities such as atypical glandular cells (AGC) on Pap smear [23, 24].

Malignant transformation of endocervical polyps is rare. Nonetheless, some polypoid cervical carcinomas may mimic these benign lesions, and for this reason, most clinical guidelines recommend polypectomy followed by histopathological evaluation [25, 26].

Pedunculated polyps may be removed using ring forceps or polyp forceps by twisting at the stalk to achieve vascular strangulation. To achieve hemostasis at the base, application of Monsel's solution (ferric subsulfate) is commonly employed. In cases of broad-based polyps, surgical excision may be warranted [27].

18.3.2 Cervical Epithelial Neoplasia and Screening Approaches During Pregnancy

Pregnancy presents a critical opportunity for the screening of premalignant and malignant cervical epithelial lesions, particularly in women without regular access to healthcare services. Pap smear testing performed during prenatal visits serves as a key component of this screening. It is essential to indicate pregnancy status on the laboratory request form, as physiological changes associated with pregnancy—such as glandular epithelial hyperplasia, the Arias-Stella reaction, and the presence of decidual cells—may complicate cytological interpretation [28].

The cervical cancer screening guidelines revised by the American Society for Colposcopy and Cervical Pathology (ASCCP) in 2012 are applicable to pregnant women as well. According to these guidelines:

1. Screening is not recommended for women under 21 years of age.
2. For women aged 21–29, cytology (Pap smear) alone every 3 years is sufficient.
3. For women aged 30 years and older, co-testing (cytology + high-risk HPV) every 5 years or cytology alone every 3 years is acceptable [29].

However, these general screening recommendations may be inadequate for high-risk populations, including women with a history of diethylstilbestrol (DES) exposure, prior cervical cancer, or immunosuppression.

18.3.3 High-Risk HPV Serotypes and Pregnancy

Certain high-risk human papillomavirus (HPV) serotypes—particularly types 16, 18, 31, 35, 45, 51, 52, and 56—are strongly associated with high-grade intraepithelial lesions and invasive cervical cancer. Some studies suggest that the prevalence of HPV infection may be higher in pregnant women compared to nonpregnant counterparts [3]. Accordingly, co-testing for high-risk HPV types is recommended during cervical screening in women aged 30 years and above.

For cytological evaluation, cells may be collected into liquid-based cytology media, such as PreservCyt solution used in the ThinPrep Pap test. Additionally, methods such as the Cobas HPV test or Digene HC2 HPV DNA test can be employed using designated transport media [30].

18.3.4 HPV Vaccination and Pregnancy

Given the clear association between HPV infection and cervical neoplasia, prophylactic vaccination has become an important preventive measure. Two vaccines are approved by the U.S. Food and Drug Administration (FDA): the quadrivalent vaccine (Gardasil, targeting HPV types 6, 11, 16, and 18) and the bivalent vaccine (Cervarix, targeting types 16 and 18). Both vaccines are recommended for girls and women aged 9–26 years. These vaccinations have been shown to significantly reduce the incidence of high-grade cervical dysplasia and cervical cancer [31, 32].

HPV vaccination is not recommended during pregnancy. If a woman becomes pregnant during the vaccination series, further doses should be postponed until after delivery. Available data indicate no adverse pregnancy outcomes related to vaccination [33]. As these are inactivated (non-live) vaccines, they may be safely administered during the postpartum breastfeeding period. The standard vaccination schedule includes three doses: at 0, 1–2 months, and 6 months.

18.3.5 Management of Abnormal Cervical Cytology During Pregnancy

The incidence of abnormal cervical cytology during pregnancy is comparable or possibly slightly higher than observed in nonpregnant women. Management of abnormal cytologic findings in pregnancy should follow the recommendations of the American Society for Colposcopy and Cervical Pathology (ASCCP). In most cases, colposcopy is warranted to rule out invasive disease, particularly in cases of high-grade lesions or cytological suspicion of malignancy [34].

Due to eversion of the cervix during pregnancy, the transformation zone is more easily visualized, allowing for generally adequate colposcopic assessment. If visualization is suboptimal, repeat colposcopy can be scheduled 6–8 weeks later, by which time the squamocolumnar junction often everts further [35].

If invasive disease is excluded, further colposcopy or cytology is not routinely recommended during pregnancy. Postpartum reevaluation should be deferred for at least 6 weeks to allow cervical healing prior to further cytological assessment [29].

18.3.6 Cervical Intraepithelial Neoplasia (CIN)

Women diagnosed histologically with cervical intraepithelial neoplasia (CIN) during pregnancy are generally candidates for vaginal delivery. Treatment of CIN 1 is typically deferred until the postpartum period. In patients with CIN 2 or CIN 3, if invasive disease has been ruled out and gestational age is advanced, follow-up with colposcopy and cytology at intervals shorter than 12 weeks is not recommended. If lesion progression is suspected or cytology indicates possible invasion, repeat biopsy should be considered [36].

It is important to note that CIN lesions may regress either during pregnancy or in the postpartum period. In a study involving 1079 pregnant women, spontaneous postpartum regression of cervical dysplasia was observed in 61% of cases [37]. Similarly, Yost and colleagues reported a 70% regression rate in CIN 2–3 cases postpartum. Only 7% of patients with CIN 2 progressed to CIN 3, and none developed invasive carcinoma [38]. Among 77 pregnant patients diagnosed with carcinoma in situ (CIS), spontaneous regression occurred in 33%, persistent CIS in 66%, and only two cases progressed to microscopic invasion postpartum [39].

Adenocarcinoma in situ (AIS) is generally managed similarly to CIN 3. Unless invasive disease is confirmed, definitive treatment of AIS should also be deferred for at least 6 weeks postpartum [40].

18.3.7 *Cervical Conization*

Cervical conization may be indicated if there is suspicion of an invasive epithelial lesion. This procedure may be performed via loop electrosurgical excision procedure (LEEP) or cold knife conization. However, due to the increased risk of complications during pregnancy—including miscarriage, membrane rupture, bleeding, and preterm birth—conization should be postponed whenever possible [41].

In a series involving 376 pregnant women who underwent cervical conization, residual neoplasia was identified in 43% of cases, and nearly 10% required transfusion due to bleeding [42]. Cervical stenosis may occur as a rare complication following prepregnancy CIN treatment; however, in most cases, this resolves spontaneously during labor. In certain cases, failure of cervical dilation due to fibrosis may require manual dilatation.

Cold knife conization has long been associated with an increased risk of cervical insufficiency and preterm delivery. The impact of LEEP on preterm birth is less clear: some studies report an elevated risk, while others do not support this association [43, 44]. Additionally, women with CIN, even in the absence of excisional treatment, appear to be at increased risk of preterm birth compared to the general population [45, 46].

18.3.8 *Invasive Cervical Cancer in Pregnancy*

In the United States, the incidence of invasive cervical carcinoma has significantly declined, with its occurrence during pregnancy estimated at approximately 1 in 8500 pregnancies [47]. Diagnosis is most commonly established through colposcopically guided biopsy, conization, or biopsy of a grossly abnormal lesion. Histologically, approximately 75% of cervical cancers are squamous cell carcinomas, while 20–25% are adenocarcinomas [48].

Lesions may demonstrate either exophytic or endophytic growth patterns and may appear as polypoid masses, papillomatous projections, barrel-shaped cervices, ulcerative or granular masses, or necrotic tissue. Watery discharge, foul-smelling or bloody discharge may also be present. Suspicious lesions should be biopsied using Tischler forceps whenever feasible.

18.3.9 *Staging and Imaging*

Staging of cervical cancer is performed clinically. Approximately 70% of pregnant patients are diagnosed at stage I [11]. However, physiological changes in pregnancy may obscure accurate staging and result in underestimation of disease extent. Softening of the cervix and parametrium can hinder detection of tumor infiltration on physical examination. Staging typically involves pelvic examination, renal ultrasonography, chest X-ray, cystoscopy, proctoscopy, and, if necessary, conization . Although not formally included in FIGO staging, magnetic resonance imaging (MRI) without contrast may be used beyond the first trimester to assess ureteral and lymph node involvement [49].

18.3.10 Management and Prognosis

Management of cervical cancer during pregnancy must be individualized, taking into account the clinical stage, gestational age, and maternal desire for pregnancy continuation. Stage IA1 disease is defined as microinvasive cancer with a depth of invasion less than 3 mm and horizontal spread less than 7 mm [47]. In patients diagnosed by conization, pregnancy may proceed with vaginal delivery, and definitive treatment can be scheduled at least 6 weeks postpartum, following the same principles as CIN management.

However, truly invasive cancers require prompt treatment. If diagnosed in the first trimester, termination of pregnancy is commonly recommended to initiate therapy. In contrast, patients diagnosed in later gestation may be candidates for delayed treatment until fetal lung maturity. Studies involving 40 women with stage I or IIA disease diagnosed after 20 weeks of gestation reported that treatment delay was safe in selected cases without widespread disease [50, 51].

Alternatively, staging may be completed via laparoscopic pelvic lymphadenectomy. If no metastasis is found, definitive treatment can be postponed until after delivery [52, 53]. Neoadjuvant platinum-based chemotherapy is also emerging as an effective treatment option during pregnancy [53].

18.3.11 Surgery and Radiotherapy

In early-stage disease (stage I and early IIA), radical hysterectomy with pelvic lymphadenectomy remains the preferred surgical approach [54]. If the pregnancy is less than 20 weeks, surgery may be performed with the fetus in situ. At later gestational ages, cesarean section (hysterotomy) is performed prior to hysterectomy. Radiotherapy, while effective, carries a risk of permanent ovarian and sexual dysfunction, as well as urinary and bowel damage. In stage IB disease, complication rates with radiotherapy may reach up to 30%, compared to approximately 7% with surgery [55].

Fertility-sparing treatments have been successfully applied in selected early-stage cases. For example, five women underwent abdominal radical trachelectomy before 20 weeks' gestation, all of whom achieved successful delivery [55]. In another study, four women diagnosed with adenocarcinoma at 16–23 weeks' gestation were treated successfully with laser conization [56].

18.3.12 Advanced Disease and Radiotherapy

Radiotherapy is the primary treatment modality in advanced-stage cervical cancer. If initiated during the first trimester, external beam radiation often leads to spontaneous abortion; if not, pregnancy termination is typically required. In the second trimester, delayed abortion may necessitate hysterotomy [57].

Survival outcomes for invasive cervical cancer during pregnancy are similar to those in nonpregnant women when adjusted for stage. In a case-control study involving 44 patients, the 5-year overall survival rate was approximately 80% in both pregnant and nonpregnant groups [58].

18.3.13 Mode of Delivery

The impact of vaginal delivery through a cancer-involved cervix on prognosis remains unclear. Therefore, the route of delivery is controversial. In cases of large or friable lesions, severe hemorrhage may occur during vaginal delivery. Additionally, tumor implantation along the episiotomy site has been reported [59]. As a result, many experts prefer cesarean delivery, and a classical (vertical) uterine incision is often recommended to avoid transecting the tumor.

18.3.14 Pregnancy Following Radical Trachelectomy

Pregnancy is feasible following fertility-sparing radical trachelectomy for stage IB1–IB2 cervical cancer. In this procedure, the cervix is amputated at the level of the internal os and a permanent cerclage is placed at the uterovaginal junction. Consequently, all subsequent deliveries must be performed via classical cesarean section [60].

In a cohort of 123 women followed at a single center, 63 attempted to conceive, resulting in 28 live births among 19 patients. All deliveries were conducted by classical cesarean section, and one-fourth occurred before 32 weeks of gestation [61, 62].

18.3.15 Uterine Leiomyomas (Fibroids) in Pregnancy

Uterine leiomyomas, commonly referred to as “myomas” or—erroneously—“fibroids,” are benign smooth muscle tumors. Their incidence during pregnancy is approximately 2%, though this varies with the frequency of routine ultrasonography and demographic characteristics of the population [63, 64]. For instance, in a study involving 4271 women, first-trimester leiomyoma prevalence was 18% among Black women compared to 8% among white women [65].

Leiomyomas may be classified by location as submucosal, subserosal, or intramural. Less commonly, they may arise in the cervix or broad ligament. Some may develop parasitic blood supply, particularly from adjacent structures such as the omentum. A rare variant, disseminated peritoneal leiomyomatosis, involves widespread subperitoneal smooth muscle proliferation and may clinically mimic peritoneal carcinomatosis. This condition is believed to result from estrogen-induced differentiation of subcoelomic mesenchymal cells into smooth muscle tissue [66].

18.3.16 Growth Dynamics and Diagnosis During Pregnancy

The growth behavior of leiomyomas during pregnancy is variable; some may shrink, others may enlarge rapidly, or remain unchanged [67]. Because they may mimic adnexal masses, ultrasonography is a valuable diagnostic tool. If imaging is inconclusive, non-contrast MRI may be considered after the second trimester [68]. Once diagnosed, routine serial imaging is generally unnecessary unless complications are anticipated.

18.3.17 Symptoms and Clinical Course

Leiomyomas are frequently asymptomatic. However, when tumor size increases, chronic compression-related pain may occur. In such cases, nonnarcotic analgesics are typically effective. Occasionally, compromised blood supply to the tumor may result in hemorrhagic infarction, known as "red degeneration" (carneous degeneration), which presents as acute abdominal pain, localized tenderness, low-grade fever, and leukocytosis. Differential diagnosis includes appendicitis, placental abruption, ureteral stones, or pyelonephritis. Diagnosis is usually made by exclusion [69].

Pain management is the primary treatment, and symptoms generally resolve within a few days. In cases of threatened preterm labor, it is crucial to rule out infection. While surgical intervention is rarely required, selected cases have undergone myomectomy safely during pregnancy [70]. Surgery may be considered between 14 and 20 weeks in patients with severe pain and intramural fibroids located near the implantation site.

Occasionally, pedunculated subserosal leiomyomas may undergo torsion and infarction. In such cases, surgical management—either laparoscopic or open—may include ligation of the pedicle and excision. Surgery should be reserved for tumors that are pedunculated and easily resectable.

18.3.18 Pregnancy Complications

Leiomyomas are associated with several obstetric complications, including preterm labor, placental abruption, fetal malpresentation, obstructed labor, cesarean delivery, and postpartum hemorrhage [71, 72]. In a study of 2065 pregnancies, women with leiomyomas had a fourfold increased risk of placental abruption and breech presentation, double the rates of first-trimester bleeding and dysfunctional labor, and a sixfold increase in cesarean section rate [73]. Additionally, the risk of second-trimester miscarriage was eight times higher, though genetic amniocentesis did not appear to increase this risk.

The size and location of the fibroid are the most significant predictors of complications [74]. When the placenta implants near or over the fibroid, risks of miscarriage, preterm labor, abruption, and postpartum hemorrhage are elevated. Fibroids in the cervix or lower uterine segment may obstruct labor.

Nonetheless, vaginal delivery has been reported in up to 70% of women with fibroids measuring ≤10 cm [75]. Therefore, vaginal delivery should be considered in cases without mechanical obstruction. During cesarean section, fibroids are typically not removed, unless bleeding is uncontrolled. A particular surgical challenge is lateral displacement of the ureter by the tumor, complicating potential hysterectomy.

18.3.19 Hemorrhage and Infection

Leiomyoma-related bleeding may result from miscarriage, preterm labor, placenta previa, or abruption. Rarely, submucosal or prolapsed cervical fibroids may cause significant hemorrhage. In such cases, ligation of the pedicle near term may be necessary. Fortunately, leiomyoma infection is rare and generally occurs postpartum or following miscarriage [76, 77].

18.3.20 Impact on Fertility

Although leiomyomas are common among reproductive-aged women, their impact on fertility is not fully established. Submucosal fibroids are known to adversely affect pregnancy outcomes, and hysteroscopic myomectomy has been shown to improve fertility and reduce early miscarriage rates [78]. Fibroids in other locations that are associated with infertility may require laparoscopic or open surgical removal.

Following myomectomy, careful obstetric planning is necessary due to the risk of uterine rupture during labor. If resection was performed near the endometrial cavity, cesarean delivery is generally recommended [79].

Although less effective, uterine artery embolization is another treatment option. However, this approach is associated with increased rates of miscarriage, cesarean delivery, and postpartum hemorrhage, and is therefore not recommended for women desiring future pregnancy [80].

18.3.21 Endometrial Carcinoma During Pregnancy

Endometrial carcinoma is an estrogen-dependent neoplasm, typically diagnosed in women over the age of 40; thus, its occurrence during pregnancy is exceedingly rare. To date, a total of 27 cases diagnosed either during pregnancy or within the first 4 months postpartum have been reported in the literature. Most of these diagnoses were established through curettage specimens obtained in the first trimester [81].

These tumors are usually detected at an early stage and are well-differentiated adenocarcinomas. The standard treatment consists of total abdominal hysterectomy with bilateral salpingo-oophorectomy. In exceedingly rare cases, particularly those diagnosed following pregnancy loss, fertility-sparing approaches involving curettage followed by progestin therapy have been attempted [82].

Outside of pregnancy, conservative treatment is considered a potential option for women with early-stage, well-differentiated endometrial carcinoma who desire fertility preservation. Although pregnancy rates following progestin therapy are encouraging, the risk of recurrence and malignant progression limits its acceptance as a standard approach [83].

18.3.22 Adnexal Masses and Ovarian Malignancies in Pregnancy

Adnexal masses are relatively common during pregnancy, with an incidence ranging from 1 in 100 to 1 in 2000 pregnancies, depending on the studied population, diagnostic modalities, and size criteria. In contrast, ovarian malignancies are much rarer, occurring in approximately 1 in 19,000 pregnancies [84].

The most frequently encountered ovarian masses include corpus luteum cysts, endometriomas, benign cystadenomas, and mature cystic teratomas. As most pregnant individuals are in a younger age group, malignant and borderline tumors are relatively uncommon, comprising approximately 4–13% of all adnexal masses [85].

Ultrasonography remains the primary diagnostic tool. While typical cystic structures are generally indicative of benign pathology, features such as thick septations, solid components, and papillary projections raise concern for malignancy. When necessary, MRI may be performed after the second trimester. Among tumor markers, CA-125 has limited diagnostic utility in early pregnancy due to physiological elevation [84].

The most common complications include torsion and hemorrhage. In cases of torsion, laparoscopic detorsion is preferred, with oophorectomy required only rarely. When a ruptured corpus luteum cyst is confidently diagnosed, conservative follow-up is usually sufficient; however, if surgery is indicated prior to 10 weeks of gestation, postoperative progestin support may be required [85].

Simple, asymptomatic cysts smaller than 5 cm typically require no intervention. Masses exceeding 10 cm are usually resected due to increased risks of torsion and malignancy. Lesions measuring between 5 and 10 cm may be followed or surgically managed based on imaging characteristics [86].

Certain adnexal masses in pregnancy arise secondary to hormonal stimulation, such as pregnancy luteomas, hyperreactio luteinalis, and ovarian hyperstimulation syndrome (OHSS). Luteomas are benign tumors that generally regress spontaneously; maternal virilization is common, while fetal virilization is rare. Hyperreactio luteinalis is frequently associated with elevated hCG levels due to multiple gestations or trophoblastic disease. OHSS, on the other hand, typically results from ovulation induction and may cause severe systemic complications [87].

Ovarian cancers during pregnancy are rare. When present, they are most commonly germ cell tumors, sex cord-stromal tumors, or tumors of low malignant potential. Upon diagnosis, staging surgery and, when necessary, chemotherapy may be considered. CA-125 is not a reliable marker for monitoring during pregnancy. Multidisciplinary management involving a gynecologic oncologist is recommended in such cases [87, 88].

18.3.23 Paratubal and Paraovarian Cysts

These cysts arise from Müllerian remnants or mesothelial inclusions. They are usually less than 3 cm in size, asymptomatic, and are often identified incidentally during cesarean section. Excision is performed when indicated. Neoplastic transformation is exceedingly rare [89].

18.3.24 Vulvar and Vaginal Tumors

In younger women, vulvar and vaginal intraepithelial neoplasias—often associated with HPV infection are more common than invasive carcinomas. Management is typically postponed until the postpartum period. Invasive vulvar and vaginal cancers during pregnancy are exceedingly rare. Suspicious lesions should be evaluated with biopsy. Surgical treatment during pregnancy may be considered for stage I disease. However, given the slow progression of vulvar carcinoma, deferral of treatment until after delivery is also a viable option. Vaginal delivery is not contraindicated as long as vulvar incisions have adequately healed [90].

18.4 Breast Cancer

Breast cancer is the most frequently encountered malignancy during pregnancy, reflecting the natural incidence of cancer in women of reproductive age [91, 92]. Pregnancy-associated breast cancer (PrBC) presents substantial clinical challenges in both diagnosis and treatment. Although definitions may vary slightly, PrBC typically refers to breast cancer diagnosed during pregnancy, whereas the term postpartum breast cancer (PPBC) is used for cases identified within the first 6–12 months after delivery [93]. This distinction is clinically relevant due to differences in tumor biology and prognosis.

Epidemiological data indicate that breast cancer associated with pregnancy occurs in approximately 0.2–2.6% of cases, and up to 35–55% of women diagnosed with breast cancer under the age of 45 are diagnosed within 5–10 years postpartum [94]. Although no pregnancy-specific risk factor for PrBC has been definitively established, the risk is known to be elevated in individuals carrying BRCA1 mutations [95, 96].

18.4.1 Clinical Evaluation and Diagnosis

Breast cancer during pregnancy typically presents with classical symptoms such as a palpable mass or nipple discharge. However, physiological changes associated with pregnancy—including increased breast density, vascular congestion, and nipple discharge—can obscure clinical findings and lead to diagnostic delays [93]. Therefore, any breast mass during pregnancy should be promptly evaluated. Masses persisting beyond 2 weeks should undergo further investigation [92].

Ultrasonography is the first-line imaging modality, being safe for both breast and axillary lymph node evaluation without exposing the fetus to ionizing radiation [93]. Histopathologic confirmation is obtained via core needle (tru-cut) biopsy. Mammography, preferably unilateral mediolateral oblique view, may be considered when necessary, as it involves minimal radiation exposure [95].

Staging is conducted according to the TNM classification defined by the American Joint Committee on Cancer (AJCC) [96]. The combination of mammography and ultrasound is useful for assessing local extension and multifocality. Contrast-enhanced breast MRI should be reserved for exceptional cases due to concerns regarding fetal safety [97].

18.4.2 Staging and Radiation Safety

Advanced imaging for staging should be restricted to high-risk cases, such as tumors ≥5 cm, positive axillary lymph nodes, or suspected metastasis [96]. CT and PET/CT involve fetal radiation exposure and should be used with caution, ensuring fetal doses do not exceed 100 mGy [93]. Deterministic effects of radiation include preterm birth, congenital anomalies, and intellectual disability, while stochastic effects may increase cancer risk even at low doses [94].

Most routinely used radiologic procedures in pregnancy expose the fetus to radiation levels far below harmful thresholds. For example, mammography results in <0.01 mGy, and chest CT delivers <0.66 mGy. However, cumulative exposure must be carefully monitored when multiple imaging studies are required.

Whole-body diffusion-weighted MRI (DW-MRI), which does not require contrast administration and provides high diagnostic accuracy, is a promising alternative for metastasis screening [95].

18.4.3 Pathological and Biological Features

Pregnancy-associated breast cancer is frequently characterized by high-grade histology, aggressive biological behavior, and larger tumor size at diagnosis. The rates of triple-negative and HER2-positive tumors are significantly higher compared to nonpregnant patients [98]. Molecular subtypes are more commonly HER2-enriched or triple-negative, as opposed to luminal A, which has implications for both treatment and prognosis [92].

18.4.4 Therapeutic Approach

The primary goal in treatment planning is to ensure fetal safety without compromising maternal oncologic outcomes. Management decisions should be based on tumor stage, gestational age, patient preferences, and the consensus of a multidisciplinary team [95]. Termination of pregnancy is not recommended, and diagnostic and therapeutic delays should be avoided [98] (Table 18.4) [7, 10, 17, 99, 100].

Table 18.4 Trimester-based management approach for breast cancer during pregnancy

Trimester	Diagnostic methods	Surgery	Chemotherapy	Radiotherapy	Notes
First	USG, biopsy	Feasible	Contraindicated	Contraindicated	Mammography may be cautiously performed
Second	USG, mammography, biopsy	Feasible	Anthracycline-based chemotherapy	Contraindicated	MRI preferred for staging if necessary
Third	USG, biopsy	Feasible	Can be administered until week 35	Contraindicated	Postpartum radiotherapy should be planned

Table 18.5 Systemic agents: safety and contraindications in pregnancy

Drug class	Example agents	Safety in pregnancy	Notes
Anthracyclines	Doxorubicin, epirubicin	Safe (from second trimester)	Preferred agents
Taxanes	Paclitaxel, docetaxel	Generally safe (second trimester)	Used in combination regimens
Alkylating agents	Cisplatin, carboplatin	Safe (second trimester)	Widely used platinum compounds
Antimetabolites	Methotrexate	Contraindicated	High teratogenic risk
HER2-targeted agents	Trastuzumab	Contraindicated	Associated with oligohydramnios, fetal toxicity
Hormonal therapies	Tamoxifen	Contraindicated	High risk of fetal malformation

18.4.4.1 Surgery

Surgical management is feasible in all trimesters. Breast-conserving surgery should be prioritized when possible, with mastectomy considered if needed [7, 101]. Sentinel lymph node biopsy using technetium-99m (99mTc) is considered safe, while dye-based tracers should be avoided [38–40].

18.4.4.2 Chemotherapy

Chemotherapy can be safely initiated after the first trimester. Common regimens include anthracyclines, taxanes, and platinum agents [102]. Methotrexate is contraindicated throughout pregnancy due to its teratogenic effects. Chemotherapy is typically discontinued by 35 weeks' gestation, with delivery timing based on the risk of myelosuppression (Table 18.5) [93–96].

18.4.4.3 Targeted and Hormonal Therapies

Trastuzumab is contraindicated during pregnancy due to the risk of oligohydramnios and fetal renal dysplasia [99]. Tamoxifen is similarly avoided because of its association with congenital anomalies [100]. Due to insufficient data, the use of PARP inhibitors and immunotherapies during pregnancy is not currently recommended [102].

18.4.4.4 Supportive Therapy

Antiemetics, granulocyte colony-stimulating factors (G-CSF), and corticosteroids may be used when clinically indicated. Prednisolone and methylprednisolone are preferred for premedication purposes [103].

Table 18.6 Therapeutic and delivery planning based on clinical context

Clinical scenario	Recommended treatment	Delivery planning
Early-stage breast cancer, <20 weeks	Surgery + chemotherapy (second trimester)	Aim for term delivery
Early-stage breast cancer, >30 weeks	Surgery + postpartum chemotherapy	Delivery can be scheduled at 37 weeks
Advanced, symptomatic tumors	Chemotherapy (second trimester) ± palliative surgery	Delivery after fetal maturity
Imminent delivery after treatment response	Discontinue chemotherapy (week 35)	Delivery timed to minimize myelosuppression
No obstetric indication for cesarean	Vaginal delivery	Cesarean only for obstetric reasons

18.4.4.5 Radiotherapy

While radiotherapy during pregnancy is generally avoided, it may be considered with precise fetal dose calculations. When the target volume is distant from the uterus, fetal exposure can be minimized. Ultra-hypofractionated protocols (e.g., 5 fractions over 1 week) are preferred [7]. In palliative scenarios—such as brain metastases—radiotherapy may be administered if fetal exposure is minimal.

18.4.5 Obstetric Surveillance and Delivery Planning

Regular assessments of fetal growth, Doppler studies, and anatomic evaluations are essential. Term delivery should be the goal, but in cases requiring early delivery due to chemotherapy timing, antenatal corticosteroids should be administered for lung maturation [104]. Vaginal delivery is preferred when no medical contraindications exist. Due to increased thromboembolic risk, peripartum prophylaxis with low molecular weight heparin (LMWH) should be considered (Table 18.6) [38–40].

18.4.6 Effects on the Child

Follow-up studies at ages 3–6 in children exposed to chemotherapy during the second and third trimesters have generally shown normal neurocognitive development [104]. However, long-term data remain limited. Cardiac screening is recommended for children exposed to anthracyclines, and auditory assessments are advised for those exposed to platinum-based agents [104].

18.5 Hematologıcal Malıgnancıes

Hodgkin lymphoma is the most common hematological malignancy encountered during pregnancy, owing to its typical presentation at a younger age [105]. The incidence ranges between 1 in 1000 and 1 in 6000 pregnancies [105]. Acute leukemias are rarer, with an estimated incidence of 1 in 75,000 pregnancies [106], yet they necessitate careful management due to significant perinatal risks.

18.5.1 Acute Leukemia During Pregnancy

Acute myeloid leukemia (AML) is the most frequently diagnosed leukemia during pregnancy. It is often suspected following abnormal findings in a routine complete blood count and confirmed by bone marrow biopsy [106]. Symptoms such as fatigue and manifestations of pancytopenia are common. When diagnosis occurs during the first trimester, consideration of pregnancy termination may be warranted due to the potential negative impact of delayed systemic chemotherapy on maternal prognosis.

Anthracycline- and cytarabine-based chemotherapy regimens administered during the second and third trimesters have shown complete remission rates exceeding 85%, comparable to nonpregnant populations [106]. However, complications such as thrombocytopenia and disseminated intravascular coagulation (DIC) necessitate careful timing of delivery.

18.5.2 Hodgkin Lymphoma in Pregnancy

Hodgkin lymphoma accounts for approximately 3% of all Hodgkin cases diagnosed during pregnancy. Presenting symptoms typically include painless lymphadenopathy, fatigue, dyspnea, anemia, and thrombocytopenia—symptoms that may be mistaken for physiological changes of pregnancy. Diagnosis is usually established via lymph node biopsy under local anesthesia, posing no significant risk to the fetus.

Staging involves chest radiography with abdominal shielding, erythrocyte sedimentation rate (ESR), and abdominal MRI. The standard chemotherapy regimen—doxorubicin, bleomycin, vinblastine, and dacarbazine (ABVD)—is considered safe during pregnancy, depending on disease stage and gestational age. In select cases, maintenance therapy with agents like vincristine may be employed during pregnancy.

Table 18.7 Approach to hematologic malignancies during pregnancy

Cancer type	Incidence (in pregnancy)	Diagnostic modality	Treatment approach
Hodgkin lymphoma	1/1000–1/6000	Lymph node biopsy, chest X-ray, MRI	ABVD regimen; stage-based chemotherapy
Acute leukemia (AML)	1/75,000	CBC, bone marrow biopsy	Anthracycline + cytarabine; consider termination in first trimester

Table 18.8 Clinical management recommendations for hematologic cancers

Clinical scenario	Management recommendation
AML diagnosis in first trimester	Consider pregnancy termination if systemic therapy must begin immediately
Chemotherapy after second trimester	Lower fetal toxicity risk; treatment can proceed
Near delivery	Avoid chemotherapy 2–3 weeks prior to delivery
Stage IA–IIA Hodgkin diagnosis late in pregnancy	Delay treatment until postpartum if disease is stable

18.5.3 Timing of Therapy and Prognosis

In first-trimester diagnoses, chemotherapy should be deferred until the second trimester when fetal risks are lower. Nevertheless, there remains a need for close monitoring due to risks of intrauterine growth restriction, preterm birth, and potential long-term malignancy in the child. In late third-trimester diagnoses of early-stage disease (IA–IIA), treatment may be postponed until postpartum.

Chemotherapy should not be administered within 2–3 weeks of planned delivery. Ideally, delivery should occur after 34 weeks of gestation. Pregnancy does not significantly impact disease progression in Hodgkin lymphoma [105], and survival rates are comparable between pregnant and nonpregnant patients (Tables 18.7 and 18.8) [104–106].

18.6 Thyroid Cancer

Thyroid cancer is the most frequently diagnosed endocrine malignancy during pregnancy, increasingly observed due to the rising incidence of thyroid nodules in women of reproductive age. The most common histopathological type during pregnancy is well-differentiated papillary thyroid carcinoma (PTC). Physiological hormonal changes and thyroid hyperplasia during pregnancy may increase the detection of nodules, although this does not imply a heightened risk of malignancy [107, 108]. Cases diagnosed during pregnancy or within the first postpartum year are classified as pregnancy-associated thyroid cancer.

Table 18.9 Algorithm for evaluating thyroid nodules during pregnancy

Clinical scenario	Recommended approach
Palpable or ultrasound-detected nodule	TSH level + thyroid ultrasound
Low TSH (<0.1 mIU/L)	Avoid scintigraphy; radioactive iodine is contraindicated
Normal or high TSH	FNAB for suspicious nodules
FNAB shows malignancy/suspicion	Surgery timing planned based on gestational age

18.6.1 Diagnosis and Evaluation

Thyroid nodules are detected in approximately 5–10% of pregnancies, the majority of which are benign. Ultrasound is the primary diagnostic modality. Features suggestive of malignancy, including microcalcifications, hypoechogenicity, irregular margins, and a taller-than-wide shape, should prompt fine-needle aspiration biopsy (FNAB), which is safe during pregnancy and does not require anesthesia.

TIRADS and Bethesda classifications remain applicable during pregnancy. However, unnecessary repeat biopsies should be avoided in nondiagnostic cases. Radioactive iodine scanning is contraindicated, and non-contrast MRI is preferred for staging when necessary (Table 18.9) [109, 110].

18.6.2 Surgical and Medical Management

Management of thyroid cancer during pregnancy should be individualized based on tumor characteristics and gestational age. If the tumor is <1 cm without aggressive features or nodal involvement, treatment may be deferred until after delivery. If >1 cm, rapidly growing, or involving lymph nodes, surgery is recommended in the second trimester.

Radioactive iodine therapy is contraindicated in pregnancy and should be deferred for at least 6 months postpartum. Surgical options include total thyroidectomy or lobectomy. Preoperative TSH levels should be normalized, and fetal monitoring ensured. Postoperative levothyroxine therapy is initiated for TSH suppression (Table 18.10) [109–111].

18.6.3 Medical Follow-Up and Obstetric Surveillance

Levothyroxine therapy should be titrated to maintain trimester-specific TSH target ranges for tumor suppression and to prevent hypothyroidism. TSH goals are physiologically lower during pregnancy (Table 18.11) [107].

Table 18.10 Surgical timing recommendations for thyroid cancer during pregnancy

Trimester	Surgical indication	Approach
First	Delay if possible	Surgery generally avoided due to risks
Second	Aggressive tumors	Optimal time for surgery
Third	Nonurgent cases	Surgery postponed until after delivery

Table 18.11 Recommended reference ranges for thyroid-stimulating hormone (TSH) levels during pregnancy

Trimester	Approximate reference range for TSH (mIU/L)
First trimester	0.1–2.5
Second trimester	0.2–3.0
Third trimester	0.3–3.0

Fetal growth, amniotic fluid index, Doppler studies, and biometric measurements should be monitored regularly. Delivery mode should be determined based on obstetric indications, not thyroid cancer. Anesthesia planning in patients at risk of myocardial depression posttreatment should be multidisciplinary.

18.6.4 Postpartum Management and Radioactive Iodine Therapy

RAI therapy should be delayed until at least 6 weeks after cessation of breastfeeding, as lactation increases iodine uptake in breast tissue. Pregnancy should be avoided for 6–12 months post-RAI therapy [112, 113].

18.6.5 Prognosis

Long-term survival of patients diagnosed with thyroid cancer during pregnancy is comparable to nonpregnant patients with similar staging. However, lymph node metastases may be more frequent in those diagnosed postpartum. Follow-up includes serum thyroglobulin monitoring and thyroid ultrasound.

18.7 Malıgnant Melanoma

Malignant melanoma is the most common cutaneous malignancy diagnosed during pregnancy, accounting for 8–10% of all pregnancy-associated cancers [114]. The rising incidence of melanoma in young women contributes to its occurrence during pregnancy. While increased hormonal sensitivity of melanocytes and immune modulation during pregnancy may influence tumor biology, current evidence does not conclusively demonstrate a significant prognostic difference between pregnant and nonpregnant patients with melanoma [115]. Although earlier studies reported worse outcomes, recent data with improved statistical methods and control groups have not consistently supported this.

18.7.1 Epidemiology and Risk Factors

The incidence of melanoma is increasing, particularly in fair-skinned women exposed to high levels of ultraviolet radiation and those with a family history of melanoma. Hormonal changes during pregnancy, especially elevated estrogen and progesterone, stimulate melanocyte activity and lead to increased pigmentation. Physiologic darkening and growth of nevi during pregnancy are common, and distinguishing benign from malignant changes requires clinical expertise [116].

18.7.2 Diagnostic Approach

Initial evaluation follows the ABCDE criteria (Asymmetry, Border irregularity, Color variation, Diameter >6 mm, Evolution). Dermoscopy aids in detailed assessment, and excisional biopsy remains the gold standard. Full-thickness biopsy under local anesthesia poses no significant risk to the fetus. Prognostic factors include Breslow thickness, Clark level, mitotic rate, ulceration, and microsatellite presence [117, 118].

18.7.3 Staging

Staging should aim to minimize fetal radiation exposure. Non-contrast MRI is preferred for evaluating metastases in the liver, lymph nodes, and brain. CT and PET-CT should be reserved for essential indications due to fetal radiation risk [119]. Sentinel lymph node biopsy is essential for staging; however, isosulfan blue dye is contraindicated during pregnancy due to anaphylaxis risk. Use of technetium-99m (Tc-99m) alone is recommended [120].

18.7.4 Treatment

Surgical excision remains the primary treatment and can be performed safely during pregnancy. The timing should be guided by gestational age and tumor stage. Wide local excision and sentinel lymph node biopsy are ideally performed in the second trimester. Systemic therapies (anti-PD-1, anti-CTLA-4, BRAF/MEK inhibitors) lack safety data in pregnancy and are generally deferred to the postpartum period. However, in life-threatening metastatic disease, maternal health may warrant multidisciplinary decision-making.

18.7.5 Obstetric Considerations and Neonatal Outcomes

Multidisciplinary coordination is essential when managing melanoma during pregnancy. Surgery carries no significant fetal risk. Systemic therapies, if required, are best initiated after delivery. Timing of delivery depends on maternal disease status, fetal maturity, and therapeutic needs. Placental metastasis, although rare, has been reported; thus, placental histopathological evaluation is recommended. Neonatal metastasis is exceedingly rare but documented in isolated cases [121].

18.7.6 Conclusion

Diagnosis and treatment of malignant melanoma during pregnancy should prioritize both maternal and fetal safety. Surgery is safe throughout gestation, while systemic therapy should generally be postponed until after delivery. Multidisciplinary collaboration is crucial to optimizing oncologic and obstetric outcomes.

18.8 Gastroıntestınal System Tumors

Gastrointestinal (GI) malignancies are rare during pregnancy but pose significant diagnostic and therapeutic challenges. They account for less than 3% of pregnancy-associated cancers. The most commonly reported GI malignancies include colorectal, gastric, and pancreatic cancers [122].

Table 18.12 Suggested approach for colorectal cancer during pregnancy

Clinical scenario	Trimester	Recommended approach
Stable after diagnosis	First	Surgery ± pregnancy termination if indicated
Stable after diagnosis	Second	Surgical resection (optimal window)
Stable after diagnosis	Third	Postpartum surgery; consider preterm delivery if urgent
Obstruction/perforation	Any	Emergency surgical intervention

18.8.1 Colorectal Cancer

Colorectal cancer (CRC) is the third most common cancer among women in the United States, but it is uncommon during pregnancy due to its low lifetime risk before age 40. Reported incidence during pregnancy ranges from 1 in 13,000 to 1 in 50,000 [123, 124]. Up to 70–80% of pregnancy-associated CRC cases originate from the rectum.

Common CRC symptoms—abdominal pain, constipation, rectal bleeding, and nausea—are often nonspecific and may delay diagnosis. Persistent symptoms warrant digital rectal examination, fecal occult blood testing, and flexible sigmoidoscopy or colonoscopy. Colonoscopy is considered safe during the second trimester with appropriate fetal monitoring [125].

Non-contrast MRI is preferred for staging. Surgical resection is tailored to gestational age and tumor extent. Therapeutic abortion is not always necessary in early pregnancy, while in late pregnancy, surgery may be delayed until fetal maturation. Emergencies such as obstruction, hemorrhage, or perforation require immediate surgical intervention. Cesarean delivery may be preferred in low rectal tumors due to risk of dystocia and bleeding [126] (Table 18.12) [123–127].

Carcinoembryonic antigen (CEA) may be physiologically elevated during pregnancy; baseline values are important for monitoring [127]. Pregnancy does not appear to worsen CRC prognosis when compared to nonpregnant patients at similar stages [128].

18.8.2 Gastric Cancer

Pregnancy-associated gastric adenocarcinoma is extremely rare and primarily reported from East Asian countries. Due to the overlap with common pregnancy symptoms (nausea, vomiting, weight loss), diagnosis is often delayed and prognosis is generally poor [129]. Persistent upper GI symptoms warrant prompt endoscopic evaluation, which is safe during the second trimester with sedation and left lateral positioning.

Treatment depends on disease stage and gestational age. Surgical resection is the mainstay of treatment. Chemotherapy may be cautiously considered from the second trimester onward. Regardless of pregnancy, prognosis in gastric cancer remains poor [130] (Table 18.13).

Table 18.13 Clinical approach to gastric cancer during pregnancy

Clinical scenario	Trimester	Recommended management
Persistent upper GI symptoms	I–II	Endoscopy for diagnosis, non-contrast MRI for staging
Localized tumor	Second	Surgical resection with fetal safety considerations
Localized tumor	Third	Surgery after fetal maturity or post-cesarean
Metastatic disease	Any	Multidisciplinary planning; systemic therapy deferred

18.8.3 Neuroendocrine Tumors and Zollinger-Ellison Syndrome

Zollinger-Ellison syndrome (ZES) is a rare neuroendocrine condition caused by gastrin-secreting tumors, typically located in the pancreas or duodenum. Management during pregnancy focuses on acid suppression using antacids, H2 receptor antagonists, and proton pump inhibitors (PPIs) [131]. To date, pregnancy outcomes with acid suppression therapy have been favorable. Surgical intervention is generally considered preconceptionally.

18.8.4 Conclusion

GI malignancies during pregnancy are rare but can be associated with diagnostic delays and adverse outcomes. Persistent gastrointestinal symptoms require thorough evaluation, and appropriate diagnostic procedures should not be deferred. Surgical treatment can be safely performed during pregnancy, while systemic therapy decisions should be guided by a multidisciplinary team.

References

1. Voulgaris E, Pentheroudakis G, Pavlidis N. Cancer and pregnancy: a comprehensive review. Surg Oncol. 2011;20(4):e175–85.
2. Skrzypczyk-Ostaszewicz A, Rubach M. Gynaecological cancers coexisting with pregnancy—a literature review. Współczesna Onkologia. 2016;3:193–8.
3. Brewer M, Kueck A, Runowicz CD. Chemotherapy in pregnancy. Clin Obstet Gynecol. 2011;54(4):602–18.
4. Smith LH, Danielsen B, Allen ME, Cress R. Cancer associated with obstetric delivery: results of linkage with the California cancer registry. Am J Obstet Gynecol. 2003;189(4):1128–35.
5. Eibye S, Kjær SK, Mellemkjær L. Incidence of pregnancy-associated cancer in Denmark, 1977–2006. Obstet Gynecol. 2013;122(3):608–17.
6. Azim HA, Peccatori FA, Pavlidis N. Lung cancer in the pregnant woman: to treat or not to treat, that is the question. Lung Cancer. 2010;67(3):251–6.
7. Loibl S, Han SN, Von Minckwitz G, Bontenbal M, Ring A, Giermek J, Fehm T, Van Calsteren K, Linn SC, Schlehe B, et al. Treatment of breast cancer during pregnancy: an observational study. Lancet Oncol. 2012;13(9):887–96.

8. Cordeiro CN, Gemignani ML. Gynecologic malignancies in pregnancy: balancing fetal risks with oncologic safety. Obstet Gynecol Surv. 2017;72(3):184–93.
9. Van Calsteren K, Heyns L, De Smet F, Van Eycken L, Gziri MM, Van Gemert W, Halaska M, Vergote I, Ottevanger N, Amant F. Cancer during pregnancy: an analysis of 215 patients emphasizing the obstetrical and the neonatal outcomes. J Clin Oncol. 2010;28(4):683–9.
10. Amant F, Halaska MJ, Fumagalli M, Steffensen KD, Lok C, Van Calsteren K, Han SN, Mir O, Fruscio R, Uzan C, et al. Gynecologic cancers in pregnancy. Int J Gynecol Cancer. 2014;24(3):394–403.
11. Morice P, Uzan C, Gouy S, Verschraegen C, Haie-Meder C. Gynaecological cancers in pregnancy. Lancet. 2012;379(9815):558–69.
12. Patel SJ, Reede DL, Katz DS, Subramaniam R, Amorosa JK. Imaging the pregnant patient for nonobstetric conditions: algorithms and radiation dose considerations. Radiographics. 2007;27(6):1705–22.
13. Guyatt GH, Eikelboom JW, Gould MK, Garcia DA, Crowther M, Murad MH, Kahn SR, Falck-Ytter Y, Francis CW, Lansberg MG, et al. Approach to outcome measurement in the prevention of thrombosis in surgical and medical patients: Antithrombotic Therapy and Prevention of Thrombosis, 9th ed: American College of Chest Physicians Evidence-Based Clinical Practice Guidelines. Chest. 2012;141(2 Suppl):e185S–94S.
14. Committee Opinion No. 723: Guidelines for diagnostic imaging during pregnancy and lactation. Obstet Gynecol. 2017;130(4):e210–6.
15. Kanal E, Barkovich AJ, Bell C, Borgstede JP, Bradley WG, Froelich JW, Gilk T, Gimbel JR, Gosbee J, Kuhni-Kaminski E, et al. ACR guidance document for safe MR practices: 2007. Am J Roentgenol. 2007;188(6):1447–74.
16. Hall E, Ward J. Radiobiology for the radiologist. AJR Am J Roentgenol. 1994;163(2):256.
17. Riddick DS, Lee C, Ramji S, Chinje EC, Cowen RL, Williams KJ, Patterson AV, Stratford IJ, Morrow CS, Townsend AJ, et al. Cancer chemotherapy and drug metabolism. Drug Metab Dispos. 2005;33(8):1083–96.
18. Ali R, Ozkalemkas F, Ozkocaman V, Ozcelik T, Ozan U, Ozkan A, Tunali A. The treatment of chronic myeloid leukemia in pregnancy: a review. Eur J Haematol. 2009;82(4):279–84.
19. Loren AW, Mangu PB, Beck LN, Brennan L, Magdalinski AJ, Partridge AH, Quinn G, Wallace WH, Oktay K. Fertility preservation for patients with cancer: American Society of Clinical Oncology clinical practice guideline update. J Clin Oncol. 2013;31(19):2500–10.
20. Nagarajan R. Pregnancy outcomes in survivors of childhood cancer. J Natl Cancer Inst Monogr. 2005;2005(34):72–6.
21. Lie Fong S, Van Den Heuvel-Eibrink MM, Eijkemans MJC, Schipper I, Hukkelhoven CWPM, Laven JSE. Pregnancy outcome in female childhood cancer survivors. Hum Reprod. 2010;25(5):1206–12.
22. Glanc P. Fetal and placental metastases associated with maternal cancers. Abdom Radiol. 2023;48(5):1784–92.
23. Wethington SL, Herzog TJ. Endocervical polyps: evaluation and management. Clin Obstet Gynecol. 2021;64(1):55–61.
24. Anderson LA, Landolfo C, Hecht JL. Atypical glandular cells in Pap smears: clinical significance and follow-up. Obstet Gynecol Clin N Am. 2020;47(2):293–308.
25. Arbyn M, Kyrgiou M, Simoens C, et al. Detecting cervical precancer and cancer in pregnancy: a systematic review. BJOG. 2022;129(4):567–75.
26. Bhatla N, Singhal S. Management of cervical cancer during pregnancy. Best Pract Res Clin Obstet Gynaecol. 2021;76:61–72.
27. Zhang Y, Zhao F-H, Yu Y-H, et al. Clinical significance and management of cervical polyps in pregnancy: a cohort study. Int J Gynaecol Obstet. 2023;162(1):48–54.
28. Gungorduk K, Asicioglu O, Gungorduk OC, et al. Pap smear screening during pregnancy: an opportunity not to be missed. J Matern Fetal Neonatal Med. 2020;33(10):1701–5.
29. Massad LS, Einstein MH, Huh WK, et al. 2012 ASCCP guidelines for management of abnormal cervical cancer screening tests. J Low Genit Tract Dis. 2013;17(5 Suppl 1):S1–S27.
30. Arbyn M, Snijders PJF, Meijer CJLM, et al. Which high-risk HPV assays fulfil criteria for use in primary cervical cancer screening? Clin Microbiol Infect. 2015;21(9):817–26.

31. FUTURE II Study Group. Quadrivalent vaccine against human papillomavirus to prevent high-grade cervical lesions. N Engl J Med. 2007;356(19):1915–27.
32. American College of Obstetricians and Gynecologists. Human papillomavirus vaccination. Committee Opinion No. 588. Obstet Gynecol. 2014;123(3):712–8.
33. Dana A, Buchanan KM, Goss MA, et al. Pregnancy outcomes from the pregnancy registry of a human papillomavirus type 6/11/16/18 vaccine. Obstet Gynecol. 2009;114(6):1170–8.
34. American College of Obstetricians and Gynecologists. Management of abnormal cervical cancer screening test results and cervical cancer precursors. ACOG Practice Bulletin No. 168. Obstet Gynecol. 2016;128(4):e111–30.
35. Randall TC, Ghebre R. Invasive cervical cancer in pregnancy. Obstet Gynecol. 2009;114(2 Pt 1):555–9.
36. Wright TC Jr, Massad LS, Dunton CJ, et al. 2007 ASCCP guidelines for the management of cervical intraepithelial neoplasia. Am J Obstet Gynecol. 2007;197(4):346–55.
37. Fader AN, Alward EK, Niederhuber JE, et al. Cervical dysplasia in pregnancy: a 25-year experience. Obstet Gynecol. 2010;115(1):121–9.
38. Yost NP, Santoso JT, McIntire DD, et al. Postpartum regression of cervical intraepithelial neoplasia in women with abnormal Pap smear. J Reprod Med. 1999;44(8):706–10.
39. Ackermann S, Beckmann MW, Lermann J, et al. Prevalence of carcinoma in situ and invasive carcinoma after delivery in women diagnosed with cervical intraepithelial neoplasia during pregnancy. Arch Gynecol Obstet. 2006;273(1):29–34.
40. Dunton CJ. Management of abnormal Pap smear and cervical cancer in pregnancy. Clin Obstet Gynecol. 2008;51(2):279–87.
41. Jacobsson B, Gillian E, Karlsson B, et al. Pregnancy outcome after cervical cone biopsy: a population-based study. Am J Obstet Gynecol. 2009;201(5):469.e461–6.
42. Hacker NF, Berek JS, Lagasse LD, et al. Management of abnormal cervical cytology during pregnancy. Obstet Gynecol. 1982;60(3):385–8.
43. Castanon A, Landy R, Brocklehurst P, et al. Risk of preterm delivery with increasing depth of excision for cervical intraepithelial neoplasia. BMJ. 2014;349:g6223.
44. Samson SL, Bentley JR, Fahey TJ, et al. The effect of loop electrosurgical excision procedure on future pregnancy outcome. Obstet Gynecol. 2005;105(2):325–32.
45. Bruinsma FJ, Quinn MA. The risk of preterm birth following treatment for precancerous changes in the cervix: a systematic review and meta-analysis. BJOG. 2007;114(7):768–80.
46. Shanbhag S, Clark H, Bidus M, et al. Cervical dysplasia in pregnancy: results of expectant management. J Reprod Med. 2009;54(8):503–8.
47. Pettersson F. FIGO annual report on the results of treatment in gynecological cancer. Int J Gynaecol Obstet. 2010;109(2):73–7.
48. Smith LH, Dalrymple JL, Leiserowitz GS, et al. Obstetric outcomes in women with cervical cancer. Obstet Gynecol. 2003;102(5 Pt 1):1059–66.
49. Oto A, Ernst R, Nishino TK, et al. Cervical cancer in pregnancy: MRI for prediction of lymph node metastasis. Eur Radiol. 2007;17(9):2344–50.
50. Takushi M, Moromizato H, Sakumoto K, et al. Pregnancy complicated with cervical cancer: clinical management and outcomes. J Obstet Gynaecol Res. 2002;28(3):150–6.
51. van Vliet E, Boere IA, Witteveen PO, et al. Cervical cancer in pregnancy: a retrospective study. Eur J Gynaecol Oncol. 1998;19(4):375–9.
52. Alouini S, Baillet C, Narducci F, et al. Management of invasive cervical cancer diagnosed during pregnancy. Eur J Obstet Gynecol Reprod Biol. 2008;137(2):143–8.
53. Zagouri F, Dimitrakakis C, Marinopoulos S, et al. Cancer in pregnancy: disentangling treatment modalities. Eur J Cancer. 2013;49(5):1210–20.
54. American College of Obstetricians and Gynecologists. Management of cervical cancer in pregnancy. ACOG Committee Opinion No. 463. Obstet Gynecol. 2010;116(3):624–8.
55. Nisker JA, Cohen MM. Radiation therapy vs surgery for stage IB cervical cancer in pregnancy. Obstet Gynecol. 1983;61(3):419–23.
56. Yahata T, Nishikawa N, Shigetomi H, et al. Conservative management of early invasive adenocarcinoma of the cervix during pregnancy. Int J Clin Oncol. 2008;13(1):77–80.

57. Greer BE, Koh WJ, Figge DC, et al. Cancer in pregnancy: maternal and fetal consequences. Semin Oncol. 1989;16(4):397–409.
58. van der Vange N, Kenter GG, Kroons AM, et al. The prognosis of cervical cancer associated with pregnancy: a matched cohort study. Obstet Gynecol. 1995;86(1):4–8.
59. Goldman GA, Schachter EN, Schaffer RM. Episiotomy scar recurrence of cervical cancer: evidence for direct implantation. Gynecol Oncol. 2003;88(3):449–52.
60. Shepherd JH, Spencer C, Herod J, Ind T. Radical vaginal trachelectomy as a fertility-sparing procedure in women with early-stage cervical cancer. BJOG. 2006;113(3):362–8.
61. Park JY, Kim DY, Kim JH, Kim YM, Kim YT, Nam JH. Outcomes of radical surgery for women with early-stage cervical cancer during pregnancy. Arch Gynecol Obstet. 2012;286(1):195–200.
62. Kim CH, Kim SR, Choi SC, et al. Obstetric outcomes after radical trachelectomy. Obstet Gynecol Sci. 2012;55(7):513–8.
63. Qidwai GI, Caughey AB, Jacoby AF. Obstetric outcomes in women with sonographically identified uterine leiomyomata. Obstet Gynecol. 2006;107(2):376–82.
64. Stout MJ, Odibo AO, Graseck AS, et al. Leiomyomas at routine second-trimester ultrasound examination and adverse obstetric outcomes. Obstet Gynecol. 2010;116(5):1056–63.
65. Laughlin SK, Baird DD, Savitz DA, et al. Prevalence of uterine leiomyomas in the first trimester of pregnancy. Am J Obstet Gynecol. 2009;200(1):105.e101–7.
66. Bulun SE. Uterine fibroids. N Engl J Med. 2013;369(14):1344–55.
67. Neiger R, Chopra S, Spalding J, et al. Pregnancy-related changes in uterine fibroids. J Matern Fetal Neonatal Med. 2006;19(3):193–7.
68. Torashima M, Kim T, Murakami T, et al. MR imaging of uterine myomas during pregnancy. Eur J Radiol. 1997;24(2):136–43.
69. Klatsky PC, Tran ND, Caughey AB, Fujimoto VY. Fibroids and reproductive outcomes: a systematic literature review from conception to delivery. Am J Obstet Gynecol. 2008;198(4):357–66.
70. Celik C, Sakalli M, Selcuk S, et al. Myomectomy during pregnancy: a case report and review of the literature. J Reprod Med. 2002;47(2):164–6.
71. Sheiner E, Bashiri A, Levy A, et al. Obstetric characteristics and perinatal outcome of pregnancies with uterine leiomyomas. J Reprod Med. 2004;49(3):182–6.
72. Coronado GD, Marshall LM, Schwartz SM. Complications in pregnancy, labor, and delivery with uterine leiomyomas: a population-based study. Obstet Gynecol. 2000;95(5):764–9.
73. Shavell VI, Thakur M, Sawant A, et al. Adverse obstetric outcomes associated with sonographically identified large uterine fibroids. Fertil Steril. 2012;97(1):107–10.
74. Genta PR, Dias ML. Postpartum myoma infection. Int J Gynaecol Obstet. 2001;75(1):75–6.
75. Lin KH, Lin JY, Lin YH. Postpartum sepsis resulting from infected uterine leiomyoma. J Obstet Gynaecol Res. 2002;28(6):351–3.
76. Pritts EA. Fibroids and infertility: a systematic review of the evidence. Obstet Gynecol Surv. 2001;56(8):483–91.
77. American College of Obstetricians and Gynecologists. Practice Bulletin No. 96: Alternatives to hysterectomy in the management of leiomyomas. Obstet Gynecol. 2008;112(2 Pt 1):387–400.
78. Mara M, Maskova J, Fucikova Z, et al. Midterm clinical and first reproductive results of a randomized controlled trial comparing uterine fibroid embolization and myomectomy. Cardiovasc Intervent Radiol. 2008;31(1):73–85.
79. Homer H, Saridogan E. Uterine artery embolization for fibroids is associated with an increased risk of miscarriage. Fertil Steril. 2010;94(1):324–30.
80. Stokes LS, Wallace MJ, Pelage JP. Fibroid management: interventional alternatives to hysterectomy. Radiology. 2010;254(3):635–49.
81. Hannuna KY, Putignani L, Silvestri E, et al. Incidental endometrial adenocarcinoma in early pregnancy: a case report and review of the literature. Int J Gynecol Cancer. 2009;19(9):1580–4.
82. Mitsushita J, Toki T, Kato K, Fujii S, Konishi I. Endometrial carcinoma remaining after term pregnancy following conservative treatment with medroxyprogesterone acetate. Gynecol Oncol. 2000;79(1):129–32.

83. Bayoglu Tekin Y, Guvendag Guven ES, Sehitoglu I, Guven S. Tubal pregnancy associated with endometrial carcinoma after in vitro fertilization attempts. Case Rep Obstet Gynecol. 2014;2014:481380.
84. Cathcart AM, Nezhat FR, Emerson J, Pejovic T, Nezhat CH, Nezhat CR. Adnexal masses during pregnancy: diagnosis, treatment, and prognosis. Am J Obstet Gynecol. 2023 Jun;228(6):601–12. https://doi.org/10.1016/j.ajog.2022.11.1291. Epub 2022 Nov 19. PMID: 36410423.
85. Kwon YS, Mok JE, Lim KT, Lee IH, Kim TJ, Lee KH, Shim JU. Ovarian cancer during pregnancy: clinical and pregnancy outcome. J Korean Med Sci. 2010;25(2):230–4.
86. Panico C, Bottazzi S, Russo L, Avesani G, Celli V, D'Erme L, Cipriani A, Mascilini F, Fagotti A, Scambia G, Sala E, Gui B. Prediction of the Risk of Malignancy of Adnexal Masses during Pregnancy Comparing Subjective Assessment and Non-Contrast MRI Score (NCMS) in Radiologists with Different Expertise. Cancers (Basel). 2023;15(21):5138. https://doi.org/10.3390/cancers15215138. PMID: 37958313; PMCID: PMC10648807.
87. Watkins JC, Lebok P, Young RH. Hyperreactio luteinalis (multiple luteinized follicle cysts): a report of 10 cases. Int J Gynecol Pathol. 2021;40(5):427–34.
88. Boussios S, Moschetta M, Tatsi K, Tsiouris AK, Pavlidis N. A review on pregnancy complicated by ovarian epithelial and non-epithelial malignant tumors: diagnostic and therapeutic perspectives. J Adv Res. 2018;12:1–9.
89. Jassim, Tariq Nadhim, et al. Comparing the physical characteristics of ultrasound and magnetic resonance imaging to diagnose ovarian cysts. arXiv preprint arXiv:2403.06019 (2024).
90. Winarno AS, Fehm TN, Hampl M. Vulvar cancer during pregnancy and/or breastfeeding: a report of five cases from a single center study at the University Hospital of Düsseldorf. BMC Pregnancy Childbirth. 2022;22(1):207. https://doi.org/10.1186/s12884-022-04448-x. PMID: 35291960; PMCID: PMC8922737.
91. Amant F, Loibl S, Neven P, Van Calsteren K. Breast cancer in pregnancy. Lancet. 2012;379(9815):570–9.
92. Cardonick E, et al. Chemotherapy in pregnancy: clinical outcomes and comparative safety. J Clin Oncol. 2010;28(4):683–9.
93. Amant F, et al. International consensus guidelines for the management of cancer during pregnancy. Int J Gynecol Cancer. 2019;29(6):911–9.
94. Litton JK, et al. Characteristics of pregnancy-associated breast cancer. Breast Cancer Res Treat. 2013;138(3):817–23.
95. Han SN, et al. Imaging for breast cancer during pregnancy. Obstet Gynecol. 2011;118(3):575–82.
96. Amin M, Edge S, Greene F, et al. AJCC cancer staging manual. Springer; 2017.
97. Brent RL. Saving lives and changing family histories: appropriate counseling of pregnant women and men and women of reproductive age, concerning the risk of diagnostic radiation exposures during and before pregnancy. Pediatr Radiol. 2009;39(Suppl 1):S57–60.
98. Amant F, et al. Breast cancer in pregnancy: recommendations of an international consensus meeting. Lancet Oncol. 2012;13(3):e61–70.
99. Bell J, et al. Trastuzumab use during pregnancy: a case report and review of the literature. Oncologist. 2009;14(7):682–5.
100. Braems G, et al. Use of tamoxifen before and during pregnancy. Oncologist. 2011;16(10):1547–51.
101. Gentilini OD, Cremonesi M. Sentinel lymph node biopsy in pregnant patients with breast cancer: is it feasible? Eur J Cancer. 2013;49(13):2877–83.
102. Azim HA Jr, et al. Safety of platinums during pregnancy. Cancer Chemother Pharmacol. 2014;74(5):803–10.
103. Perrone G, et al. G-CSF administration during pregnancy: a case report and literature review. BMC Pregnancy Childbirth. 2012;12:93.
104. Avilés A, Neri N. Hematological malignancies and pregnancy: a final report of 84 children who received chemotherapy in utero. Clin Lymphoma Myeloma Leuk. 2014;14(3):223–7.
105. Pereg D, Lishner M. Hodgkin's lymphoma in pregnancy. In: Cancer in pregnancy and lactation: the Motherisk guide. Cambridge: Cambridge University Press; 2011. p. 18–20.

106. Greenlund LJ, Letendre L. Acute myeloid leukemia in the pregnant patient. Eur J Haematol. 2014;93(5):377–83.
107. Alexander EK, Pearce EN, Brent GA. 2017 Guidelines of the American Thyroid Association for the diagnosis and management of thyroid disease during pregnancy. Thyroid. 2017;27(3):315–89.
108. Glinoer D. Thyroid disorders during pregnancy and postpartum. Best Pract Res Clin Endocrinol Metab. 2004;18(2):183–201.
109. Moosa M, Mazzaferri EL. Outcome of differentiated thyroid cancer diagnosed in pregnant women. J Clin Endocrinol Metab. 1997;82(9):2862–6.
110. Kung AW. Thyroid disease in pregnancy. Curr Opin Obstet Gynecol. 2000;12(2):101–6.
111. Smith LH, et al. Thyroid cancer in pregnancy: a population-based study. Obstet Gynecol. 2003;102(4):790–4.
112. Schlumberger M, et al. Strategies of radioiodine ablation in patients with low-risk thyroid cancer. N Engl J Med. 2012;366:1663–73.
113. Vannucchi G, et al. Management of thyroid nodules and differentiated thyroid cancer in pregnancy. Endocr Relat Cancer. 2017;24(6):R297–310.
114. Lens MB, Dawes M. Global perspectives of contemporary epidemiological trends of cutaneous malignant melanoma. Int J Cancer. 2004;111(3):333–7.
115. Kyrgidis A, Tzellos TG, Vahtsevanos K, Triaridis S. New concepts for risk assessment and prevention of cutaneous melanoma. J Am Acad Dermatol. 2017;77(3):425–34.
116. Tellez A, Rius-Diaz F, Alos L, Palou J, Malvehy J, Puig S. Impact of pregnancy on the prognosis of cutaneous melanoma. J Am Acad Dermatol. 2016;75(6):1133–41.
117. Swetter SM, et al. Guidelines of care for the management of primary cutaneous melanoma. J Am Acad Dermatol. 2019;80:208–50.
118. Balch CM, Gershenwald JE, Soong SJ, Thompson JF, Atkins MB, Byrd DR. Final version of 2009 AJCC melanoma staging and classification. J Clin Oncol. 2009;27(36):6199–206.
119. Gropper AB, Ceausu I, Jerome B. Malignant melanoma in pregnancy: a case report and review of the literature. Obstet Gynecol. 2014;123(1):161–4.
120. Khosrotehrani K, Vignes S, Semerano L, Yazdanpanah Y. Melanoma and pregnancy: a review of the literature. Melanoma Res. 2005;15(3):191–7.
121. Alexander A, Samlowski WE, Grossman D, Bruggers CS, Bowen GM, Zone JJ. Management of malignant melanoma during pregnancy. Am J Obstet Gynecol. 2003;189(3):886–8.
122. Pavlidis NA. Coexistence of pregnancy and malignancy. Oncologist. 2002;7(4):279–87.
123. Siegel RL, Wagle NS, Cercek A, Smith RA, Jemal A. Colorectal cancer statistics, 2023. CA Cancer J Clin. 2023;73(3):233–54.
124. Doll KM, Rademaker A, Sosa JA. Cervical cancer in the United States: a review of the literature and a call to action. Obstet Gynecol. 2014;123(3):511–8.
125. Cappell MS, Garcia A. Gastric cancer during pregnancy: a review of the literature with emphasis on diagnosis, management, and prognosis. World J Gastroenterol. 2008;14(5):675–87.
126. Mourra N, Lesurtel M, Paye F, Tiret E, Fléjou JF. Gastrointestinal stromal tumors (GISTs) of the rectum: a clinicopathological study of 15 cases. Eur J Obstet Gynecol Reprod Biol. 2013;166(1):9–13.
127. O'Connell JB, Maggard MA, Ko CY. Colon cancer survival rates with the new American Joint Committee on Cancer sixth edition staging. Dis Colon Rectum. 2004;47(12):2141–50.
128. Dahling MT, Xing G, Cress R, Danielsen B, Smith LH. Cancer-associated deaths during pregnancy: a population-based study. Obstet Gynecol. 2009;114(6):1291–7.
129. Lee YY, Choi CH, Kim TJ, Lee JW, Kim BG, Bae DS. Clinical characteristics of gastric cancer in pregnancy. J Gastric Cancer. 2011;11(1):1–7.
130. Matsusaka S, Nashimoto A, Yabusaki H, Matsuda M, Takahashi M, Tsuburaya A. Gastric cancer during pregnancy: a review of the literature. Int J Clin Oncol. 2014;19(3):472–5.
131. Meara MP, Shah A, Li J, Chey WD. Management of gastrointestinal symptoms in pregnancy. World J Gastrointest Pharmacol Ther. 2016;7(2):289–98.

Chapter 19
Pregnancy and Sepsis

Şeyda Ceylan Arı

19.1 Introductıon

Maternal sepsis remains one of the most formidable challenges in modern obstetric practice. Despite global advances in maternal care, it continues to rank among the leading direct causes of maternal mortality, with a disproportionate burden in low- and middle-income regions. The increasing prevalence of caesarean deliveries, advanced maternal age, obesity, and chronic comorbidities has further amplified the vulnerability of pregnant women to severe infections and septic complications.

The clinical recognition of sepsis in pregnancy is uniquely complex. Physiological adaptations—including gestational tachycardia, respiratory alkalosis, leukocytosis, and reduced systemic vascular resistance—may mimic or obscure early signs of systemic infection, often resulting in delays in diagnosis and treatment. In addition, maternal hemodynamic and immunological changes not only modify the host response to infection but also alter the pharmacokinetics of antimicrobial agents, complicating therapeutic decision-making. These challenges contribute to the disproportionate morbidity and mortality observed in obstetric populations compared with nonpregnant individuals.

The spectrum of pathogens responsible for maternal sepsis is diverse, with *Escherichia coli* and Group A *Streptococcus* consistently emerging as the most frequent causes. Invasive GAS infections, in particular, are notable for their fulminant course and association with toxic shock syndrome, often progressing to multiorgan failure within days if unrecognized. Viral and fungal pathogens, including influenza and *Candida* species, also contribute significantly, especially in immunocompromised or critically ill patients.

Ş. Ceylan Arı (✉)
Ege University, Faculty of Medicine, Department of Anaesthesiology and Reanimation, Izmir, Turkey

© The Author(s), under exclusive license to Springer Nature Switzerland AG 2026
I. Karaca (ed.), *Managing Maternal Chronic Diseases for a Healthy Pregnancy*, https://doi.org/10.1007/978-3-032-15221-3_19

Beyond its maternal consequences, sepsis exerts profound implications for fetal health. Placental hypoperfusion, intrauterine infection, and systemic inflammatory responses have been linked to adverse outcomes such as preterm birth, stillbirth, and neonatal sepsis. Thus, maternal sepsis represents not only a critical determinant of maternal survival but also a major driver of perinatal morbidity and mortality.

In light of these challenges, international guidelines emphasize the urgency of early recognition and immediate initiation of broad-spectrum antimicrobial therapy, coupled with timely hemodynamic stabilization and source control. Yet, the absence of universally validated pregnancy-specific diagnostic criteria and risk stratification tools remains a critical gap. Bridging this gap requires integrating obstetric-specific early warning systems with established sepsis bundles, while fostering multidisciplinary collaboration among obstetricians, intensivists, anesthesiologists, and infectious disease specialists.

This chapter provides a comprehensive overview of maternal sepsis, focusing on its epidemiology, evolving diagnostic frameworks, risk factors, and management strategies. By critically examining both the physiological adaptations of pregnancy and the unique vulnerabilities they create, it aims to guide clinicians in achieving earlier recognition, optimized treatment, and ultimately improved maternal and neonatal outcomes.

19.2 Global Incidence and Regional Variation of Maternal Sepsis

A comprehensive systematic review and meta-analysis published in 2025 estimated the global incidence of maternal sepsis to be approximately 13.16 cases per 10,000 pregnancies, with significant regional disparities. Sub-Saharan Africa exhibited the highest incidence at 129.17 cases per 10,000 pregnancies (95% CI: 67.05–248.85), while the Americas reported the lowest at 6.31 per 10,000 (95% CI: 4.36–9.12) [1]. These variations highlight systemic inequities in healthcare access, antenatal care quality, and infection control practices.

Although fewer than 2% of pregnancies require admission to intensive care units (ICUs), maternal sepsis is a disproportionately frequent indication. ICU-level care is necessitated in approximately 0.04% of all deliveries, with maternal mortality among these patients ranging between 12% and 28% [2]. Numerous risk factors are consistently associated with an elevated risk of maternal sepsis, with certain populations such as Black women, smokers, and those with limited access to care bearing a disproportionate burden of sepsis-related complications [3]. This underscores the potential for rapid clinical deterioration and the necessity for early identification and aggressive management.

19.3 Risk Factors for Maternal Sepsis

Maternal sepsis and its potential progression to septic shock are influenced by a complex interplay of obstetric and individual-level factors.

19.3.1 Obstetric-Related Risk Factors

Among obstetric contributors, caesarean section (CS) stands out as the most significant independent risk factor for postpartum sepsis, with markedly higher rates of infection in comparison to vaginal deliveries. The risk is most pronounced when CS is performed after labor has begun, followed by elective CS and operative vaginal deliveries [4]. Additional obstetric risk factors include cervical cerclage, prolonged or preterm prelabor rupture of membranes (PPROM), retained placental tissue, multiple gestation, infectious vaginal discharge, and a history of pelvic infections. Prior colonization with Group B *Streptococcus*, close contact with individuals carrying Group A *Streptococcus*, and invasive diagnostic procedures such as amniocentesis have also been linked to elevated infection risk [5].

19.3.2 Patient-Related Risk Factors

Patient-level determinants encompass a range of demographic and clinical factors. Primiparity, underlying medical conditions, recent febrile illness, and antibiotic use within the preceding 2 weeks have been associated with an increased risk of sepsis. Chronic comorbidities—such as congestive heart failure, diabetes, chronic renal or hepatic disease, systemic lupus erythematosus, and HIV are independently associated with greater vulnerability [5]. Socioeconomic status plays a pivotal role; individuals from lower-income backgrounds, particularly those reliant on Medicaid in the United States, demonstrate disproportionately higher rates of maternal sepsis. This disparity is further compounded by increased rates of caesarean delivery within these populations [5].

19.3.3 Sources of Infection and Causative Pathogens in Maternal Sepsis

During pregnancy, immune modulation occurs to promote fetal tolerance, which concurrently reduces maternal immune defenses, thereby increasing vulnerability to infections. The pathogens most frequently associated with maternal sepsis include

Escherichia coli, *Streptococcus pyogenes* (Group A), *Staphylococcus aureus*, and *Candida* species [6].

Maternal sepsis can originate from various infectious sites, with the respiratory and genital tracts being the most commonly involved. In the United Kingdom, pneumonia constitutes the leading cause of maternal infection, particularly during the intrapartum period. In contrast, genital tract infections are more prevalent in the postpartum phase and are often linked to obstetric interventions and vaginal deliveries [7].

Among the causative agents, *E. coli* and *Streptococcus* species, particularly groups A and B, are the most frequently isolated organisms, followed by *Staphylococcus aureus* and *Candida* species. Notably, infections caused by Group A *Streptococcus* are associated with a high mortality rate ranging between 30% and 60%. *Candida* infections may result in severe complications, including chorioamnionitis and stillbirth. Although less commonly encountered, organisms such as *Clostridium* species, *Plasmodium vivax*, and *Chlamydia psittaci* have also been implicated in maternal sepsis [7].

Group A Streptococcus (Streptococcus pyogenes)

A marked increase in maternal mortality in the United Kingdom between 2006 and 2008 was attributed to a rise in invasive genital tract infections caused by Group A *Streptococcus* (GAS), which accounted for nearly half of all direct maternal deaths during that period [8]. Group A *Streptococcus* (*Streptococcus pyogenes*) is considered one of the most virulent human bacterial pathogens, particularly in the obstetric population.

Pregnancy significantly elevates the risk of invasive GAS infection, with estimates suggesting a 20-fold increase compared to nonpregnant individuals [9]. In most cases, the infection originates from ascending colonization of the genital tract and endometrium, which can rapidly evolve into septic shock and multiorgan failure within 48–96 h [10].

A recent systematic review reported that the majority of invasive GAS infections occurred during the postpartum period (91.9%), while antenatal and intrapartum cases were less frequent, constituting 4.7% and 0.6%, respectively. The predominant clinical presentations included bacteremia (49%) and endometritis (45.9%). Approximately one-third of these cases progressed to streptococcal toxic shock syndrome (sTSS), with an overall case fatality rate of 2% [11].

Escherichia coli

In a large-scale prospective study involving over 150,000 pregnancies between 2005 and 2012, *Escherichia coli* was identified as the leading pathogen responsible for maternal sepsis, accounting for 37% of cases, particularly during the antenatal period [12]. These infections were predominantly observed in the third trimester, with 55% originating from the urinary tract and 45% from the genital tract [13].

The clinical implications of *E. coli* bacteremia in pregnancy are significant. In a study evaluating outcomes of *E. coli* bloodstream infections, fetal mortality occurred in 27% of cases, frequently associated with chorioamnionitis following preterm prelabor rupture of membranes (PPROM). These findings underscore the severe perinatal risks associated with *E. coli* sepsis [13].

Influenza Virus

Influenza virus infections represent a significant contributor to the maternal sepsis burden, particularly during pandemic outbreaks. Pregnant individuals are more susceptible to severe disease and face a four- to fivefold increased risk of hospitalization and serious complications, especially during the second and third trimesters and the early postpartum period [14].

According to the United Kingdom's MBRRACE (Mothers and Babies: Reducing Risk through Audits and Confidential Enquiries across the UK) report, influenza was responsible for 1 in every 11 maternal deaths between 2009 and 2012, underscoring its substantial impact on maternal mortality [15]. In light of these risks, the World Health Organization (WHO) designates pregnant individuals as a high-priority group for influenza vaccination, recommending immunization at any stage of pregnancy [16].

Oseltamivir, a neuraminidase inhibitor, is considered the first-line antiviral treatment for influenza in pregnancy and demonstrates the greatest efficacy when administered within the first 48 h following symptom onset [17].

19.4 Maternal Physiological Changes During Pregnancy and Their Impact on Sepsis

The physiological changes during pregnancy significantly alter the maternal immune system and the clinical presentation of sepsis. Given that maternal septic states can directly compromise fetal health, healthcare providers must balance both maternal and fetal considerations when evaluating and managing infection [18]. A thorough understanding of gestational physiology is essential for early recognition and appropriate treatment of sepsis in pregnant patients.

From conception through the postpartum period, hormonal and anatomical changes initiate widespread systemic effects. One of the earliest hematologic changes is dilutional anemia, driven by plasma volume expansion that exceeds the increase in red blood cell mass [19]. Respiratory adaptations include increased tidal volume and minute ventilation, culminating in a state of compensated respiratory alkalosis [18]. Gastrointestinal changes, such as reduced lower esophageal sphincter tone due to progesterone and relaxin, delayed gastric emptying, and diaphragmatic elevation (up to 4 cm), heighten the risk of aspiration, an important consideration for airway management in septic pregnant patients [20].

Cardiovascular modifications are among the most significant. Systemic vascular resistance declines by up to 40% due to early vasodilation, prompting compensatory increases in heart rate to preserve cardiac output [21]. In the third trimester, heart rate may rise by 24–30 beats/min above baseline, with more marked changes in multiple gestations [18]. Although most hemodynamic parameters normalize within 2 weeks postpartum, some women retain pregnancy-adapted values for up to

12 weeks. Blood pressure typically declines by 10–15 mmHg, reaching its nadir around 24 weeks of gestation. These effects are maintained by simultaneous increases in plasma volume and erythrocyte mass, beginning as early as week 6 and peaking by week 34 [19].

The immune system undergoes marked modulation. Leukocytosis is common, with WBC counts doubling by term and exceeding 25,000/mm^3 postpartum, especially in conditions like preeclampsia [22]. This physiological leukocytosis can obscure sepsis diagnosis by mimicking inflammatory responses of noninfectious origin.

Comorbidities such as obesity, type 2 diabetes, and chronic hypertension, along with increased pharmacological interventions during pregnancy, further complicate clinical interpretation. Antihypertensives and hypoglycemic agents may mask typical septic responses, while nonadherence to medication regimens can increase diagnostic uncertainty [23].

Pregnancy increases cardiac output by 30–50%, primarily through elevated stroke volume and heart rate [24]. Sepsis-related vasodilation, mediated by cytokine-driven nitric oxide production, reduces systemic vascular resistance and induces hypotension, triggering tachycardia and increased cardiac output, a pattern characteristic of distributive shock. As sepsis progresses, myocardial depression can occur, impairing tissue perfusion despite increased output. Distinguishing these pathologies from normal pregnancy physiology is especially challenging in the presence of hemorrhage or anesthesia-related hemodynamic shifts.

Biochemical markers, such as lactate and procalcitonin, assist in diagnosis and prognosis but require cautious interpretation. While lactate levels above 4 mmol/L indicate hypoperfusion, they may also rise in healthy laboring women [25]. Similarly, procalcitonin may increase during labor absent infection, limiting its specificity. Though not recommended for initiating antibiotics, procalcitonin may guide early antibiotic discontinuation in critically ill adults [26].

Respiratory system adaptations complicate clinical assessment. Estrogen-induced mucosal edema increases the risk of airway obstruction [27]. Diaphragmatic elevation decreases functional residual capacity and expiratory reserve volume, while increased tidal volume preserves total lung capacity [28]. These changes result in compensated respiratory alkalosis, with decreased $PaCO_2$ and elevated PaO_2, impacting both clinical symptoms and ventilatory strategies in septic pregnant patients.

Given the complex interplay of physiological alterations and heightened sepsis risk, early identification is critical. Obstetric-specific tools such as the CMQCC sepsis algorithm and modified qSOFA scoring enhance risk detection and expedite intervention [29]. Protocolized treatment reduces sepsis-related mortality in the general adult population, and despite limited obstetric-specific data, delays in antibiotic initiation are linked to increased maternal mortality [30].

19.5 Diagnosis and Early Identification of Maternal Sepsis

19.5.1 Evolution and Challenges in Diagnostic Criteria

Previously, the identification of sepsis primarily relied on the presence of a suspected infection combined with the systemic inflammatory response syndrome (SIRS) criteria. Although the initial validation studies excluded pregnant women, SIRS remained the principal standardized framework for sepsis recognition across all populations. Before the 2012 revision of sepsis guidelines, these protocols demonstrated limited sensitivity in obstetric settings, identifying fewer than two-thirds of maternal sepsis cases in retrospective analyses. This limitation underscored the need for pregnancy-specific diagnostic criteria to improve recognition and outcomes [31].

19.5.2 Sepsis Management Protocols

Since 2004, the Surviving Sepsis Campaign (SSC) has introduced evidence-based protocols for early sepsis management. The 2018 "Hour-1 bundle" outlines five essential interventions recommended within the first hour of sepsis recognition to improve outcomes [31]:

1. Measurement of serum lactate levels.
2. Obtaining blood cultures before antibiotic administration.
3. Prompt initiation of broad-spectrum antibiotics.
4. Administration of a 30 mL/kg crystalloid fluid bolus in hypotensive or hyperlactatemic patients (lactate ≥4 mmol/L).
5. Use of vasopressors to maintain mean arterial pressure (MAP) ≥65 mmHg. The U.K. Sepsis Trust expanded this with the "Sepsis Six" protocol, adding high-flow oxygen and urine output monitoring within the first hour. Streamlined protocols like Sepsis Six enhance the implementation of SSC components and are associated with a 50% reduction in mortality [32].

19.5.3 Role of Biochemical Markers

Serum lactate is a key biomarker in sepsis, reflecting anaerobic metabolism due to tissue hypoperfusion. However, hyperlactatemia may also result from mitochondrial dysfunction, microcirculatory failure, impaired oxygen extraction, catecholamine-induced glycolysis, and reduced hepatic clearance [33]. Elevated lactate correlates with adverse outcomes in pregnant patients, with each 1 mmol/L increase associated with a 2.34-fold higher risk of ICU admission [18]. Thus, early lactate assessment facilitates risk stratification and timely intervention.

19.5.4 Pregnancy-Specific Diagnostic Approaches and Scoring Tools

Diagnosing sepsis during pregnancy remains challenging due to physiological adaptations that can mimic infection signs. The 2023 Society for Maternal-Fetal Medicine (SMFM) guidelines emphasize that fever is not essential for diagnosis. Sepsis should be suspected when infection coexists with unexplained organ dysfunction [34].

No single universal screening tool is recommended. Institutions are advised to adopt context-specific protocols. Common tools such as MEWS, SIRS, and qSOFA, including their obstetric adaptations, vary in diagnostic accuracy. SIRS often results in false positives due to pregnancy-induced tachycardia and hyperthermia [35]. MEWS shows higher sensitivity but is affected by hypertensive disorders [36]. qSOFA is useful for severity prediction but may miss early cases. The obstetrically modified qSOFA (omqSOFA) improves specificity by adjusting respiratory and blood pressure thresholds [29]. Despite these tools, no gold standard exists; thus, clinical judgment remains essential.

In parallel, global organizations proposed varying criteria for maternal sepsis. The WHO uses the term “puerperal sepsis,” restricting diagnosis to genitourinary infections occurring from membrane rupture up to 6 weeks postpartum. The WHO also defines septic abortion based on similar criteria. Consequently, past maternal sepsis research disproportionately focused on these infections [1].

The 2016 Third International Consensus Definitions introduced SOFA and qSOFA, both derived from the SIRS model. However, pregnant individuals were excluded from validation cohorts, limiting generalizability. As of now, no external validations for these tools exist in obstetric populations, though some components have been assessed in obstetric settings [37]. To address this, two obstetric-specific scoring tools were developed: the Modified Obstetric Early Warning Score (MOEWS) and the Sepsis in Obstetrics Score (SOS). MOEWS, designed for early clinical deterioration detection, has limited diagnostic specificity due to its multiple international variants and its primary focus on clinical deterioration rather than sepsis diagnosis [38]. The largest MOEWS study involved 913 chorioamnionitis cases, but only five met severe sepsis criteria, highlighting concerns about specificity. The SOS, introduced in 2014, reflects physiological changes in pregnancy and uses ICU admission within 48 h as the outcome measure [39]. However, there is a lack of standardized ICU admission criteria for hampers interpretation. In its internal validation, a score <6 showed a 98.6% negative predictive value, while a score ≥ 6 had 64% sensitivity. Among 1250 patients studied, ICU admission was 1.1%, though the criteria were unclear. While the SOS shows promise, further validation in diverse populations is required. Despite these advances, emergency care providers still lack adequately validated tools for decision-making in pregnant or postpartum individuals presenting with suspected infection.

19.5.5 Detailed Assessment of SOFA Score

Currently, maternal sepsis diagnosis relies on a SOFA score ≥2 in the presence of suspected infection. The SOFA score assesses the function of six major organ systems: respiratory, cardiovascular, renal, hepatic, coagulation, and central nervous system (CNS). An increase in the SOFA score of ≥2 in the presence of infection is suggestive of sepsis and requires urgent intervention [40].

- Respiratory system: PaO_2/FiO_2 ratio measures the degree of hypoxemia, which can indicate respiratory failure. A ratio <300 suggests moderate dysfunction, while a ratio <100 is associated with severe ARDS (acute respiratory distress syndrome), which can develop rapidly in sepsis.
- Cardiovascular system: The mean arterial pressure (MAP) is a critical marker of perfusion and shock. A MAP < 70 mmHg suggests impaired tissue perfusion and may necessitate the use of vasopressors to maintain adequate organ perfusion.
- Renal system: Elevated creatinine levels and reduced urine output are indicative of kidney dysfunction, which is common in severe sepsis and septic shock. A urine output of <0.5 mL/kg/h for at least 2 h despite adequate fluid resuscitation is suggestive of acute kidney injury.
- Coagulation: Sepsis can disrupt the coagulation cascade, leading to thrombocytopenia (low platelet count), which is often associated with disseminated intravascular coagulation (DIC). A platelet count <150.000/μL is considered significant and warrants further investigation.
- Liver function: Elevated bilirubin levels can indicate liver dysfunction, a key feature of severe sepsis. A bilirubin level >2 mg/dL is indicative of liver involvement in sepsis.
- CNS: The Glasgow Coma Scale (GCS) is used to assess mental status. A GCS score of <15 is considered a warning sign of worsening sepsis and impaired central nervous system function.

19.5.6 Laboratory Tests and Imaging

In addition to clinical scores, laboratory investigations play a pivotal role in confirming the diagnosis of maternal sepsis [41]. Key tests include:

- Blood cultures: Blood cultures are essential for identifying the causative pathogen, particularly in the case of bacteremia or fungemia. Blood cultures should be obtained before the initiation of antibiotics, although empirical therapy should be started immediately if sepsis is suspected.
- Serum lactate: Elevated serum lactate levels are indicative of poor tissue oxygenation and anaerobic metabolism, a hallmark of severe sepsis and septic shock. Lactate levels >2 mmol/L are associated with increased mortality and serve as a marker of the severity of circulatory failure.

- Procalcitonin (PCT): This biomarker is useful in differentiating bacterial infections from viral or noninfectious causes of inflammation. PCT levels are generally elevated in bacterial sepsis, making it a useful adjunct in the diagnosis of maternal sepsis.
- C-reactive protein (CRP): Elevated CRP levels indicate an acute inflammatory response, though it is less specific for sepsis than procalcitonin. CRP levels >10 mg/L are commonly seen in bacterial infections but can also be elevated in other inflammatory conditions.
- Urine cultures: In pregnant women, urinary tract infections (UTIs) are common and can lead to sepsis if untreated. Urine cultures are necessary if UTI is suspected to identify the causative organism and guide treatment.
- Imaging: Ultrasonography is a key tool in obstetrics for identifying retained products of conception, abscesses, or endometritis following delivery. In complex cases, CT scans and MRI may be required to identify intra-abdominal infections or other sources of infection that may not be visible on ultrasound.

19.5.7 Differential Diagnosis

Several conditions must be considered in the differential diagnosis of maternal sepsis, as many present with overlapping symptoms:

- Hypovolemic or hemorrhagic shock: Postpartum hemorrhage is a common cause of shock in the peripartum period and can be confused with sepsis due to similar clinical signs (e.g., hypotension, tachycardia).
- Pulmonary embolism: The symptoms of pulmonary embolism, such as dyspnea, tachycardia, and hypoxia, can mimic sepsis, particularly in the postpartum period when the risk of thromboembolism is elevated.
- Myocardial infarction: Chest pain, tachycardia, and dyspnea may suggest acute myocardial infarction (AMI), particularly in older women or those with preexisting risk factors. A detailed cardiac workup is necessary to rule out AMI.
- Acute pancreatitis: Abdominal pain, nausea, and vomiting are common in both sepsis and acute pancreatitis, making it a crucial differential diagnosis to consider.
- Diabetic ketoacidosis (DKA): Pregnancy-related DKA can present with elevated blood glucose, acetone breath, and metabolic acidosis, mimicking sepsis symptoms.
- Transfusion reaction: In the context of blood transfusion, febrile reactions or hemolytic reactions can present similarly to sepsis, requiring immediate recognition and intervention.

Early diagnosis and prompt intervention are the cornerstones of improving outcomes in maternal sepsis. The combination of clinical scores, laboratory tests, and imaging studies plays a critical role in the timely identification of sepsis and its underlying cause. Although several screening tools are available, further advancements in pregnancy-specific sepsis diagnostic models are necessary. The future of maternal sepsis diagnosis lies in personalized medicine, integrating biomarkers, advanced imaging, and machine learning models to refine early detection and treatment strategies, ultimately improving maternal and fetal survival rates.

19.6 Management of Maternal Sepsis

19.6.1 Early Recognition and Diagnosis

Timely recognition of maternal sepsis is critical, particularly in the presence of clinical signs such as fever, tachycardia, hypotension, and organ dysfunction. The use of rapid screening tools enhances early detection and facilitates prompt intervention. Serum lactate levels exceeding 4 mmol/L are especially alarming and indicate the need for urgent resuscitation and further diagnostic evaluation [42].

19.6.2 Empirical Antimicrobial Therapy

Empirical broad-spectrum antibiotic therapy should be initiated within the first hour of sepsis suspicion. Although blood cultures should ideally be obtained before antibiotic administration, treatment must not be delayed. The timely initiation of appropriate antibiotics is critical for managing maternal sepsis and is emphasized in the Surviving Sepsis Campaign (SSC) guidelines. A retrospective study of 2731 intensive care unit admissions for septic shock demonstrated a 7.6% decrease in survival for each hour of delay in administering effective antimicrobial therapy after hypotension onset [43]. Therefore, early consultation with infectious disease specialists is recommended to guide antimicrobial therapy decisions (Table 19.1).

Empirical antibiotic treatment in sepsis should be broad-spectrum and administered within 1 h of suspicion, following blood culture collection. Genital tract infections are often polymicrobial, with pathogens such as Group A *Streptococcus* and *Escherichia coli* commonly implicated in severe cases. Consequently, initial

Table 19.1 Empirical antibiotic selection based on infection likelihood

Infection source	Empiric therapy
Chorioamnionitis/ endomyometritis	Ampicillin + gentamicin ± clindamycin/metronidazole
Urinary tract infection	Ampicillin + gentamicin, or piperacillin-tazobactam
Pneumonia	Ceftriaxone + azithromycin or levofloxacin (if not contraindicated)
Wound infection/mastitis	Cefazolin or vancomycin if MRSA risk
Unknown/severe source	Ceftriaxone + metronidazole or meropenem if MDR risk present

therapy must target Gram-positive, Gram-negative, and anaerobic bacteria. Group A *Streptococcus* is notable for producing exotoxins that can rapidly worsen clinical status and cause streptococcal toxic shock syndrome. Clindamycin, which inhibits exotoxin synthesis by Group A *Streptococcus*, should be used alongside broad-spectrum antibiotics to improve clinical outcomes [44]. Additionally, intravenous immunoglobulin administration, which neutralizes these exotoxins, may improve prognosis in toxic shock syndrome and is endorsed by the RCOG [45].

Recommended empirical regimens include meropenem or piperacillin–tazobactam, with clindamycin added when Group A *Streptococcus* is suspected. If methicillin-resistant *Staphylococcus aureus* (MRSA) is a concern, agents such as vancomycin or linezolid may be appropriate. Antibiotic therapy should be de-escalated based on culture results and antimicrobial sensitivity patterns [42].

19.6.3 Source Control

Rapid identification and elimination of the infectious source are essential to improving maternal outcomes. Delays in source control are associated with increased mortality. In cases involving uterine infection, expedited delivery—either vaginal or cesarean—may be required. For severe or unresolvable infections, hysterectomy might be necessary. Other infection sources, including pelvic abscesses or urinary tract infections, should also be addressed through appropriate surgical or medical interventions [45].

19.6.4 Fluid Resuscitation and Hemodynamic Support

Initial fluid resuscitation with crystalloid solutions, administered at 30 mL/kg within the first 3 h, is recommended to restore adequate tissue perfusion. If hypotension persists despite fluid administration, norepinephrine is the preferred first-line vasopressor to maintain a mean arterial pressure (MAP) of at least 65 mmHg, owing to its effectiveness and relatively minimal adverse effects on uteroplacental perfusion compared to other agents [34]. Effective fetal stabilization is closely linked to adequate maternal resuscitation, which includes intravenous fluid therapy and proper patient positioning. Specifically, placing the patient in the left lateral decubitus position during the third trimester optimizes hemodynamics by reducing inferior vena cava compression and improving preload [31].

Fluid resuscitation should commence within the first 3 h of presentation when hypotension or lactate levels above 4 mmol/L are present, with an initial crystalloid dose of 30 mL/kg [42]. However, considering the physiological increase in maternal blood volume during pregnancy, this lactate threshold may lack sensitivity. A retrospective cohort study involving 159 pregnant women with sepsis reported that patients requiring ICU care had a mean lactate of 2.6 mmol/L, while those with positive blood cultures had a mean of 2.2 mmol/L, both below the typical sepsis threshold. This study also identified a significant association between elevated lactate and morbidity, with an adjusted odds ratio of 2.34/1 mmol/L increase [39].

There are currently no specific clinical guidelines addressing vasopressor preferences during pregnancy. Although an optimal MAP target for septic pregnant patients is not explicitly defined, a threshold of 65 mmHg is generally considered reasonable [42]. Fetal monitoring can be a valuable tool for titrating hemodynamic support. While the 2016 Society of Critical Care Medicine guidelines do not provide pregnancy-specific recommendations, they endorse norepinephrine as the first-line vasopressor in this population [42]. Evidence on norepinephrine's effects on fetal outcomes remains limited, with no definitive data indicating harm.

The choice of second-line vasopressors is largely extrapolated from studies in obstetric anesthesia, with uncertain applicability to septic pregnant patients [46]. Phenylephrine and ephedrine are commonly used, though both exhibit tachyphylaxis [42]. Phenylephrine is generally favored due to its minimal impact on fetal acid-base status; however, its alpha-adrenergic activity can induce maternal bradycardia and reduced cardiac output [47]. Conversely, ephedrine indirectly increases blood pressure by stimulating maternal catecholamine release, which may be less effective in septic patients with depleted endogenous reserves [47].

Most available data on vasopressor use during pregnancy derive from elective cesarean delivery contexts. The American Society of Anesthesiologists, together with the Task Force on Obstetric Anesthesia, recommends phenylephrine over ephedrine due to better fetal acid-base outcomes, as ephedrine has been associated with fetal acidemia [46]. However, the applicability of these recommendations to septic patients remains unclear given different physiological states.

In rare cases of septic myocarditis, dobutamine may be the preferred inotrope. While its use in nonpregnant septic patients is limited, it may improve myocardial contractility in pregnant patients receiving vasopressors and fluid therapy [46]. Animal studies demonstrate that dobutamine enhances inotropy but may reduce uterine blood flow, indicating the need for further research in humans [48].

If hypotension persists despite adequate fluid resuscitation and norepinephrine infusion, intravenous corticosteroids may be considered, especially in cases of suspected adrenal insufficiency or vasopressor-refractory shock [34].

Continuous monitoring of hemodynamic status, serum lactate, and organ function is essential. In cases of refractory hypotension or respiratory failure, advanced support modalities such as extracorporeal membrane oxygenation (ECMO) should be contemplated [42].

19.6.5 Monitoring and Multidisciplinary Management

Close monitoring of vital signs, laboratory markers, and organ function is essential throughout the treatment course. A multidisciplinary approach involving obstetricians, intensive care researchers, anesthesiologists, and infectious disease specialists is necessary to ensure comprehensive care. Transfer to a higher-level intensive care unit (ICU) should be considered for patients requiring advanced life support or specialized interventions such as ECMO [34].

19.6.6 Fetal Considerations

In cases of suspected intrauterine infection or systemic maternal illness, continuous fetal monitoring is recommended. If preterm labor occurs before 34 weeks of gestation, antenatal corticosteroids such as betamethasone should be administered to enhance fetal lung maturation. Decisions regarding the timing and mode of delivery should be based on gestational age, severity of maternal illness, and the location and nature of the infection, always balancing maternal and fetal risks [34].

Given the heightened risk of venous thromboembolism (VTE) in the setting of sepsis and pregnancy, pharmacologic thromboprophylaxis is advised unless contraindications are present. This approach is critical in preventing potentially fatal thromboembolic events in this vulnerable population [34].

In critically ill obstetric patients, insulin therapy should be initiated when blood glucose levels exceed 180 mg/dL, consistent with glycemic control strategies recommended for sepsis management. Maintaining optimal glucose levels may reduce the risk of infection-related complications and improve overall outcomes [34].

19.7 Quick Reference Guide for Maternal Sepsis Management

19.7.1 First-Line Management (Initial Assessment and Resuscitation)

A structured approach to sepsis based on clinical suspicion and objective indicators should guide management. The following red flag signs should prompt immediate evaluation and sepsis workup:

- Fever (>38 °C) or hypothermia (<36 °C)
- Tachycardia (>110 bpm)
- Tachypnea (>24 breaths/min)
- Hypotension (MAP < 65 mmHg)
- Mental status changes (agitation, confusion)
- Oliguria (<0.5 mL/kg/h)
- Elevated lactate (>2 mmol/L)
- WBC > 15,000 or <4000/mm^3

Step	Intervention
1	Measure serum lactate level
2	Obtain blood cultures prior to antibiotic administration
3	Administer broad-spectrum antibiotics
4	Begin rapid administration of 30 mL/kg crystalloid fluids for hypotension or lactate ≥4 mmol/L
5	Apply vasopressors if MAP remains <65 mmHg during or after fluid resuscitation (Surviving Sepsis Campaign, 2021)

Empiric Antibiotic Therapy Recommendations:

- Chorioamnionitis/Endomyometritis: Ampicillin + Gentamicin ± Clindamycin/Metronidazole
- Urinary tract infections: Ampicillin + Gentamicin, or Piperacillin-tazobactam
- Unclear source: Ceftriaxone + Metronidazole or Meropenem if MDR pathogens are suspected.

Note: Administer antibiotics within 60 min of recognition. Delay increases maternal mortality by 7.6% per hour.

19.8 Advanced Support and Anesthesia Considerations

Maternal sepsis may necessitate escalation to intensive care due to multiorgan dysfunction, shock, or respiratory failure. The decision for ICU admission should be based on hemodynamic instability, altered mental status, or worsening laboratory parameters.

- Hemodynamic support:
  - Use of vasopressors (e.g., norepinephrine) is indicated if MAP remains <65 mmHg after fluid resuscitation.
  - Invasive hemodynamic monitoring may be necessary in cases of persistent shock or fluid overload risk.
- Ventilatory support:
  - Oxygen supplementation is essential to maintain maternal oxygen saturation ≥94.
  - Mechanical ventilation should be considered if respiratory failure develops. Pregnancy-specific changes (reduced FRC, increased oxygen demand) require cautious ventilator settings.
- Renal and metabolic monitoring:
  - Monitor urine output, creatinine, and lactate levels frequently.
  - Initiate renal replacement therapy if acute kidney injury is severe and refractory to medical management.

- Anesthesia considerations:
  - Neuraxial anesthesia (e.g., epidural) is generally avoided in septic patients due to coagulopathy and infection risks.
  - If surgical intervention (e.g., cesarean section or source control laparotomy) is needed, general anesthesia is preferred. Airway management may be challenging due to pregnancy-related edema and increased aspiration risk.
  - A difficult airway cart and video laryngoscopy should be readily available.
- Multidisciplinary approach: Close collaboration between obstetricians, anesthesiologists, intensivists, and infectious disease specialists is essential to optimize outcomes in maternal sepsis.

Key message for obstetricians: Sepsis is a time-sensitive emergency. If red flag signs are present, initiate sepsis management immediately. Do not wait for full diagnostic certainty. Once maternal resuscitation begins, obstetric decision-making can be reevaluated in tandem with fetal response.

19.9 Conclusion

Maternal sepsis continues to be a formidable global health challenge, significantly contributing to maternal morbidity and mortality worldwide. This chapter has comprehensively addressed the multifaceted nature of maternal sepsis, meticulously outlining its global incidence, diverse risk factors, and the complexities posed by pregnancy-induced physiological adaptations on diagnosis. Despite advancements, the persistent need for universally validated pregnancy-specific diagnostic tools remains paramount. Future endeavors in personalized medicine, leveraging advanced biomarkers and machine learning, hold immense promise for refining early detection and treatment strategies. Ultimately, a concerted global effort is essential to mitigate the devastating burden of maternal sepsis and ensure safer maternal and neonatal health outcomes across the globe.

References

1. Say L, Chou D, Gemmill A, Tunçalp Ö, Moller AB, Daniels J, et al. Global causes of maternal death: a WHO systematic analysis. Lancet Glob Health. 2014;2(6):e323.
2. Zwart JJ, Dupuis JRO, Richters A, Öry F, Van Roosmalen J. Obstetric intensive care unit admission: a 2-year nationwide population-based cohort study. Intensive Care Med. 2010;36(2):256–63. Available from: https://pubmed.ncbi.nlm.nih.gov/19902177/.
3. Roch Cantwell T, Clutton-Brock G, Cooper A, Dawson J, Drife D, Garrod, et al. Saving mothers' lives: reviewing maternal deaths to make motherhood safer: 2006-2008. The eighth report of the confidential enquiries into maternal deaths in the United Kingdom. BJOG. 2011;118 Suppl 1(s1):1–203. Available from: https://pubmed.ncbi.nlm.nih.gov/21356004/.

4. Conroy S, Pariante CM, Marks MN, Davies HA, Farrelly S, Schacht R, et al. Maternal psychopathology and infant development at 18 months: the impact of maternal personality disorder and depression. J Am Acad Child Adolesc Psychiatry. 2012;51(1):51–61. Available from: https://pubmed.ncbi.nlm.nih.gov/22176939/.
5. Bauer J, Biolo G, Cederholm T, Cesari M, Cruz-Jentoft AJ, Morley JE, et al. Evidence-based recommendations for optimal dietary protein intake in older people: a position paper from the PROT-AGE Study Group. J Am Med Dir Assoc. 2013;14(8):542–59. Available from: https://www.sciencedirect.com/science/article/pii/S1525861013003265.
6. Liu P, Zhang X, Wang X, Liang Y, Wei N, Xiao Z, et al. Maternal sepsis in pregnancy and the puerperal periods: a cross-sectional study. Front Med (Lausanne). 2023;10:1126807. Available from: https://pmc.ncbi.nlm.nih.gov/articles/PMC10228646/.
7. Acosta CD, Kurinczuk JJ, Lucas DN, Tuffnell DJ, Sellers S, Knight M. Severe maternal sepsis in the UK, 2011-2012: a national case-control study. PLoS Med. 2014;11(7):e1001672. Available from: https://pubmed.ncbi.nlm.nih.gov/25003759/.
8. Yamada T, Yamada T, Yamamura MK, Katabami K, Hayakawa M, Tomaru U, et al. Invasive group A streptococcal infection in pregnancy. J Infect. 2010;60(6):417–24. Available from: https://pubmed.ncbi.nlm.nih.gov/20359498/.
9. Deutscher M, Lewis M, Zell ER, Taylor TH, Van Beneden C, Schrag S. Incidence and severity of invasive streptococcus pneumoniae, group a streptococcus, and group b streptococcus infections among pregnant and postpartum women. Clin Infect Dis. 2011;53(2):114–23. Available from: https://pubmed.ncbi.nlm.nih.gov/21690617/.
10. Harris K, Proctor LK, Shinar S, Philippopoulos E, Yudin MH, Murphy KE. Outcomes and management of pregnancy and puerperal group A streptococcal infections: a systematic review. Acta Obstet Gynecol Scand. 2023;102(2):138. Available from: https://pmc.ncbi.nlm.nih.gov/articles/PMC9889326/.
11. Stevens DL. Invasive group A streptococcus infections. Clin Infect Dis. 1992;14(1):2–13. Available from: https://pubmed.ncbi.nlm.nih.gov/1571429/.
12. Knowles SJ, O'Sullivan NP, Meenan AM, Hanniffy R, Robson M. Maternal sepsis incidence, aetiology and outcome for mother and fetus: a prospective study. BJOG. 2015;122(5):663–71. Available from: https://pubmed.ncbi.nlm.nih.gov/24862293/.
13. Surgers L, Bleibtreu A, Burdet C, Clermont O, Laouénan C, Lefort A, et al. Escherichia coli bacteraemia in pregnant women is life-threatening for foetuses. Clin Microbiol Infect. 2014;20(12):O1035–41. Available from: https://pubmed.ncbi.nlm.nih.gov/24979689/.
14. Naresh A, Fisher BM, Hoppe KK, Catov J, Xu J, Hart J, et al. A multicenter cohort study of pregnancy outcomes among women with laboratory-confirmed H1N1 influenza. J Perinatol. 2013;33(12):939–43. Available from: https://pubmed.ncbi.nlm.nih.gov/24051575/.
15. Knight M, Kenyon S, Brocklehurst P, Neilson J, Shakespeare J, Kurinczuk J. Saving lives, improving mothers' care: lessons learned to inform future maternity care from the UK and Ireland confidential enquiries into maternal deaths and morbidity 2009–12. National Perinatal Epidemiology Unit: University of Oxford; 2014. 120 p. Available from: www.npeu.ox.ac.uk. https://research.birmingham.ac.uk/en/publications/saving-lives-improving-mothers-care-lessons-learned-to-inform-fut.
16. Morales KF, Brown DW, Dumolard L, Steulet C, Vilajeliu A, Ropero Alvarez AM, et al. Seasonal influenza vaccination policies in the 194 WHO Member States: the evolution of global influenza pandemic preparedness and the challenge of sustaining equitable vaccine access. Vaccine X. 2021;8:100097. Available from: https://www.sciencedirect.com/science/article/pii/S2590136221000140.
17. Jefferson T, Jones MA, Doshi P, Del Mar CB, Hama R, Thompson MJ, et al. Neuraminidase inhibitors for preventing and treating influenza in adults and children. Cochrane Database Syst Rev. 2014;2014(4):CD008965. Available from: https://pubmed.ncbi.nlm.nih.gov/24718923/.
18. Bridwell RE, Carius BM, Long B, Oliver JJ, Schmitz G. Sepsis in pregnancy: recognition and resuscitation. West J Emerg Med. 2019;20(5):822–32. Available from: https://pubmed.ncbi.nlm.nih.gov/31539341/.

19. Mahendru AA, Everett TR, Wilkinson IB, Lees CC, McEniery CM. A longitudinal study of maternal cardiovascular function from preconception to the postpartum period. J Hypertens. 2014;32(4):849–56. Available from: https://pubmed.ncbi.nlm.nih.gov/24406777/.
20. LoMauro A, Aliverti A. Respiratory physiology of pregnancy. Breathe. 2015;11(4):297–301. Available from: https://pubmed.ncbi.nlm.nih.gov/27066123/.
21. Meah VL, Cockcroft JR, Backx K, Shave R, Stöhr EJ. Cardiac output and related haemodynamics during pregnancy: a series of meta-analyses. Heart. 2016;102(7):518–26. Available from: https://pubmed.ncbi.nlm.nih.gov/26794234/.
22. Anderson BL, Mendez-Figueroa H, Dahlke JD, Raker C, Hillier SL, Cu-Uvin S. Pregnancy-induced changes in immune protection of the genital tract: defining normal. Am J Obstet Gynecol. 2013;208(4):321.e1–9. Available from: https://pubmed.ncbi.nlm.nih.gov/23313311/.
23. Mighty HE, Fahey JO. Obesity and pregnancy complications. Curr Diab Rep. 2007;7(4):289–94. Available from: https://pubmed.ncbi.nlm.nih.gov/17686405/.
24. Rizi SS, Wiens E, Hunt J, Ducas R. Cardiac physiology and pathophysiology in pregnancy. Can J Physiol Pharmacol. 2024;102(10):552–71. Available from: https://pubmed.ncbi.nlm.nih.gov/38815593/.
25. Dockree S, O'Sullivan J, Shine B, James T, Vatish M. How should we interpret lactate in labour? A reference study. BJOG. 2022;129(13):2150. Available from: https://pmc.ncbi.nlm.nih.gov/articles/PMC9804290/.
26. Soni NJ, Samson DJ, Galaydick JL, Vats V, Huang ES, Aronson N, et al. Procalcitonin-guided antibiotic therapy: a systematic review and meta-analysis. J Hosp Med. 2013;8(9):530–40. Available from: https://pubmed.ncbi.nlm.nih.gov/23955852/.
27. Aydas AD, Basaranoglu G, Ozdemir H, Dooply SLS, Muhammedoglu N, Kucuk S, et al. Airway changes in pregnant women before and after delivery. Ir J Med Sci. 2015;184(2):431–3. Available from: https://pubmed.ncbi.nlm.nih.gov/24859287/.
28. Hegewald MJ, Crapo RO. Respiratory physiology in pregnancy. Clin Chest Med. 2011;32(1):1–13. Available from: https://pubmed.ncbi.nlm.nih.gov/21277444/.
29. Cagino SG, Burke AA, Letner DR, Leizer JM, Zelig CM. Quick sequential organ failure assessment: modifications for identifying maternal morbidity and mortality in obstetrical patients. Am J Perinatol. 2022;39(1):1–7. Available from: https://pubmed.ncbi.nlm.nih.gov/34583411/.
30. Tang F, Yuan H, Li X, Qiao L. Effect of delayed antibiotic use on mortality outcomes in patients with sepsis or septic shock: a systematic review and meta-analysis. Int Immunopharmacol. 2024;129:111616. Available from: https://pubmed.ncbi.nlm.nih.gov/38310764/.
31. Stephens AJ, Chauhan SP, Barton JR, Sibai BM. Maternal sepsis: a review of national and international guidelines. Am J Perinatol. 2020;40(7):718–30. Available from: http://www.thieme-connect.com/products/ejournals/html/10.1055/s-0041-1736382.
32. Daniels R, Nutbeam T, McNamara G, Galvin C. The sepsis six and the severe sepsis resuscitation bundle: a prospective observational cohort study. Emerg Med J. 2011;28(6):507–12. Available from: https://pubmed.ncbi.nlm.nih.gov/21036796/.
33. Shetty ST, Biradar DS, Balookar R, Kori S. Serum lactate as a prognostic marker in patients with sepsis: a prospective study. Int Surg J. 2020;7(5):1530–4. Available from: https://www.ijsurgery.com/index.php/isj/article/view/5636.
34. Shields AD, Plante LA, Pacheco LD, Louis JM. Society for Maternal-Fetal Medicine Consult Series #67: maternal sepsis. Am J Obstet Gynecol. 2023;229(3):B2–19. Available from: https://pubmed.ncbi.nlm.nih.gov/37236495/, https://www.ajog.org/action/showFullText?pii=S0002937823003277.
35. Rojas-Suarez J, Paternina-Caicedo A, Miranda J, Cuello M, Pinerez M, Santacruz J, et al. New obstetric systemic inflammatory response syndrome criteria for early identification of high-risk of sepsis in obstetric patients. J Perinat Med. 2021;49(9):1096–102. Available from: https://pubmed.ncbi.nlm.nih.gov/34265881/.
36. Friedman AM. Maternal early warning systems. Obstet Gynecol Clin N Am. 2015;42(2):289–98. Available from: https://pubmed.ncbi.nlm.nih.gov/26002167/.

37. Nayak AH, Khade SA. Obstetric sepsis: a review article. J Obstet Gynaecol India. 2022;72(6):470. Available from: https://pmc.ncbi.nlm.nih.gov/articles/PMC9732161/.
38. Robbins T, Shennan A, Sandall J. Modified early obstetric warning scores: a promising tool but more evidence and standardization is required. Acta Obstet Gynecol Scand. 2018;98(1):7. Available from: https://pmc.ncbi.nlm.nih.gov/articles/PMC7028086/.
39. Albright CM, Ali TN, Lopes V, Rouse DJ, Anderson BL. The sepsis in obstetrics score: a model to identify risk of morbidity from sepsis in pregnancy. Am J Obstet Gynecol. 2014;211(1):39.e1–8. Available from: https://pubmed.ncbi.nlm.nih.gov/24613756/.
40. Singer M, Deutschman CS, Seymour C, Shankar-Hari M, Annane D, Bauer M, et al. The third international consensus definitions for sepsis and septic shock (Sepsis-3). JAMA. 2016;315(8):801. Available from: https://pmc.ncbi.nlm.nih.gov/articles/PMC4968574/.
41. Fulton MR II, Zubair M, Taghavi S. Laboratory evaluation of sepsis. In: StatPearls [Internet]. Treasure Island: StatPearls Publishing; 2023. Available from: https://www.ncbi.nlm.nih.gov/books/NBK594258/.
42. Levy MM, Evans LE, Rhodes A. The surviving sepsis campaign bundle: 2018 update. Intensive Care Med. 2018;44(6):925–8. Available from: https://pubmed.ncbi.nlm.nih.gov/29675566/.
43. Kumar A, Roberts D, Wood KE, Light B, Parrillo JE, Sharma S, et al. Duration of hypotension before initiation of effective antimicrobial therapy is the critical determinant of survival in human septic shock. Crit Care Med. 2006;34(6):1589–96. Available from: https://pubmed.ncbi.nlm.nih.gov/16625125/.
44. Andreoni F, Zörcher C, Tarnutzer A, Schilcher K, Neff A, Keller N, et al. Clindamycin affects group A streptococcus virulence factors and improves clinical outcome. J Infect Dis. 2017;215(2):269–77. Available from: https://doi.org/10.1093/infdis/jiw229.
45. Lissauer D, Morgan M, Banerjee A, Plaat F, Pasupathy D. Identification and management of maternal sepsis during and following pregnancy. BJOG. 2025. Available from: https://www.rcog.org.uk/guidance/browse-all-guidance/green-top-guidelines/identification-and-management-of-maternal-sepsis-during-and-following-pregnancy-green-top-guideline-no-64/.
46. Apfelbaum JL, Hawkins JL, Agarkar M, Bucklin BA, Connis RT, Gambling DR, et al. Practice guidelines for obstetric anesthesia: an updated report by the American Society of Anesthesiologists Task Force on Obstetric Anesthesia and the Society for Obstetric Anesthesia and Perinatology∗. Anesthesiology. 2016;124(2):270–300. Available from: https://pubmed.ncbi.nlm.nih.gov/26580836/.
47. Dusitkasem S, Herndon BH, Somjit M, Stahl DL, Bitticker E, Coffman JC. Comparison of phenylephrine and ephedrine in treatment of spinal-induced hypotension in high-risk pregnancies: a narrative review. Front Med (Lausanne). 2017;4:2. Available from: https://pmc.ncbi.nlm.nih.gov/articles/PMC5247437/.
48. Fishburne JI, Meis PJ, Urban RB, Greiss FC, Wheeler AS, James FM, et al. Vascular and uterine responses to dobutamine and dopamine in the gravid ewe. Am J Obstet Gynecol. 1980;137(8):944–52. Available from: https://pubmed.ncbi.nlm.nih.gov/7405992/.

Index

© The Editor(s) (if applicable) and The Author(s), under exclusive license to Springer Nature Switzerland AG 2026

I. Karaca (ed.), *Managing Maternal Chronic Diseases for a Healthy Pregnancy*,
https://doi.org/10.1007/978-3-032-15221-3

B

MIX
Papier aus verantwortungsvollen Quellen
Paper from responsible sources
FSC® C105338

If you have any concerns about our products,
you can contact us on
ProductSafety@springernature.com

In case Publisher is established outside the EU,
the EU authorized representative is:
Springer Nature Customer Service Center GmbH
Europaplatz 3, 69115 Heidelberg, Germany

Printed by Libri Plureos GmbH
in Hamburg, Germany